CASE REVIEW
Nuclear Medicine

ELSEVIER
MOSBY

Harvey A. Ziessman, MD
Professor of Radiology
Director of Nuclear Medicine Imaging
Division of Nuclear Medicine
Russell H. Morgan Department of Radiology and
  Radiological Sciences
The Johns Hopkins University
Baltimore, Maryland

Patrice Rehm, MD
Associate Professor of Radiology
Director of Nuclear Medicine
University of Virginia Health Science Center
Charlottesville, Virginia

Associate Editors

Twyla B. Bartel, DO, MBA
Assistant Professor of Radiology
PET Director, Chief of Nuclear Medicine Imaging
University of Arkansas for Medical Sciences
Little Rock, Arkansas

Tracy L.Y. Brown, MD, PhD
Assistant Professor of Radiology
Program Director of Nuclear Medicine Residency
University of Arkansas for Medical Sciences
Little Rock, Arkansas

CASE REVIEW

Nuclear Medicine

SECOND EDITION

CASE REVIEW SERIES

1600 John F. Kennedy Boulevard
Suite 1800
Philadelphia, PA 19103-2899

NUCLEAR MEDICINE: CASE REVIEW, SECOND EDITION   ISBN: 978-0-323-05308-2

Previous edition copyrighted 2001.

International Standard Book Number: 978-0-323-05308-2

Acquisitions Editor: Rebecca Gaertner
Publishing Services Manager: Pat Joiner-Myers
Project Manager: Marlene Weeks
Designer: Steven Stave

Printed in the United States of America

Last digit is the print number: 9 8 7 6 5 4 3 2 1

To Karen and Bob

In the last decade, no field has made more monumental clinical strides in radiology than nuclear medicine. The explosion of PET/CT scanners has been instrumental in retooling how oncologic specialists decide who receives therapy, how that therapy is affecting the patient, whether to continue treatment, and if there is evidence of residual or recurrent disease. As a head and neck radiology aficionado, I see these cases frequently in the clinic and admire the value of the functional FDG PET component of the study. Similar advances in cardiac imaging, sestamibi scanning for parathyroid adenomas, and molecular imaging have had a great impact in medicine.

The second edition of *Nuclear Medicine: Case Review* by Drs. Ziessman, Rehm, Bartel, and Brown builds on the success of the first edition. It brings the reader up to date with the advances in technology as it supplies 200 excellent quality cases with poignant questions and discussions. The authorship team has been successful in maintaining a balance of nuclear medicine physics, radiation safety information, and clinically based material to produce a valuable Case Review Series book for trainees and practitioners in nuclear medicine. The style of the Case Review Series continues to be the best means to learn material in an interactive fashion with selected images, provocative questions, short answers, great discussions, pertinent references, and links back to *Nuclear Medicine: THE REQUISITES* for those who prefer more didactic textual material.

Congratulations to Drs. Ziessman, Rehm, Bartel, and Brown for furthering the success of *Nuclear Medicine: Case Review* with their exceptional second edition.

David M. Yousem, MD, MBA

The second edition of *Nuclear Medicine: Case Review* builds on the successful first edition and emphasizes the many advances that have taken place since its publication in 2002. This new edition extensively updates the case study material to reflect these advances and encompasses the current practice of nuclear medicine. We have two new associate editors, Drs. Twyla Bartel and Tracy Brown from the University of Arkansas, who contributed many excellent cases for this new edition. It has been a challenge to limit the number of cases to 200 because we had so much good new material, but I think we have succeeded in selecting the best. Much of the material is completely new, particularly the cases on PET/CT, SPECT/CT, and radiation safety. With the first edition, F-18 FDG PET was just beginning to become a clinical imaging modality after decades of investigation and development. It was primarily indicated for oncologic imaging. FDG PET was a major advance and changed the practice of oncology and nuclear imaging. Since then, hybrid PET/CT instruments became commercially available and their clinical use grew at a rapid rate, becoming the standard PET imaging modality. FDG PET/CT is now routinely reimbursed for many different oncologic indications and increasingly for neurologic and cardiac indications. Cardiac stress imaging using rubidium-82 PET is now used at many imaging centers because of its excellent image quality. Because it is generator produced, an on-site cyclotron is not needed. Cardiac viability imaging with F-18 FDG and Rb-82 is also increasing. Brain PET/CT is growing and expected soon to achieve its long-anticipated clinical utility, particularly for Alzheimer's disease, epilepsy, and Parkinson's disease. The great success of PET/CT led to the introduction of hybrid SPECT/CT for single photon imaging (e.g., somatostatin receptor imaging, I-123 MIBG, Tc-99m sestamibi parathyroid imaging, infection imaging). SPECT/CT is now showing the rapid clinical growth shown previously by PET/CT. Both hybrid technologies are leading us into the future of molecular imaging. Radiation safety, long an important topic but not emphasized in the first edition, is discussed in many cases presented in the second edition. Any case study retained from the first edition continues to prove its clinical importance and has been updated to reflect current practice. We think that the second edition will surpass the success of the first edition.

Harvey A. Ziessman, MD
Patrice Rehm, MD

We wish to acknowledge the important contributions to this second edition by Harry W. Schultz, CNMT, David Chien, MD, Frank Bengel, MD, Isaac Filat, CNMT, Terri Alpe, CNMT, and Tammy Thompson. They contributed time, images, and needed technical support to make the second edition possible.

Opening Round

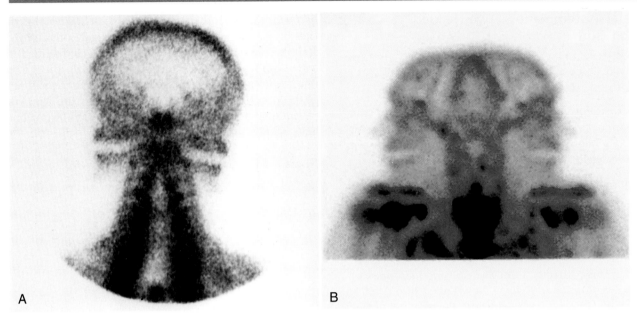

A   B

1. What radiopharmaceutical was used for these two studies?

2. Describe the scintigraphic findings. Interpret the limited studies.

3. Name the mythological Roman god that these images suggest.

4. What is the difference between a radioisotope, a radionuclide, a radionucleotide, radioactivity, and a radiotracer?

Skeletal System: Janus—Two-Headed Roman God

1. Bone scan radiopharmaceuticals in clinical use are usually diphosphonates (e.g., technetium-99m [^{99m}Tc] methylene diphosphonate).

2. Two patients, both with apparently two heads looking in opposite directions. A, The patient moved his/her head while being imaged; the technologist did not move his/hers. B, Right lateral and left lateral fused.

3. Janus.

4. These terms are frequently misused and confused. See the discussion under Comment.

References

Burr E (trans): Chapter J. In: *The Chiron Dictionary of Greek & Roman Mythology*. New York: Chiron, 1994.

Cherry SR, Sorenson JA, Phelps ME: *Physics in Nuclear Medicine*, 3rd ed. Philadelphia: WB Saunders, 2003.

Cross-Reference

Nuclear Medicine: THE REQUISITES, 3rd ed, pp 5, 113–158.

Comment

Janus is the two-faced Roman god of beginnings and endings, the god of gates and doors, from which the month of January and janitor get their names. He is depicted with two faces gazing in opposite directions. Looking back at the short history of nuclear medicine, there have been many major advances in the field—in instrumentation and radiopharmaceuticals and in their clinical use. Fluorodeoxyglucose (FDG) positron emission tomography (PET) is a relatively recent and excellent example of this progress. The radiotracer has transformed the practice of nuclear medicine and oncology. Like Janus, we should not only look back to know from where we have come, but we must look forward to the many opportunities ahead.

Nucleotides are basic structural building blocks of DNA and RNA, i.e., ribose or deoxyribose sugar, joined to a purine or pyrimidine base and a phosphate group. As different types of atomic structures are called elements, different types of nuclei are termed *nuclides*. *Radionuclides* are unstable radioactive elements. Radioactivity is the spontaneous emission radiation due to unstable atomic nuclei. Nuclides with the same number of protons are *isotopes* (e.g., ^{131}I, ^{123}I). An element is characterized by its atomic number (Z) alone, whereas a nuclide is characterized by its mass number (A) and its atomic number (Z). Radionuclides refer to radioactive elements of all types, whether natural or man-made. Technetium was the first man-made radionuclide. *Radio-*

pharmaceuticals are radionuclides attached to chemicals, drugs, or molecules used to investigate physiologic and biochemical processes (e.g., ^{99m}Tc labeled to methylene diphosphonate). Radiopharmaceuticals often are referred to as *radiotracers* because only trace amounts of the drugs are used, indicating that they are markers of physiologic processes (e.g., bone metabolism), but have no pharmacologic effect.

Notes

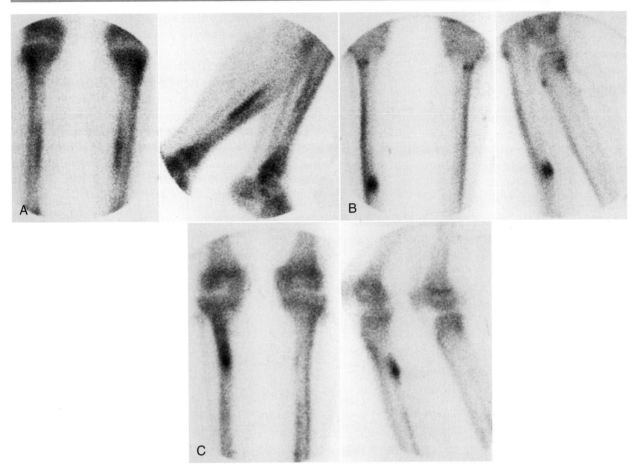

Three patients (A, B, C) have lower extremity pain. All are members of a high school track team.

1. Describe the findings in patient A.

2. What is the most likely diagnosis?

3. Describe the findings in patients B and C.

4. Provide the most likely diagnosis for patients B and C.

Skeletal System: Stress Fractures and Shin Splints

1. Increased activity in a linear pattern along the posterior and medial aspect of both mid-tibias.

2. Shin splints.

3. Patient B: focal ovoid activity posteromedial right tibia at the junction of the proximal two thirds and distal one third. Patient C: focal fusiform activity posteromedially in the right proximal tibia and linear activity along the posteromedial left tibia proximally which is more prominent distally.

4. Patient B: stress fracture. Patient C: stress fracture on the right and shin splints on the left.

References

Etchebehere EC, Etchebehere M, Gama R, et al: Orthopedic pathology of the lower extremities: scintigraphic evaluation of the thigh, knee, and leg, *Semin Nucl Med* 28:41–61, 1998.

Love C, Din AS, Tomas MB, et al: Radionuclide bone imaging: an illustrative review, *Radiographics* 23:341–358, 2003.

Cross-Reference

Nuclear Medicine: THE REQUISITES, 3rd ed, pp 138–139.

Comment

Bone is a dynamic tissue in which intermittent forces stimulate remodeling of the bone architecture to withstand applied stresses. Stress injury stimulates osteoclasts that cause small areas of resorption and microfractures and remodeling within lamellar bone. When bone formation cannot keep up with bone resorption, bone weakening results. In response to the temporarily weakened bone, periosteal reaction, endosteal proliferation, or both occur at the site of stress. If the stress is not reduced, the repair mechanisms may become overwhelmed, resulting in fracture.

Stress fractures on a bone scan have uptake due to the increased bone turnover described. They are focal, usually oval or fusiform, and based at the cortex with the axis of the abnormality parallel to that of the bone. Sometimes stress fractures may appear as a transverse band of increased activity. The scan abnormality typically precedes radiographic changes by 1 to 2 weeks, if they are seen on radiographs at all. Tibial stress fractures are most commonly seen posteromedially at the junction of the middle and distal thirds of the tibia, as in patient B.

The term *shin splints* is used for another type of leg pain, sometimes called an anterior tibial stress syndrome. Although there is no identifiable inciting event, pain often occurs after athletic activity and is typically relieved by rest. Scan findings vary, but there is bilateral linear tibial uptake involving the cortex in multiple areas or even diffusely. Uptake may be asymmetrical. The pattern differs from the pattern of a stress fracture. Because of the nature of the inciting stresses, stress fractures commonly coexist with shin splints. The difference has clinical significance because stress fractures are treated more aggressively, usually with discontinuance of the inciting physical activity for 6 weeks because of the potential for a through-and-through fracture. Shin splints are only treated symptomatically.

Notes

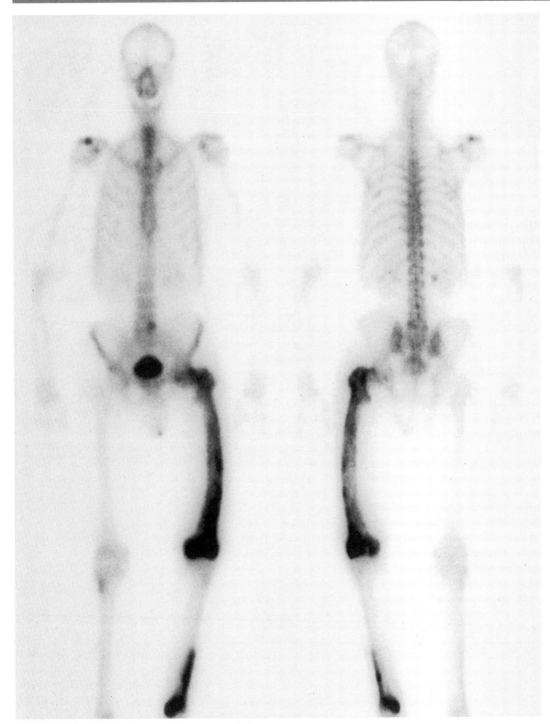

1. Describe the bone scan abnormalities.

2. Describe the characteristic pattern of uptake in the tibia.

3. Provide the differential diagnosis.

4. Patients with this disease may experience clinical symptoms related to another organ system. What is the mechanism?

Skeletal System: Paget's Disease

1. Abnormal increased uptake involving the entire left femur, which appears bowed and expanded, as well as the distal third of the left tibia.

2. A sharp leading edge that appears tapered, referred to as "flame-shaped" or "blade of grass," which may be seen in the lytic phase on radiographs and on bone scintigraphy.

3. Paget's disease versus osteosarcoma, but also fibrous dysplasia, chronic osteomyelitis, and primary bone tumors.

4. High-output congestive heart failure. Once believed to be the result of arteriovenous shunting within a bone lesion, increased blood flow through the lesion is now thought to be the cause.

References

Brown ML: Bone scintigraphy in benign and malignant tumors, *Radiol Clin North Am* 31:731–738, 1993.

Manaster BJ, May DA, Disler DG: *Musculoskeletal Imaging: THE REQUISITES*, 3rd ed. St. Louis: Mosby, 2007, pp 397–404.

Cross-Reference

Nuclear Medicine: THE REQUISITES, 3rd ed, pp 132, 144–145.

Comment

Paget's disease is a benign disorder characterized by excessive and abnormal bone remodeling. Common after the age of 40, Paget's disease is recognized because of bone pain, tenderness, or increase in bone size, but frequently is identified incidentally by an elevated serum alkaline phosphatase level or on radiographs or bone scans ordered for other reasons. The radiographic appearance has three phases: lytic, sclerotic, and mixed lytic-sclerotic. The classic appearance is one of bone enlargement, increased density, and a coarsened trabecular pattern. Lesions typically start at the end of a long bone; 20% are monostotic. The disease is characterized by an initial phase of excess bone resorption with a lytic front, followed by an intense osteoblastic reaction with deposition of woven bone. Skeletal architecture becomes disorganized with a mixed pattern of lytic and sclerotic disease. This imbalance of bone remodeling in favor of formation leads to cortical thickening and bone expansion. Bone scintigraphy demonstrates abnormal intense radiotracer uptake extending from the subcortical region for the length of the lesion, which may be most or all of the bone. The lesion may be three-phase positive in the active phase of the disease, although Paget's disease is most commonly identified on the delayed or bone phase.

A three-phase study is not necessary for diagnosis. Bone scans can be used to evaluate therapy, e.g., calcitonin or bisphosphonates. Response to therapy is indicated by a uniform or nonuniform decrease in radiotracer uptake.

Notes

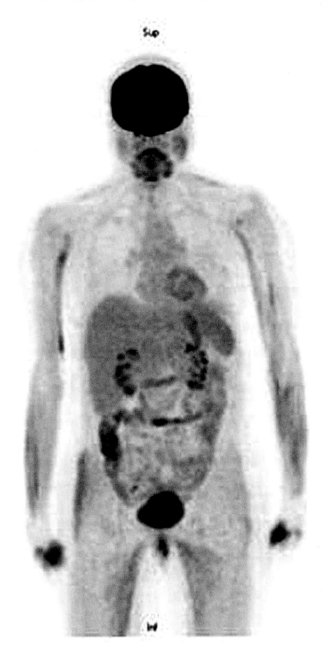

1. Name the radiopharmaceutical used for this study.

2. What is the radiopharmaceutical's mechanism of uptake?

3. Is this a normal distribution and excretion of this radiopharmaceutical?

4. Is this study normal? If not, explain.

C A S E 4

FDG-PET: Fluorine-18 (^{18}F)-Fluorodeoxyglucose (FDG) Uptake, Distribution, and Excretion

1. ^{18}F-FDG.

2. FDG is a glucose analogue transported into cells by the glucose transporter (GLUT) family of membrane transporters, GLUT-1 (non–insulin-sensitive tissues) and GLUT-4 (insulin-responsive tissues, e.g., striated muscle). FDG undergoes phosphorylation by hexokinase, and in most cell types is trapped as FDG-6-phosphate (FDG-6-P). This is different from glucose, which, once phosphorylated, is then metabolized by glucose-6-phosphatase and can leave the cell.

3. FDG normally distributes to organs/tissues in the body according to the degree that they metabolize glucose. The greatest uptake is in the brain, followed by the liver and spleen. Salivary glands, heart, and intestines have variable uptake. Unlike glucose, FDG is predominantly excreted through the kidneys and bladder.

4. Yes, except for increased uptake in the arms and thighs due to muscular use.

References

Cherry SR, Sorenson JA, Phelps ME: *Physics in Nuclear Medicine*, 3rd ed. Philadelphia: Saunders, 2003, pp 358–359.

Fanti S, Farsad M, Mansi L: *Atlas of PET/CT: A Quick Guide to Image Interpretation*. Berlin/ Heidelberg: Springer-Verlag, 2009.

Cross-Reference

Nuclear Medicine: THE REQUISITES, 3rd ed, pp 304–307.

Comment

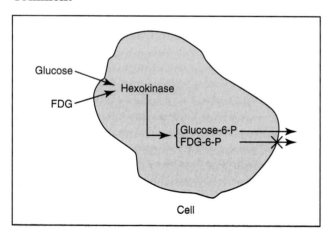

After ^{18}F-FDG injection, imaging is usually performed 1 hour later. FDG uptake increases progressively over this period of time. Although uptake continues after this time point, the 1-hour time period is usually considered the optimal time for imaging based on the degree of uptake, ^{18}F decay ($t_{1/2}$ of 120 minutes), and the logistics of a busy clinic. The relative amount of uptake in tissues/cells is dependent on the concentration of glucose-6-phosphatase within a particular cell type. The more a cell uses glucose, the greater the accumulation of FDG within that cell. The brain is an obligate glucose user, and thus uptake is high. Cardiac uptake is variable and depends on whether the patient is fasting. Under good fasting conditions, there is relatively low cardiac uptake. Patients are asked to fast from 4 to 12 hours before the study. Intestinal uptake is probably related to smooth muscle contraction, although there is some FDG excretion via the bowel. FDG uptake occurs in areas of inflammation and muscle tension. Note upper and lower extremity uptake due to muscle overuse or recent stress. Patients are asked to refrain from exercise before the study.

Notes

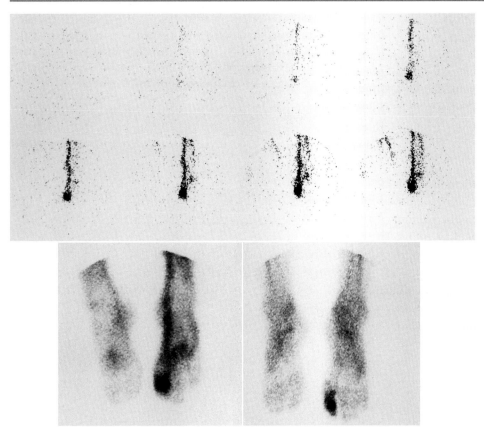

A 60-year-old diabetic patient with cellulitis of the distal foot. The patient was referred to rule out osteomyelitis of the left great toe. The radiograph was not diagnostic.

1. Describe the physiology of each of the three phases shown.

2. Describe the scintigraphic findings.

3. What is the differential diagnosis?

4. What is the most likely diagnosis and the sensitivity and specificity of the three-phase bone scan for diagnosis?

Skeletal System: Pedal Osteomyelitis—Three-Phase Positive Bone Scan

1. First phase: arterial blood flow (1- to 3-second frames). Second phase: "blood pool" or extracellular space distribution immediately following the flow phase. Third phase: bone uptake and background clearance at 3 hours after injection.

2. Increased flow, blood pool, and delayed imaging uptake to the left first digit distal phalanx.

3. Osteomyelitis versus fracture. The radiograph did not show a fracture.

4. Osteomyelitis. Sensitivity and specificity of approximately 95% if the radiograph is normal.

References

Donovan A, Schweitzer ME: Current concepts in imaging diabetic pedal osteomyelitis, *Radiol Clin North Am* 46:1105–1124, 2008.

Palestro CJ, Love C: Nuclear medicine and diabetic foot infections, *Semin Nucl Med* 39:52–65, 2009.

Cross-Reference

Nuclear Medicine: THE REQUISITES, 3rd ed, pp 147, 151, 155–157.

Comment

Foot ulcers frequently serve as the portal of entry for infection and osteomyelitis in patients with diabetes. Radiographic findings may be negative or nonspecific in early phases. A negative three-phase bone scan rules out osteomyelitis with a high degree of certainty. With osteomyelitis, bone scintigraphy is usually three-phase positive. With cellulitis, only the first two phases are positive. However, patients with vascular insufficiency may have decreased flow and blood pool phases. Checking for foot warmth and pedal pulses aids interpretation. A cold region in the distal extremity on all three phases suggests gangrene and nonviability. Differentiating joint infection from bone infection is important. With inflammatory synovitis, uptake is seen in distal bone on both sides of the joint.

The specificity of the three-phase scan is considerably lower in patients with violated or chronically diseased bone. Any cause of bone remodeling (e.g., healing fracture, recent orthopedic implants, gouty arthritis, and neuropathic osteoarthropathy) may result in a false-positive study result. However, radiographs often reveal these potential problems. In uncertain cases, radiolabeled leukocytes can be helpful. Differentiating bone from overlying soft-tissue infection can sometimes be difficult with ^{111}In oxine leukocytes because of its limited resolution. ^{99m}Tc-hexamethylpropyleneamine oxime (HMPAO) offers an advantage in the distal foot in such situations, and soft-tissue uptake usually can be distinguished from bone uptake. Single-photon emission computed tomography (SPECT)/CT can be very helpful in confirming or excluding bone involvement.

Notes

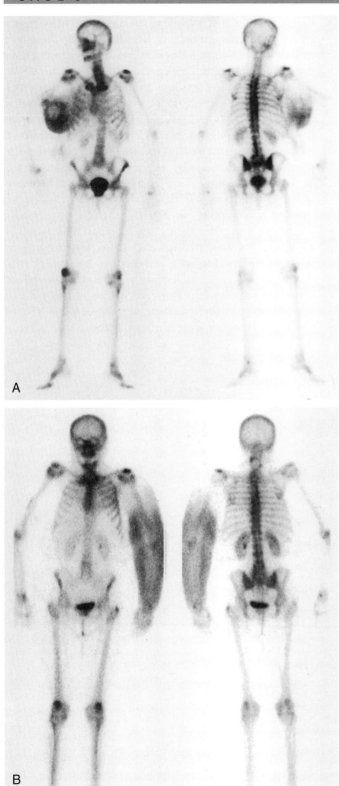

A

B

1. Describe the scintigraphic findings in patient A.

2. Describe the scintigraphic findings in patient B.

3. Provide a differential diagnosis for patient A.

4. Name three general processes that could account for the findings in patient B. What is the most likely?

Skeletal System: Inflammatory Breast Cancer and Lymphedema

1. Nonuniform abnormal soft-tissue uptake exists in the soft tissue overlying the chest, likely in the right breast.

2. The soft tissues of the left arm are enlarged and show abnormal increased activity; the left anterior ribs are uniformly more intense than the right.

3. Breast cancer, aseptic or septic mastitis, primary skin disease such as psoriasis, vascular and lymphatic obstruction, radiation therapy.

4. Venous or lymphatic obstruction, soft-tissue neoplasm, soft-tissue injury.

References

Hamaoka T, Madewell JE, Podoloff, et al: Bone imaging in metastatic breast cancer, *J Clin Oncol* 22:2942-2953, 2004.

Maffiioli L, Florimonte L, Pagani, et al: Current role of bone scan with phosphonates in the followup of breast cancer, *Eur J Nucl Med Mol Imaging* 31:S143-S148, 2004.

Yang WT, Le-Petross HT, Macapinlac H, et al: Inflammatory breast cancer: PET/CT, MRI, mammography, and sonography findings, *Breast Cancer Res Treat* 109:417-426, 2008.

Cross-Reference

Nuclear Medicine: THE REQUISITES, 3rd ed, pp 125-126.

Comment

Breast uptake on bone scans can be a normal finding. The greater the amount of uptake and degree of asymmetry, the more likely a pathologic condition exists. Bilateral uptake is usually seen with fibroadenomas, mammary dysplasia, cystic mastitis, and with lactation. Malignant uptake usually is unilateral. Patient A reported that the breast had been inflamed for weeks and a biopsy performed. The combination of the bone scan findings and clinical history limit the diagnosis to inflammatory carcinoma or mastitis. Inflammatory carcinoma consists of diffuse early invasion of the dermal lymphatics by an aggressive form of infiltrating carcinoma. An underlying primary lesion may not be evident. Inflammatory carcinoma occurs in less than 1% of invasive breast cancers. Its prognosis is worse than infiltrating ductal carcinoma that has secondarily invaded the skin. Soft-tissue involvement by malignant neoplasms, primary or metastatic, may show abnormal uptake of bone radiotracer. The most common causes are primary or metastatic breast cancer, lung cancer, metastatic colon cancer, and melanoma.

The finding of soft-tissue uptake in an enlarged upper extremity is characteristic of lymphedema as a result of axillary lymph node dissection and mastectomy. Other causes of lymphatic or venous obstruction should be considered, such as previous lymphadenectomy for melanoma, tumor replacement of lymph nodes causing obstruction to lymph flow, and venous obstruction from idiopathic thrombus or a previous indwelling catheter. Processes primarily related to the arm that could cause this appearance, such as sarcoma and electrical, frostbite, or crush injuries, are considerations but are seen much less frequently. In patients with breast cancer, the axillary lymph node dissection generally is primarily diagnostic and prognostic. It is controversial whether surgical excision of involved nodes also provides a therapeutic benefit. However, excision is associated with morbidity, such as transient or lifelong discomfort, abnormal sensation, or lymphedema, as in this patient. Lymphedema in the ipsilateral arm develops in 15% of women with breast cancer after therapy.

Notes

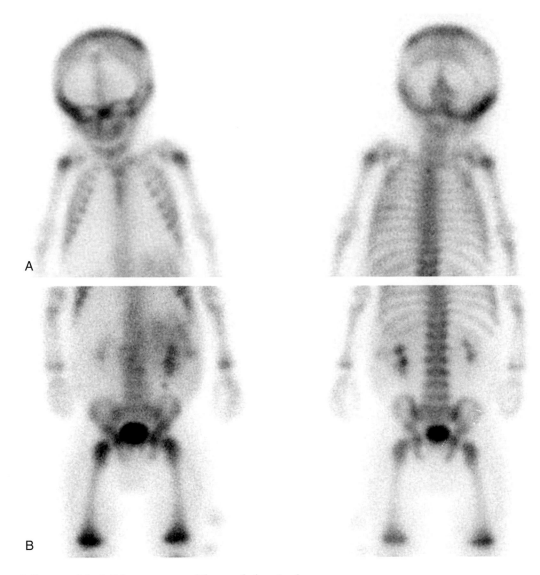

A

B

A 2-year-old child presents with an abdominal mass.

1. Describe the scintigraphic bone scan findings.

2. Name a likely organ of origin.

3. What is the most likely diagnosis?

4. What other exams are commonly used for staging of the patient's illness?

Skeletal System: Neuroblastoma

1. A large region of nonuniform abnormal soft-tissue uptake is seen in the left side of the abdomen, seen best on an anterior image. Uptake in the skull adjacent to right orbit, probably left orbit as well, and left occipitotemporal cortex.

2. Adrenal gland.

3. Primary neuroblastoma with metastases to bones.

4. I-123 *meta*-iodobenzylguanidine imaging, MRI.

References

Connolly LP, Drubach LA, Treves ST: Applications of nuclear medicine in pediatric oncology, *Clin Nucl Med* 27:117–125, 2002.

Kushner BH: Neuroblastoma: a disease requiring a multitude of imaging studies, *J Nucl Med* 45:1172–1188, 2004.

Cross-Reference

Nuclear Medicine: THE REQUISITES, 3rd ed, p 126.

Comment

Neuroblastoma is a malignant tumor of the sympathetic nervous system and occurs most frequently in early childhood. More than 85% of the tumors secrete variable amounts of catecholamines and their metabolites. Most neuroblastomas take up bone radiopharmaceuticals to varying degrees. The intensity of uptake does not correlate with the degree of malignancy or prognosis. Even primary tumors without radiographic evidence of calcification often have increased bone radiopharmaceutical uptake. The bone scan is a sensitive detector of neuroblastoma metastatic to bone and is abnormal weeks before radiographic changes are present. The combination of bone scan and I-123 or I-131 MIBG has the highest sensitivity for detection of bone involvement, and both are often used in evaluating response to therapy.

Staging requires determination of the extent of disease, necessitating anatomic imaging with CT, MRI, and histologic evaluation of the bone marrow. The Evans staging system is used most commonly. In this system, stage I disease is confined to the structure of origin. Stage II disease involves tumor extension in continuity but not across the midline or tumors arising in the midline. Stage III disease extends in continuity across the midline. Stage IV disease is disseminated disease with metastases involving the skeleton, soft tissues, distant lymph nodes, or organs. Stage IV-S disease occurs in patients whose primary tumor would be stage I or II except for metastatic disease to the liver, skin, or bone marrow but not the skeleton.

Notes

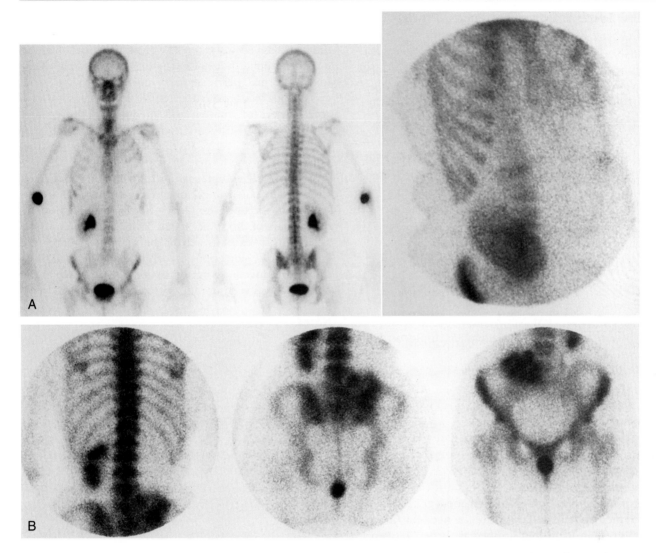

1. Describe and interpret the abnormal soft-tissue findings in patient A. Supine (*left*) and upright anterior oblique (*right*) images.

2. Describe the findings in patient B.

3. Provide the general classification for this finding in patient B and the likely diagnosis.

4. Name other conditions that fall in the same spectrum of abnormalities.

C A S E 8

Skeletal System: Extrarenal Pelvis, Ptotic, and Ectopic Kidneys

1. Solitary right kidney with a prominent renal pelvis. This is likely an extrarenal pelvis that clears radiotracer on standing, excluding obstruction. The kidney also descends in the upright position. There is no functioning left kidney. Incidental uptake is noted at the antecubital injection site.

2. The right kidney is not seen in the renal fossa. Non-uniform activity is noted in the right sacroiliac region, which extends beyond the expected superior margin of the bone.

3. Congenital renal anomaly, pelvic kidney.

4. Anomalies of number (supernumerary kidney), position (malrotation), or fusion (horseshoe).

References

Dunnick NR, Sandler CM, Newhouse JH, et al: *Textbook of Uroradiology*, 3rd ed. Philadelphia: Lippincott Williams & Wilkins, 2001.

Zagoria RJ: *Genitourinary Radiology: The REQUISITES,* 2nd ed. St Louis: Mosby, 2004.

Cross-Reference

Nuclear Medicine: THE REQUISITES, 3rd ed, pp 215–216.

Comment

Case A demonstrates how a simple maneuver can clarify scintigraphic findings and eliminate the need for further evaluation. If imaging had stopped with the full renal pelvis, the differential diagnosis would have included obstruction and likely prompted further diagnostic evaluation. Review of the completed scan by the physician before the patient leaves the department allows for tailoring of the scan protocol, which can lead to a more definitive interpretation and avoidance of further unnecessary testing. This case is a good example of renal mobility because the image was obtained initially in the supine and then erect position.

Renal anomalies involve the following factors: (1) number, which includes agenesis or the rare condition of supernumerary kidney; (2) position, which includes nonrotation, malrotation, and ectopia; and (3) fusion, which includes horseshoe kidney and cross-fused ectopia. Renal ectopia is an anomaly that arises from alteration of the normal caudal to cranial movement of the kidneys during development. Under ascent is much more common than over ascent (which gives rise to the thoracic kidney). In these cases, adjacent vessels usually provide the blood supply to the ectopic kidney. Renal ectopia may be associated with anomalies of fusion and contralateral renal anomalies. Under ascent of the kidney ranges from pelvic kidneys that lie in the true pelvis, in the iliac fossa opposite the iliac crest, to a location in the lower abdomen, but not at the expected level adjacent to L2. Normal pelvic kidneys do not have the same appearance as normally located kidneys because of variable degrees of rotation and alteration in the calices. Pelvic kidneys usually are asymptomatic, although they are at increased risk of ureteropelvic junction obstruction, reflux, stone formation, and trauma.

Cross-fused ectopia is an uncommon congenital anomaly in which one kidney crosses the midline and fuses with the opposite kidney, so that both kidneys lie on one side of the spine. Its ureter inserts in the normal position, but extends across the midline to enter the bladder on the side opposite to the kidney. Fused kidneys usually produce no symptoms but are susceptible to the complications seen in other ectopic kidneys.

Notes

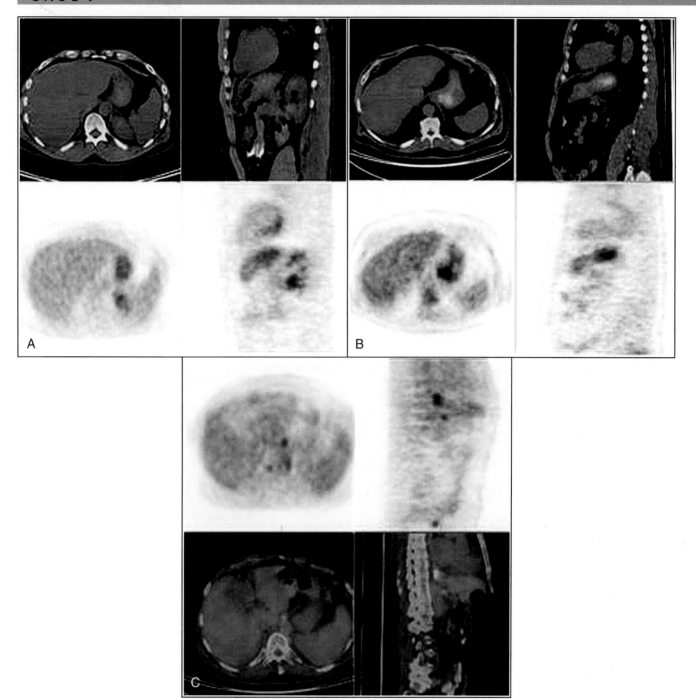

1. Describe the pattern of gastrointestinal FDG uptake in patients A and B.

2. What are the most common causes for *focal* FDG uptake in the stomach?

3. What are the most common causes for *diffuse* increased gastric FDG uptake?

4. What is the most likely cause of focal FDG uptake in patient C?

FDG-PET/CT: Gastric Uptake

1. Patient A: diffuse increased gastric uptake. Patient B: intense focal uptake in the gastric fundus with a background of moderate diffuse gastric uptake. Both have mild intestinal activity.

2. Malignant tumors, including adenocarcinoma, carcinoid, gastrointestinal stromal tumor, lymphoma, and benign tumors (e.g., polyps), as well as ulcer and focal inflammation. Patient B was diagnosed with a gastrointestinal stromal tumor.

3. Infection (e.g., *Helicobacter pylori*), gastritis, and infiltrative gastric neoplasms. However, diffuse gastric uptake is variable and often physiologic.

4. Focal uptake at the gastroesophageal junction and in lymph nodes inferior to the stomach (sagittal slice). The apparent metastatic lymph node suggests a distal esophageal/gastroesophageal junction carcinoma. Uptake at the gastroesophageal junction alone is not uncommon due to sphincter contraction or benign inflammation.

References

Lim JS, Hun MJ, Kim MJ, et al: CT and PET in stomach cancer: preoperative staging and monitoring of response to therapy, *Radiographics* 26:143–156, 2006.

Wong WL, Chambers RJ: Role of PET/PET CT in the staging and restaging of thoracic oesophageal cancer and gastro-oesophageal cancer: a literature review, *Abdom Imaging* 33:183–190, 2008.

Cross-Reference

Nuclear Medicine: THE REQUISITES, 3rd ed, pp 326–336.

Comment

In past years, squamous cell carcinoma was the most common histopathology, arising in the upper/middle esophagus. However, adenocarcinoma, arising in the distal esophagus, is increasing in incidence; 95% arise from Barrett's esophagus. In Asia, adenocarcinoma has long been the most common histology. In the stomach, adenocarcinoma is the most frequent histopathology.

Gastric adenocarcinoma often has a focal or masslike appearance on FDG-PET. Gastrointestinal stromal tumors demonstrate variable uptake. Two thirds originate in the stomach. Pretherapy studies are recommended to document FDG avidity to assess subsequent treatment response. Infiltrating tumors of the stomach (e.g., diffuse type or signet ring adenocarcinoma) can have low FDG uptake. Poorly differentiated adenocarcinoma, nonintestinal subtype tumors, and mucosa-associated lymphoid tissue lymphoma (Malt lymphoma) have only moderate and nonfocal FDG-PET.

PET is superior to CT for the detection of primary esophageal/esophagogastric junction tumors (80–85% vs. 65–70%) but has comparable accuracy for the detection of regional lymph nodes (63% vs. 66%). Both CT and PET are less accurate than endoscopic ultrasonography, with 75% accuracy for locoregional lymph node metastases. In newly diagnosed esophageal cancer patients, FDG-PET is most useful for the detection of distant solid organ metastases. PET sensitivity (67–82%) is superior to CT sensitivity (29–64%). FDG-PET more frequently correctly identifies inoperable patients than CT in esophageal and gastric malignancies. PET has also been shown to be effective in monitoring therapy response; changes in FDG uptake during therapy have prognostic implications.

Notes

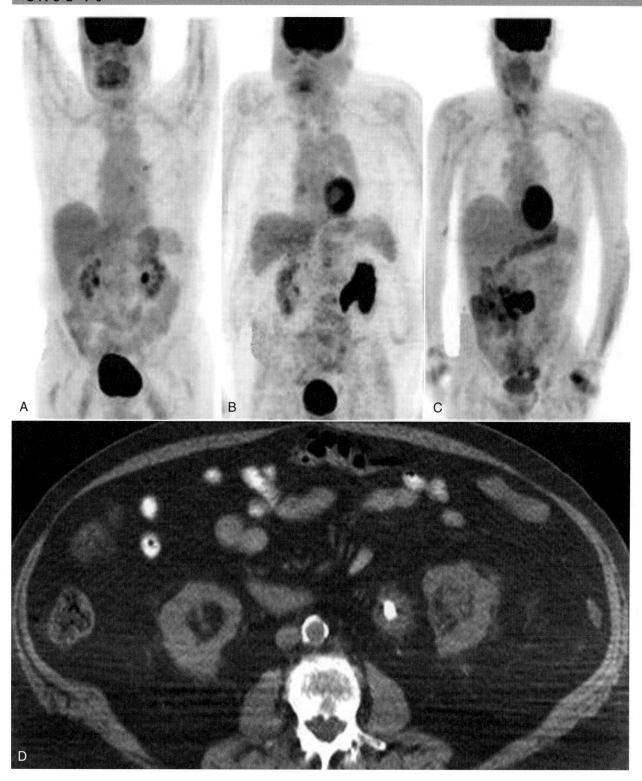

1. Describe the renal pattern of FDG uptake in patient A.

2. Why is there increased activity in the left kidney of patient B? Image D is patient B's CT.

3. What could be the cause of the renal uptake pattern in patient C?

4. How can radiation exposure to the kidneys and bladder be reduced during FDG-PET imaging?

FDG-PET: Renal Dysfunction, Renal Cancer

1. Patient A: Normal pattern. FDG is excreted via the kidneys, and, thus, activity is normally seen in the kidneys and often in the ureters and bladder.

2. Patient B: Intensely increased activity in the left kidney and proximal ureter. The cause of the abrupt cutoff is seen in the corresponding abdominal CT slice. A renal stone is present in the proximal ureter causing obstruction.

3. Patient C: No definite activity is seen in the kidneys, and little activity is seen in the bladder, likely indicating renal disease. This patient had biopsy-proven chronic interstitial nephritis and interstitial fibrosis.

4. Patients should empty their bladder before image acquisition. Intravenous furosemide is sometimes used.

References

Delbeke D, Coleman RE, Guiberteau MJ, et al: *Procedure Guideline for Tumor Imaging with F-18-FDG PET/ CT 1.0.* Reston, VA: Society of Nuclear Medicine, 2006.

Laffon E, Cazeau AL, Monet A, et al: The effect of renal failure on F-18-FDG uptake: a theoretic assessment, *J Nucl Med Technol* 36:200–202, 2008.

Scheipers C: *PET and PET/CT in Kidney Cancer.* Berlin/ Heidelberg: Springer-Verlag, 2006, pp 89–101.

Cross-Reference

Nuclear Medicine: THE REQUISITES, 3rd ed, pp 344–345.

Comment

FDG is filtered through the kidneys and cleared into the bladder. This is different from glucose, in which glycosuria is abnormal. Radioactive urine often makes it difficult to evaluate the kidneys or bladder for possible malignancy. Hydroureteronephrosis is an anatomic diagnosis. Retention in the collecting system shown on FDG-PET may not be due to obstruction, but rather to dehydration, stasis, duplicated collecting system, etc.

Careful evaluation on the correlative CT portion of the exam is important. FDG has variable uptake in renal cell carcinoma. This is likely due to a lower expression of GLUT. However, FDG-PET can be helpful in identifying distant metastatic disease of renal cell carcinoma.

The total effective radiation dose to an adult from FDG-PET is approximately 1 rem. The highest dose is to the bladder. The CT increases the PET/CT radiation dose to 2.5 rem. Obstruction will increase the renal dose; renal dysfunction will increase the total body effective dose. Furosemide is used in some imaging centers to reduce the patient or bladder radiation dose, improve renal cortical images, shorten the examination time, and avoid Foley catheter placement in some patients.

Notes

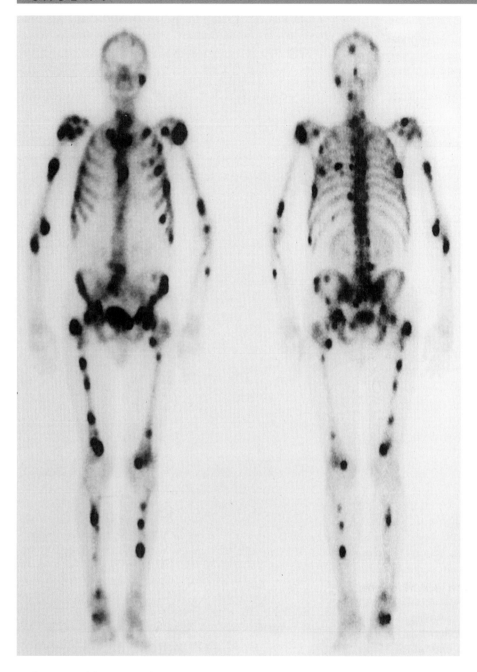

A 67-year-old man with prostate cancer.

1. Describe the findings on this bone scan and interpret the study.

2. What would you predict the serum prostate-specific antigen (PSA) level to be?

3. Which metastatic cancers produce predominantly lytic lesions in bone and, thus, are less likely to be detected (lower sensitivity) by bone scanning?

4. If a patient with prostate cancer has a significantly elevated serum PSA level postoperatively but negative bone scan findings, what other radionuclide imaging options might be helpful?

Skeletal System: Metastatic Prostate Cancer

1. Abnormal focal uptake throughout the axial and appendicular skeleton strongly suggestive of metastatic disease. The many distal appendicular lesions are uncommon and are usually seen with late-stage disease.

2. Greater than 20 ng/mL. Metastases are rarely seen with the serum PSA less than 10 ng/mL.

3. Multiple myeloma, followed by thyroid cancer, renal cell carcinoma, and lymphoma.

4. An [111]In ProstaScint study. CT and MRI have a poor sensitivity for detection of prostate cancer soft-tissue/nodal metastases (<20%).

References

Dasgeb B, Mulligan MH, Kim CK: The current status of bone scintigraphy in malignant diseases, *Semin Musculoskelet Radiol* 11:301–311, 2007.

Jacobson AF, Fogelman I: Skeletal scintigraphy in breast and prostate cancer: past, present, and future. In Freeman LM (ed): *Nuclear Medicine Annual 1999.* Philadelphia: Lippincott Williams & Wilkins, 1999.

Cross-Reference

Nuclear Medicine: THE REQUISITES, 3rd ed, pp 120, 290.

Comment

Bone scans are very sensitive for the detection of bone metastases in most cancers, considerably more sensitive than radiographs. At least 50% of the bone mineral content must be lost before a metastasis is detectable on radiographs. Although bone scans are not routinely indicated in patients with PSA levels less than 20 ng/mL, baseline scans are appropriate in patients with high Gleason scores, skeletal symptoms, abnormal radiographic findings, and patients with preexisting skeletal conditions that might render interpretation of scans difficult. PSA levels greater than 100 ng/mL suggest widespread skeletal involvement. Eighty percent of metastatic lesions are in the axial skeleton. In patients with known metastases, the incidence of extremity or skull involvement increases to 50%. The sensitivity of the bone scan for the detection of bone lesions caused by multiple myeloma is considerably lower (~50%) because these lesions are often lytic (i.e., predominantly osteoclastic).

Bone scans are used to determine the effectiveness of therapy, although serum PSA levels are increasingly used for this purpose. Nonetheless, the bone scan still is useful for the evaluation of symptomatic patients or when a change in management is contemplated. The serum PSA level may not be as useful in patients who have had hormone therapy. Patients with anti-androgen therapy may have metastases, yet normal levels of PSA.

Notes

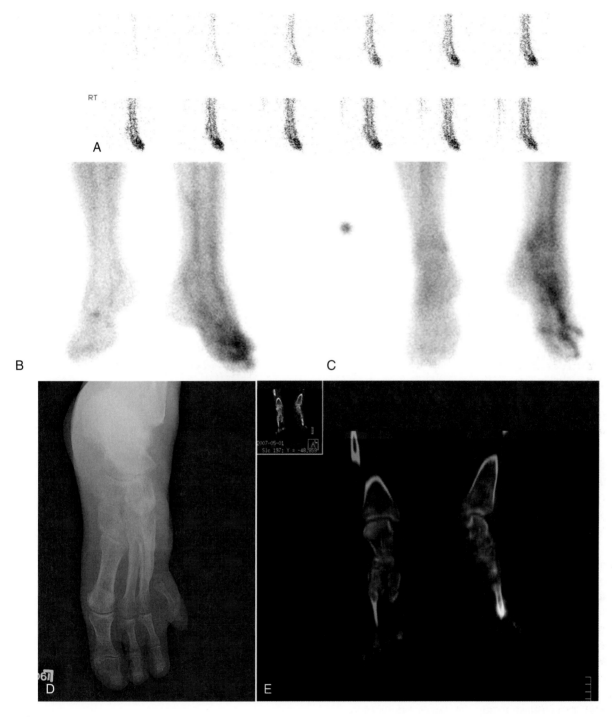

RT

A

B

C

D

E

A 65-year-old diabetic patient with left foot cellulitis with a history of distal amputations is referred to rule out osteomyelitis. Blood flow (A), blood pool (B), delayed bone images (C), radiograph (D), and SPECT/CT images (E) are shown.

1. What are potential diagnostic problems associated with interpretation of this three-phase bone scan for the diagnosis of osteomyelitis?

2. What is the added value of a flow study?

3. Describe the image findings in this study.

4. What is the added value of SPECT/CT? What is the likely diagnosis?

Skeletal System: Osteomyelitis, SPECT/CT

1. Bone scan uptake is nonspecific. It could be due to previous operations or fracture. Overlying soft-tissue infection and edema may make differentiation between bone and soft-tissue uptake somewhat difficult.

2. Improves specificity. Old fractures, surgery, degenerative changes will not usually have increased flow.

3. X-ray shows amputation of the entire left fifth digit and fourth metatarsal (D). Increased blood flow to the distal left foot (A). Increased blood pool in the distal foot (B). Considerable blood pool retention (C). Suspected uptake in the third metatarsal. Difficult for patient to position foot. SPECT/CT shows third metatarsal uptake (E).

4. SPECT provides improved contrast to eliminate overlying soft-tissue activity. CT provides improved anatomic localization (i.e., there is indeed uptake within bone).

References

Palestro CJ, Love C: Nuclear medicine and diabetic foot infections, *Semin Nucl Med* 39:52–65, 2009.

Scharf S: SPECT/CT imaging in general orthopedic practice, *Semin Nucl Med* 39:293–307, 2009.

Cross-Reference

Nuclear Medicine: THE REQUISITES, 3rd ed, pp 147–153.

Comment

The bone scan is used to detect and diagnose not only malignant disease, but also benign bone disease (e.g., occult fractures, stress fractures, osteoid osteomas, and osteomyelitis). Osteomyelitis is particularly problematic because it commonly occurs in the diabetic foot, which is often complicated by involvement with multiple pathologies, including Charcot joints, fractures, postsurgical inflammation with remolding, and degenerative disease, all of which can be third-phase bone scan positive. Thus, diagnosis and interpretation are often challenging. The three-phase study improves specificity. However, overlying soft-tissue infection and edema result in considerable radioactivity that clears slowly. A fourth phase is sometimes acquired to allow time for soft-tissue activity to clear, but this maneuver is often not adequate for differentiation of bone and soft tissue uptake. SPECT/CT makes it possible to differentiate cellulitis from osteomyelitis. SPECT improves contrast resolution by removing overlapping bone and soft-tissue activity. However, anatomic localization is limited, particularly in the setting of abnormal anatomy. Therefore, combining CT with SPECT enables better anatomic localization of abnormal foci. Similarly, SPECT/CT has been found useful for confirmatory studies using radiolabeled leukocytes. Leukocytes will go to both the soft-tissue infection and bone infection. SPECT/CT can differentiate these two (i.e., whether there is bone localization).

Notes

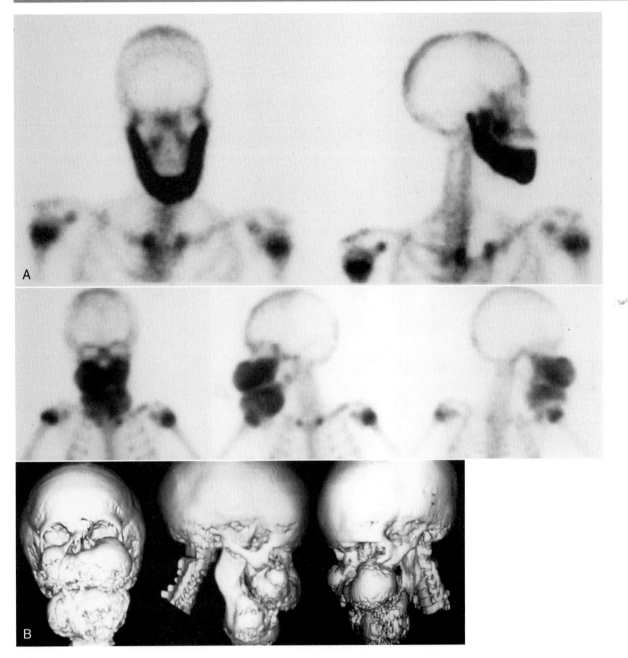

Because of a "jaw problem," a bone scan (A) and a bone scan/CT-3D reconstruction (B) were obtained in two children.

1. Describe the bone scan findings.

2. What additional information would be helpful?

3. Provide a short differential diagnosis.

4. The mother says there is no known disease in the child (B) or family. What is the most likely diagnosis?

Skeletal System: Fibrous Dysplasia

1. A shows increased uptake in the entire mandible. B shows intense increased uptake in the mandible and maxilla, which appear deformed and overgrown.

2. Check the rest of the bone scan for other sites; obtain a history of known underlying or familial disease.

3. Fibrous dysplasia, cherubism.

4. Fibrous dysplasia.

References

Blickman H, Parker BR, Barnes PD: *Pediatric Imaging: THE REQUISITES*, 3rd ed. St. Louis: Mosby, 2009.

Sartoris DJ: *Musculoskeletal Imaging: THE REQUISITES*, 3rd ed. St. Louis: Mosby, 2007, pp 460–465.

Cross-Reference

Nuclear Medicine: THE REQUISITES, 3rd ed, pp 131–133.

Comment

Fibrous dysplasia is a common congenital, nonhereditary skeletal disorder of unknown origin. It is characterized by a developmental anomaly of bone formation in which the marrow is replaced by fibrous tissue. Fibrous dysplasia occurs during periods of bone growth in older children and adolescents and slowly enlarges for life. Seventy-five percent of cases are monostotic. Other frequently affected sites include the proximal femur (35%), tibia (20%), and facial bones and ribs (15%). Sclerotic thickening caused by involvement of the facial bones is called leontiasis ossea ("resembling a lion's face").

Cherubism is a rare but different entity and results in bilateral swelling in the jaw with multilobular expansile bone lesions, which may simulate fibrous dysplasia. In contrast to fibrous dysplasia, cherubism is a familiar disorder. Skeletal deformities also can occur as a result of repeated pathologic fractures.

CT is most useful to determine the extent of involvement in a particular skeletal region. Identification of polyostotic involvement is one of the main indications for skeletal scintigraphy because many of these sites are asymptomatic. Hypertrophy of soft tissues and bones can be seen in several other conditions, including neurofibromatosis, macrodystrophia lipomatosa, hemangiomas as in Klippel-Trénaunay-Weber disease, and lymphangiomatosis.

Notes

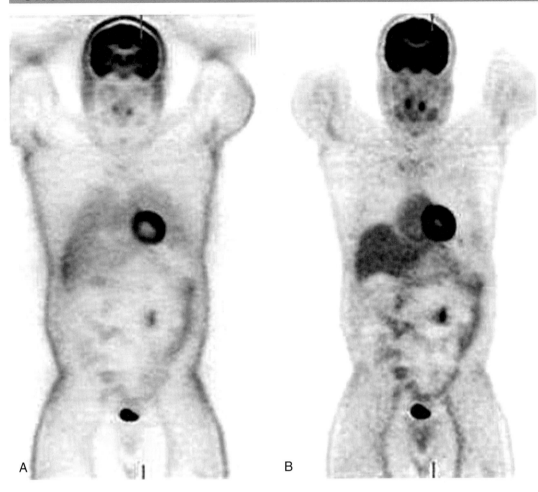

A   B

1. Describe the difference in the pattern of ^{18}F-FDG activity in A and B.

2. A and B are the same patient. What is the difference in processing?

3. For what purpose is each image used?

4. What is the origin of the two foci of increased uptake in the oral area?

C A S E 1 4

PET: Attenuation Correction

1. Patient A has higher uptake at the skin surface and lesser uptake in internal organs compared to patient B.

2. A is a nonattenuation-corrected PET image with greater intensity seen at the body surface where photons are least attenuated. B is an attenuation-corrected image that allows for a truer representation of FDG distribution, particularly for internal organs.

3. The attenuation-corrected image (B) is generally used for routine clinical interpretation. The nonattenuation-corrected image (A) is most useful when there is a question of pathology versus artifact producing "hot" areas on the attenuation-corrected images. Superficial structures (e.g., nodules in the periphery of the lung or cutaneous lesions) may be better seen without correction.

4. Uptake within the palatine tonsils. More lateral and inferior is normal submandibular uptake.

References

Saha GB: *Basics of PET Imaging*. New York: Springer, 2005, pp 48–53.

von Schulthess GK, Steiner HC, Hany TF: Integrated PET/CT: current applications and future directions, *Radiology* 238:405–422, 2006.

Cross-Reference

Nuclear Medicine: THE REQUISITES, 3rd ed, pp 60, 317.

Comment

For PET-only cameras, a radioactive transmission source, usually germanium-68, is rotated around the patient to generate a transmission scan for attenuation correction. In hybrid PET/CT cameras, the CT provides the transmission scan. While the high count density provided by CT is not required for good correction, currently sold commercial cameras are combined PET/CT systems.

For PET/CT, attenuation correction of the PET data occurs by generating a map of tissue attenuation coefficients (μ) determined by CT using x-rays at a given energy (usually 40–140 kVp). Different scale factors for bone and nonbone materials are applied with bilinear scaling methods. Because the PET data represent photons detected at 511 keV, the CT-based attenuation map is then transformed to represent the attenuation that would be seen with 511-keV photons. This "map" is then applied to the nonattenuation-corrected PET data, yielding an attenuation-corrected PET data set. The major advantage of CT rather than a radioactive transmission source for attenuation correction is faster data acquisition, by 25% to 30%. Of course, the CT images are used for organ localization of PET activity.

Correct interpretation of PET/CT images requires alignment of the PET and CT. In hybrid PET/CT cameras, the scans are acquired sequentially; first CT, followed by the PET study. The two image sets are then aligned using inherent fiducial/hardware markers. Because they are not obtained simultaneously, misalignment can occur if the patient moves or there is physiologic motion (e.g., intestinal) between the PET and CT acquisitions. When PET and CT images are misregistered or misaligned, the attenuation-corrected PET images will contain errors that can sometimes be corrected with software-based coregistration algorithms. Combining proper software- and hardware-based coregistration is an important aspect of attenuation correction.

Notes

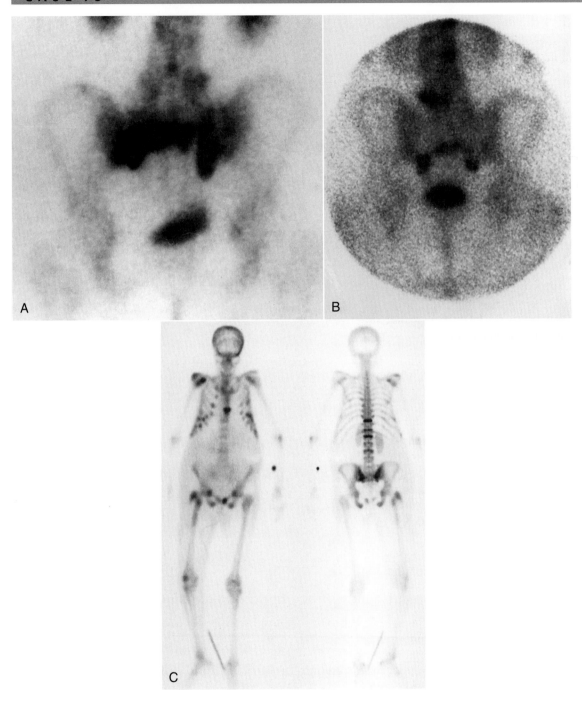

Patient A has low back pain. Patient B has a history of hip fracture and now reports pelvic pain and inability to walk.

1. Describe the bone scan abnormalities in patient A and provide likely diagnoses.

2. Describe the scintigraphic abnormalities in patient B.

3. Provide a differential diagnosis and most likely diagnosis for patient B.

4. Name three medical conditions that predispose patients to this underlying disease process.

Skeletal System: Insufficiency Fractures of Sacrum and Pelvis

1. Patient A has increased uptake bilaterally in the region of the sacroiliac joints and across the sacrum (H pattern). Patient B has abnormal increased uptake in a curvilinear pattern across the lower sacrum. These are characteristic of sacral insufficiency fractures. Malignancy has to be excluded.

2. Multiple focal areas of increased radiotracer uptake are noted in several ribs and multiple sites in the pelvis, including both pubic rami, lower sternum, and multiple vertebrae. Bilateral uptake in the region of the sacroiliac joints and low-grade activity between them in the sacrum.

3. Multifocal involvement by benign or malignant tumor, multifocal osteomyelitis, fractures. Multiple insufficiency fractures secondary to osteoporosis is most likely. Degenerative change is present in the right shoulder and postoperative change related to previous right hip orthopedic fixation.

4. Hypercortisolism, hyperparathyroidism, hyperthyroidism.

References

Balseiro J, Brower AC, Ziessman HA: Scintigraphic diagnosis of sacral fractures, *AJR Am J Roentgenol* 148:111, 1987.

Fujii M, Abe K, Hayashi K, et al: Honda sign and variants in patients suspected of having a sacral insufficiency fracture, *Clin Nucl Med* 30:165–169, 2005.

Cross-Reference

Nuclear Medicine: THE REQUISITES, 3rd ed, pp 132–133, 144.

Comment

Insufficiency fractures are an important and common complication of osteoporosis, a condition resulting from diminished bone quantity seen in postmenopausal women, hyperparathyroidism, and patients on steroid therapy. In many cases, fractures occur with minimal or no known trauma. Common sites of osteoporosis-related insufficiency fractures outside the pelvis are the vertebral bodies, femoral neck and intertrochanteric region, distal radius, humeral neck, proximal and distal tibia, ribs, and sternum. Dual-energy x-ray absorptiometry (DEXA) studies are used to predict fracture risk. Although multiple bone abnormalities may suggest tumor metastases, close review of the character and location of the findings usually leads to the correct diagnosis. Radiographs can be confirmatory. The spine abnormalities have a linear appearance that suggests fracture (either wedge compression fracture or vertebral end-plate deformity). Rib abnormalities occur in adjacent ribs in a linear pattern that strongly suggests fractures.

Because of the increased radiolucency of affected bone, fractures may be difficult to identify on radiographs. However, usually they are easily detectable on bone scintigraphy because of its high sensitivity for identification of sites of increased bone turnover and osteoblastic activity. Insufficiency fractures in the pelvis typically involve the sacrum, symphysis pubis, or pubic rami. Sacral fractures are associated with characteristic bone scan appearances, such as the H pattern with vertical involvement of sacral ala and horizontal involvement of the sacrum. Only portions of the H may be seen. Another pattern is that of linear, curvilinear, or a "dot and dash" appearance seen in case B. Postradiation-induced fractures can have a similar appearance.

Notes

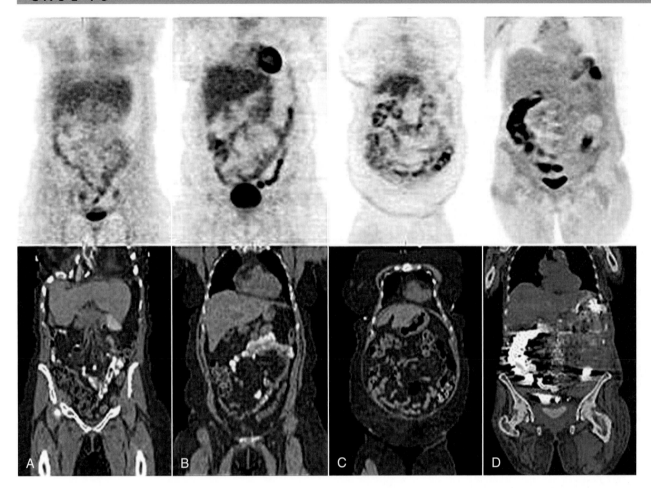

Coronal PET (*top*) and CT (*bottom*) images of four patients.

1. Describe the varying intestinal FDG activity in these four different patients.

2. Which of the patients has normal or abnormal distribution?

3. Explain the cause for the different patterns of uptake/distribution.

4. What is the effect of oral contrast in bowel on FDG-PET/CT imaging?

FDG-PET: Intestinal Activity

1. All patients show FDG activity in the intestinal tract and small and/or large bowel to varying degrees and in different patterns. Some increased activity corresponds to regions with oral contrast. The oral contrast can cause attenuation reconstruction artifacts and affect attenuation correction.

2. All have physiologic distribution. There is considerable normal variation in the pattern of intestinal FDG uptake.

3. Variability may be due to smooth muscle peristalsis, increased density of lymphoid tissue, smooth muscle uptake in the ileocecal valve, oral contrast-induced irritation, or some combination, and some FDG physiologic excretion.

4. Oral contrast can cause apparent increases in physiologic FDG uptake. This may be due to bowel irritation secondary to the oral contrast and/or a reconstruction artifact as counts in the region of dense contrast are artificially increased on attenuation-correction images, although not on nonattenuation-corrected images. The PET and CT images to the far right demonstrate a case in which barium contrast causes count overcorrection. Dilute oral contrast is administered to minimize this effect.

References

Antoch G, Jentzen W, Freudenberg LS, et al: Effect of oral contrast agents on computed tomography-based positron emission tomography attenuation correction in dual-modality positron emission tomography/computed tomography imaging, *Invest Radiol* 28:784–789, 2003.

Otsuka H, Graham MM, Kubo A, Nishitani H: The effect of oral contrast on large bowel activity in FDG-PET/CT, *Ann Nucl Med* 19:101–108, 2005.

Rabhakar HB, Sahani DV, Fischman AJ, et al: Bowel hot spots at PET-CT, *Radiographics* 27:145–159, 2007.

Cross-Reference
Nuclear Medicine: THE REQUISITES, 3rd ed, p 306.

Comment

There are several causes of increased normal FDG bowel activity on PET, including artifact from surgical clips or contrast, muscle uptake, and tracer excreted in the bowel. One should be cautious in overinterpreting increased bowel activity and be familiar with the different and variable patterns seen. Having the correlative anatomic CT image for review can help differentiate between the various causes. Segmental or diffuse FDG activity in the bowel suggests inflammation. However, when intense focal activity is noted in the bowel, it is important to correlate this finding with the corresponding CT to determine whether there are soft-tissue abnormalities such as stranding, edema, or mass that would explain the uptake. Current recommendations are to follow-up intense focal uptake with endoscopy to exclude an underlying malignant or premalignant lesion.

The presence of oral contrast typically causes an overestimation of radiotracer activity concentration when using CT-based attenuation correction and more so, the denser it is. The oral contrast used with PET/CT is relatively dilute and not as likely to cause artifacts as contrast from a recent barium enema. Artifacts are seen because of the correction algorithm's misclassification of contrast as bone. The overestimation is directly related to the contrast concentration. In cases in which this overestimation is suspected, careful examination of the nonattenuation-corrected images should be done as the artifact should be absent on these images.

Notes

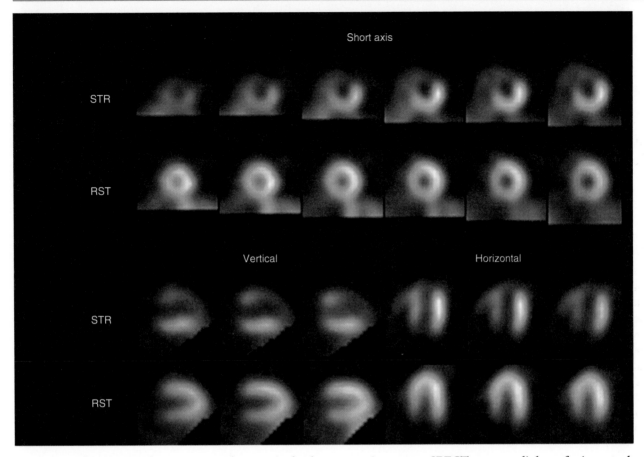

A 55-year-old man with recurrent chest pain had an exercise stress SPECT myocardial perfusion study.

1. Describe the perfusion abnormalities and give your interpretation.

2. Name the likely culprit vessel or vessels.

3. List any ancillary scan findings.

4. List symptoms or findings of the stress test relevant to interpretation of the scan.

Cardiovascular System: Left Anterior Descending Artery Ischemia

1. Severely decreased perfusion in much of the anterior wall, apex, and septum, which normalizes on the rest image, indicating severe ischemia.

2. Left anterior descending coronary artery.

3. Transient stress-induced cavity dilation.

4. Stress-induced angina, ST-segment abnormalities, decrease in systolic blood pressure, ventricular tachyarrhythmias, and level of exercise achieved.

Reference

Yao SS, Rozanski A: Myocardial perfusion scintigraphy in conjunction with exercise and pharmacologic stress: prognostic applications in the clinical management of patients with coronary artery disease. In DePuey EG, Garcia EV, Berman DS (eds): *Cardiac SPECT Imaging,* 2nd ed. Philadelphia: Lippincott Williams & Wilkins, 2001, pp 263–296.

Cross-Reference

Nuclear Medicine: THE REQUISITES, 3rd ed, pp 459–470.

Comment

Although stress myocardial perfusion studies are sensitive for the detection of coronary artery disease (CAD; >85%), the sensitivity for diagnosis of multivessel disease is lower. Ischemia in multiple vascular distributions may not be evident on the perfusion study. This is because the most severe lesion produces symptomatic ischemia and exercise is discontinued before producing ischemia in myocardial regions of less diseased vessels.

Both transient ischemic dilation and stress-induced pulmonary ^{201}Tl uptake are important indicators of multivessel disease. Stress-induced left ventricular cavity dilation is apparent by comparison of stress (STR) and rest (RST) images. This finding may be the result of an increase in the left ventricular volume, indicating stress-induced ventricular dysfunction. Alternatively, this finding may be due to diffuse subendocardial ischemia, making the ventricular cavity appear larger.

Angina-type chest pain and depression of the ST segment on electrocardiographic evaluation during stress are suggestive of ischemia. Indicators of severe ischemia include a decrease in the patient's systolic blood pressure, 2 mm or greater ST wave segment depression, and ventricular arrhythmia (frequent premature ventricular contractions, ventricular tachycardia). These findings are reasons to stop the exercise, allowing, if possible, 1 minute after the stress dose injection for radiopharmaceutical uptake so that diagnostic images can still be obtained.

Notes

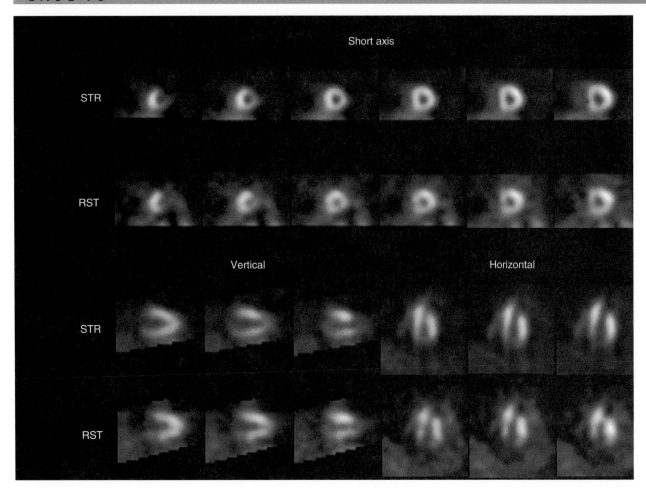

Short axis

STR

RST

Vertical   Horizontal

STR

RST

A 60-year-old thin man with a history of a remote myocardial infarction and coronary artery bypass graft surgery. A Persantine (dipyridamole) stress test was performed. Echocardiography results were normal.

1. Describe the SPECT findings.

2. Provide the differential diagnosis.

3. What is the most likely diagnosis?

4. Explain the discrepancy between the echocardiography and SPECT studies.

Cardiovascular System: Apical Infarct

1. Fixed stress (STR) and rest (RST) moderate size severe apical lateral perfusion defect of small size. Heart and cavity size appear normal.

2. Myocardial infarction, apical thinning, attenuation.

3. Small apical scar.

4. Possible factors: technical factors, operator error, interpretation error.

References

Berman DS, Hayes SW, Germano G: Assessment of myocardial perfusion and viability with ^{99m}Tc perfusion agents. In DePuey EG, Garcia EV, Berman DS (eds): *Cardiac SPECT Imaging,* 2nd ed. Philadelphia: Lippincott Williams & Wilkins, 2001, pp 179–210.

Jain D, Zaret BL: Nuclear imaging in cardiovascular medicine. In Rosendorf C (ed): *Essential Cardiology: Principles and Practice*, 2nd ed. Totowa, NJ: Humana Press, 2005, pp 221-244.

Cross-Reference

Nuclear Medicine: THE REQUISITES, 3rd ed, pp 463–466, 470-474.

Comment

This fixed apical perfusion defect in a thin man is unlikely to be caused by attenuation. The appearance of apical thinning is thought to be related to the normal lesser myocardial mass at the apex and perhaps partial volume effect. In a normal-sized heart, apical thinning is most commonly seen on the horizontal long-axis view but uncommonly on the vertical long-axis and short-axis views, as in this case. With ventricular dilation, apical thinning becomes more prominent and may be seen on more than the horizontal long-axis slices. This ventricle is not dilated in this patient. The lack of improvement in perfusion at rest confirms that this is an infarction, not ischemia. A septal wall motion abnormality (hypokinesis or dyskinesis) is often seen in patients with previous coronary artery bypass graft surgery. The subdiaphragmatic liver activity just inferior to the heart suggests that the patient had either pharmacologic stress or inadequate exercise. Exercise shifts blood flow away from abdominal viscera to the exercising muscles.

Echocardiography would also show the akinesis in this patient. Echocardiography is operator dependent and stress echocardiography even more so (i.e., operator skills and effort on a given case can affect the results). In some patients, particularly those with chronic obstructive pulmonary disease, the acoustic window may be suboptimal and limit the examination. If a gated wall motion study had been performed, it might have shown hypokinesis in this region; however, because of the small size, motion could appear normal. Normal wall motion or hyperkinesis of the adjacent myocardial regions can obscure a small hypokinetic segment of myocardium.

Notes

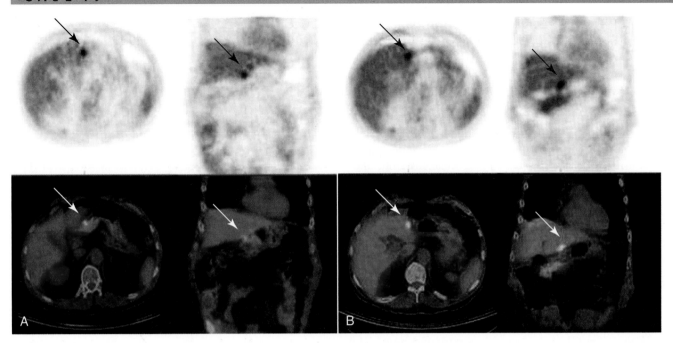

A 64-year-old patient with stage IIIA adenocarcinoma of the rectosigmoid colon is referred for treatment strategy. A, Selected FDG-PET images (*top*) and fused PET/CT images (*bottom*) from the initial study. B, Follow-up images at 3 months. No therapy in the interval.

1. What is the differential diagnosis for the focal uptake (*arrows*) on both studies?

2. What are common clinical indications for FDG-PET scanning in patients with colorectal cancer?

3. What quality control issues should be considered during interpretation of PET/CT images?

4. In what ways do CT images obtained during a hybrid PET/CT study for the purpose of attenuation correction differ from diagnostic CTs of the abdomen?

PET/CT: Misregistration and Fusion of FDG-PET and CT

1. Metastasis to the stomach or bowel wall, peritoneal metastasis, liver metastasis, gastric ulcer, or polyp.

2. (1) Staging before curative surgical resection of primary colorectal cancer or limited metastases, (2) localization of recurrence in patients with increasing serum carcinoembryonic antigen levels and equivocal/negative findings on conventional imaging, and (3) assessment for active disease in residual masses after treatment.

3. Review images for evidence of poor patient preparation (e.g., nonfasting) and errors of reconstruction. CT should be checked for artifacts (e.g., hardware, inadequate field-of-view). PET/CT fusion images should be checked for misregistration due to patient, respiratory, or cardiac motion.

4. Diagnostic abdominal CT is obtained during breath hold. This CT was obtained as part of whole-body FDG. PET/CT is acquired during "quiet" tidal breathing. Tube current (mAs) and voltage (kVp) used for attenuation-correction CT scans are often lower than those used for a diagnostic CT in an effort to minimize radiation exposure.

References

De Geus-Oei LF, Vriens D, van Laarhoven HW, et al: Monitoring and predicting response to therapy with 18F-FDG PET in colorectal cancer: a systematic review, *J Nucl Med* 50(Suppl 1):43S–54S, 2009.

Nehmeh SA, Erdi YE: Respiratory motion in positron emission tomography/computed tomography: a review, *Semin Nucl Med* 38:167–176, 2008.

Cross-Reference

Nuclear Medicine: The REQUISITES, 3rd ed, pp 311–312.

Comment

Review of the fusion images in part A reveals that PET and CT images are misregistered, with PET translated inferiorly and posteriorly relative to CT. A, Focal uptake in the right upper quadrant is localized to the stomach. With better registration (B), uptake is localized to the liver, suggesting liver metastasis.

Liver metastases from colorectal cancer are typically intensely FDG avid. FDG-PET in the pretherapy detection of metastasis has increased sensitivity compared with conventional staging (CT, MRI) and can identify disease that was occult or unsuspected clinically in 25% of patients. Sensitivity and specificity for the detection of liver metastases from recurrent colorectal cancer are greater than 96%. In the setting of increasing carcinoembryonic antigen and negative findings on conventional imaging, FDG-PET can identify sites of recurrence with a sensitivity of 92% to 100%.

Due to the relatively long imaging time required at each bed position, PET images are acquired during tidal breathing. The diaphragm and adjacent structures (e.g., liver, kidneys, lung bases) may translate as much as 8 to 25 mm along the z axis. To maximize registration between PET and CT images, CT images with PET/CT are also acquired during tidal breathing. Organs may be shifted on CT relative to PET because the CT acquisition time is brief. Thus, images may still be misregistered. This results in underestimation of uptake because of partial volume effect. Respiratory gating can be used to minimize this effect.

Notes

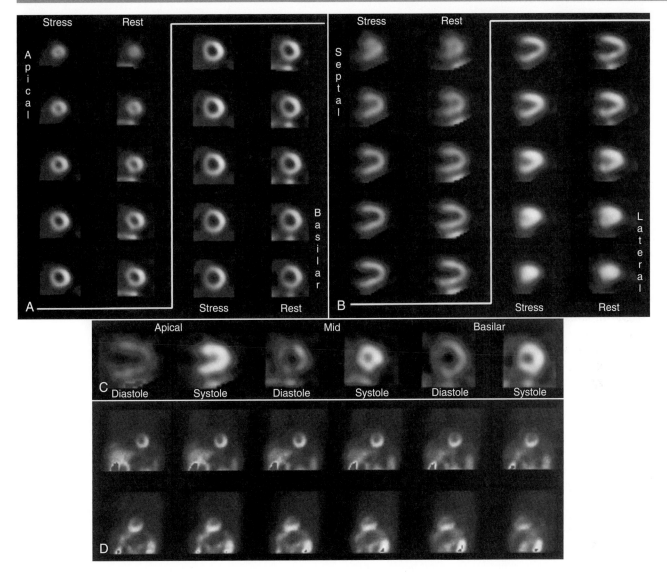

A 50-year-old woman presented with atypical chest pain. The exercise treadmill cardiogram result was interpreted as negative. SPECT perfusion images (A, gated short-axis; B, vertical long-axis; C, SPECT wall thickening; D, sequential raw data projection acquisition images) are provided.

1. Describe the SPECT myocardial perfusion and gated image findings.

2. What information is available from the raw data sequential projection images?

3. What is the most likely diagnosis?

4. List the advantages of electrocardiogram-synchronization (gating) to SPECT.

Cardiovascular System: Breast Attenuation, Wall Thickening

1. Fixed mildly decreased anteroseptal radioactivity that demonstrates uniform wall motion and brightening on gated SPECT, the latter indicating normal myocardial wall thickening.

2. Decreased radiotracer in the upper portions of the heart is most obvious on the left anterior oblique and lateral frames. No obvious patient motion.

3. Normal perfusion study with normal wall thickening and breast attenuation.

4. Assessment of regional wall motion/wall thickening and calculation of left ventricular ejection fraction (LVEF).

Reference

Go V, Bhatt MR, Hendel RC: The diagnostic and prognostic value of ECG-gated SPECT myocardial perfusion imaging, *J Nucl Med* 45:912–921, 2004.

Cross-Reference

Nuclear Medicine: THE REQUISITES, 3rd ed, pp 470–472.

Comment

Gated SPECT analysis allows for assessment of regional wall motion, wall thickening, and calculated LVEF. For gated SPECT, the cardiac cycle is usually divided into 8 frames (in contrast to 16 or more frames for planar equilibrium ventriculography) because of the lower count rate. The lower number of frames has somewhat poorer accuracy for LVEF calculation because of the more limited temporal resolution. For example, true end-systole and end-diastole may not be detected because of summation of counts in the longer time frames. The higher count rates available with ^{99m}Tc agents compared with ^{201}Tl and the use of multiheaded cameras are advantageous in maximizing the count rate for gated SPECT. Myocardial thickening is estimated by apparent brightening at end-systole due to the same number of counts in a smaller volume myocardial wall.

Stress myocardial perfusion imaging is considerably more accurate for assessment of CAD than stress electrocardiography. Stress electrocardiography has a sensitivity and specificity of approximately 70%, thus 30% false-negative and false-positive rates. False-positive results are a particular problem in female patients, to some degree, because of variable breast attenuation due to different breast positioning. In contrast, stress myocardial perfusion studies have an overall accuracy rate of approximately 85%. Individuals with normal scan results have less than 1% annual incidence of a major cardiac event.

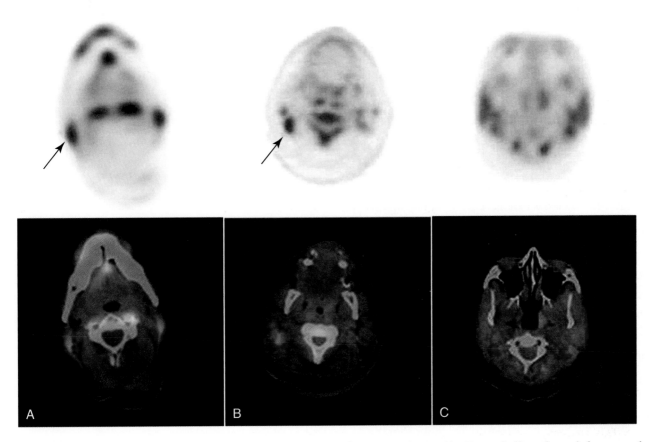

Head and neck FDG-PET and fused PET/CT obtained in 3 patients (A, B, and C) referred for oncologic restaging.

1. Describe the pattern of uptake in each of the three patients (A, B, and C). *Upper images* are PET and *lower images* are fused PET/CT.

2. What is the most likely etiology for this pattern in each case?

3. What is the mechanism of FDG uptake in patient C versus patient A?

4. Focal uptake in patient B has a maximum standard uptake value (SUV) of 2.8, whereas focal uptake in the neck in patient A has a maximum SUV of 3.3 (*arrow*). What SUV cutoff can differentiate benign from malignant disease in the head and neck?

FDG-PET: Cervical Uptake, Brown Fat, Adenopathy

1. There are multiple foci of intense FDG uptake bilaterally that appear fairly symmetrical in all 3 patients, perhaps slightly less so in patient B.

2. A, Physiologic uptake in muscles in lymphoma patient. B, Pathologic FDG-avid lymph nodes in a patient with head and neck cancer. C, Physiologic uptake predominantly in brown fat in a breast cancer patient.

3. Uptake in brown adipose tissue (C) is related to thermoregulation. In contrast to white fat, which stores energy, brown fat has extensive β-adrenergic innervation. Norepinephrine stimulation increases blood flow and glucose utilization. The uptake in muscles in patient A is caused by increased metabolism due to tension.

4. No absolute SUV cutoff has been shown to be reliable in differentiating benign from malignant uptake in the head and neck. Asymmetry, chronology, and CT correlation should be considered during study interpretation.

References

Cypess AM, Lehman S, Williams G, et al: Identification and importance of brown adipose tissue in adult humans, *N Engl J Med* 360:1509–1517, 2009.

Nakamoto Y, Tatsumi M, Hammoud D, et al: Normal FDG distribution patterns in the head and neck: PET/CT evaluation, *Radiology* 234:879–885, 2005.

Cross-Reference

Nuclear Medicine: THE REQUISITES, 3rd ed, pp 306–307.

Comment

FDG uptake in brown fat is seen most commonly in the neck and supraclavicular regions, less frequently in the mediastinum, axillae, paraspinal, perirenal and perisplenic regions. Prominent brown fat uptake in the neck is seen in 2.5% to 4% of patients. Although it is readily appreciated on PET/CT, it can potentially obscure uptake in pathologic lymph nodes, particularly subcentimeter ones. Although uptake in both muscle and brown fat is typically symmetrical and often elongated, it may appear focal. Brown fat is most commonly seen in patients during cold weather, often in patients who are shivering, nervous, or anxious, and frequently in young women and children. It is also seen after nicotine or ephedrine administration.

The advent of hybrid PET/CT scanners has significantly improved the accuracy and specificity of PET imaging in a variety of tumors and patient settings. With the addition of CT, focal brown fat or muscle uptake may now be easily attributed to the appropriate physiologic processes when previously it posed a greater diagnostic challenge. Current strategies to minimize brown fat uptake include a warm injection and imaging room, warming blankets, and benzodiazepine or β-blocker administration.

Notes

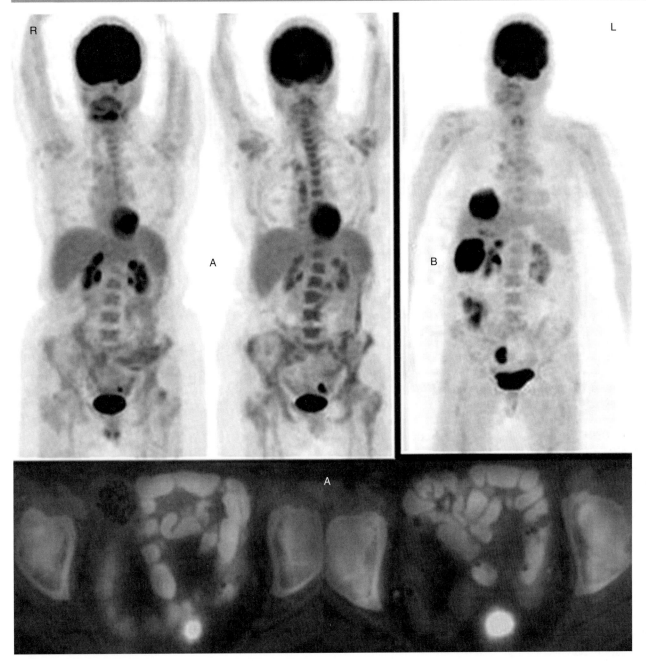

Patients A (*left*) and B (*right*) have colon cancer. Patient A underwent two PET/CT studies, the initial one (*left*) and the follow-up 7 months later (*middle*).

1. For patient A, name at least two differences between the study findings in the PET-only studies and explain possible causes.

2. After viewing the CT images for patient A and assuming there is no soft-tissue stranding, edema, or bowel contrast located where the enlarging posterior hypermetabolic focal uptake is, what is the likely diagnosis?

3. What are the likely causes of the abnormalities noted for patient B?

4. How often is focal activity in the bowel seen on PET found to be malignant?

PET/CT: Focal Pelvic Uptake in Colon Cancer

1. The focal uptake above the left portion of bladder is more intense and larger on the follow-up study. The differential diagnosis includes radioactive urine retention in the left ureter, diverticulitis, and tumor. The diffuse intense uptake seen in the spine more on the later images is compatible with red marrow activation.

2. Enlarging soft-tissue lesion in bowel. Diverticulitis or artifact from bowel contrast would be excluded with the information given.

3. Two large FDG-avid lesions are seen in the liver. There is focal uptake to the right of midline and above the bladder, likely due to a primary colon cancer with metastatic disease to the liver. The uptake in the right lateral abdomen fused to the ileocecal region on CT without evidence of a mass; it is likely physiologic.

4. Approximately 20% to 35%. Focal uptake due to premalignant adenomas is also occasionally seen.

References

Pandit-Taskar N, Schoder H, Gonen M, et al: Clinical significance of unexplained abnormal focal FDG uptake in the abdomen during whole-body PET, *AJR Am J Roentgenol* 183:1143–1147, 2004.

Tatlidil R, Jadvar H, Bading JR, et al: Incidental colonic fluorodeoxyglucose uptake: correlation with colonoscopic and histopathologic findings, *Radiology* 224:783–787, 2002.

Cross-Reference

Nuclear Medicine: THE REQUISITES, 3rd ed, pp 330–331.

Comment

Uptake seen on FDG-PET imaging in the ileocecal region is usually considered benign when there is no abnormality seen on CT in this region. This uptake is thought to be related to the higher concentration of lymphoid tissue in this region and/or physiologic muscle activity of the ileocecal valve. In patients who have undergone chemotherapy, the ileocecal uptake can be due to inflammatory typhlitis (cecitis).

Diffuse bone marrow activity with increased FDG uptake is commonly seen in the red marrow after chemotherapy, most commonly in the vertebral bodies, pelvis, hips, proximal long bones, and sternum. It should not be confused with malignant marrow involvement, which is more focal. Often, increased FDG marrow uptake is caused by drugs given to stimulate white blood cell production (e.g., granulocyte colony-stimulating factor). Uptake may last approximately 4 weeks or longer after discontinuation of the drug. Increased red marrow uptake can also be seen with anemia and other marrow expansion process. Radiation therapy will focally decrease marrow uptake.

Notes

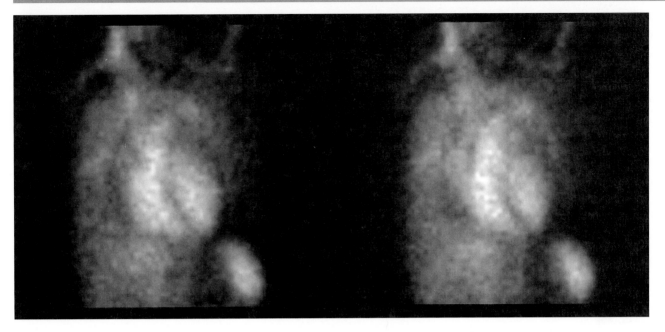

A 45-year-old man has dyspnea on exertion. Recent cardiac catheterization found no coronary disease. Planar images at end-diastole (*left*) and end-systole (*right*) are shown.

1. Name the radiopharmaceutical, the exam being performed, and describe the findings.

2. Which cardiac view is shown? Why was it selected to calculate an LVEF? Name other views often obtained.

3. List the terms used to describe myocardial wall motion.

4. Provide a classification for cardiomyopathies.

Cardiovascular System: Cardiomyopathy on Gated Blood Pool Ventriculography

1. ^{99m}Tc-labeled erythrocytes. Equilibrium-gated radionuclide ventriculography (RVG) or multigated acquisition. End-diastole and end-systole frames look similar, thus, there is globally decreased LVEF.

2. The left anterior oblique view provides the best septal separation of the two ventricles. Often, anterior and left lateral or posterior oblique views are also obtained to judge wall motion.

3. Global or regional akinesis, hypokinesis, dyskinesis, tardokinesis.

4. Classification according to the functional status of the ventricle: restrictive, dilated, or hypertrophic; or according to cause: alcoholic, infectious, metabolic, toxic, drug-induced, or ischemia/CAD, idiopathic.

References

Guido G, Borer JS, Berman DS: Myocardial function assessment by nuclear techniques. In: Dilsizian V, Narula J (eds): *Atlas of Nuclear Cardiology*, 2nd ed. Philadelphia: Current Medicine Group, 2006, pp 115–142.

Sheiner J, Sinusas A, Wittry MD, et al: Procedure guideline for gated equilibrium radionuclide ventriculography. Society of Nuclear Medicine Procedure Guidelines Manual, June 2002.

Cross-Reference

Nuclear Medicine: THE REQUISITES, 3rd ed, pp 492–502.

Comment

Radionuclide ventriculography is a time-proven and accurate technique for evaluating wall motion and calculating the LVEF. The rationale is that the number of counts in the left ventricle is proportional to the ventricular volume. Thus, a ratio of the stroke volume (end-diastolic volume minus end-systolic volume) divided by the end-diastolic volume is used to calculate the LVEF. Today, this is most commonly done in patients receiving cardiotoxic chemotherapy. Wall motion abnormalities may be global, as in this patient, or regional. Regional abnormalities are often caused by CAD (e.g., infarction) or occur with stress-induced acute ischemia. Terms to describe cardiac wall motion are normal, akinesia (complete absence of wall motion), hypokinesia (residual but diminished contraction), dyskinesia (paradoxical wall motion, opposite to the direction of expected motion, seen in the septum of patients after a coronary artery bypass graft due to disruption of the pericardium and in patients after myocardial infarctions with aneurysmal wall dysmotility), and tardokinesia (motion present but delayed compared with adjacent segments).

Cardiomyopathies can be classified functionally: restrictive, dilated, or hypertrophic, according to the cause, or as primary or secondary. When the cause is known, cardiomyopathy is labeled as alcoholic, infectious, metabolic, toxic, drug induced, or ischemic; otherwise, it is idiopathic. Dilated cardiomyopathies usually are associated with a dilated left ventricle and a depressed LVEF. In contrast, hypertrophic and restrictive cardiomyopathies usually are associated with a small or normal left ventricle.

Notes

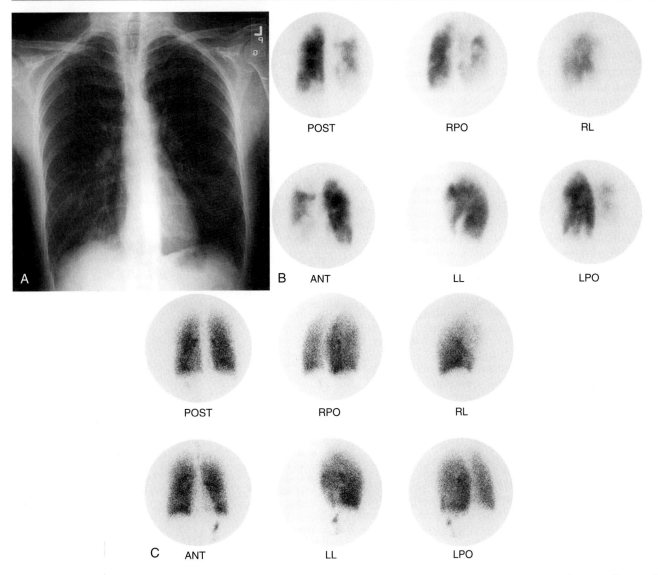

A 62-year-old patient has right-sided chest pain and shortness of breath. A posteroanterior chest radiograph (A), perfusion lung scan (B), and ventilation scan (C) are shown.

1. What are the radiopharmaceuticals used in this study? Describe their mechanism of uptake and distribution.

2. Describe the ventilation-perfusion image findings.

3. Interpret the study. What is the likelihood of pulmonary embolus in this patient?

4. What are the most common chest radiographic findings in patients with pulmonary emboli?

Pulmonary System: High Probability of Pulmonary Embolus

1. ^{99m}Tc-macroaggregated albumin (MAA). These macro-aggregated particles are 30 to 60 µm in size and lodge in the arterioles and capillaries of the lung according to blood flow after intravenous injection. ^{99m}Tc-diethylenetriaminepentaacetic acid (DTPA) aerosol is inhaled and distributed in the lungs to the aerated alveoli in normal lungs.

2. Perfusion is markedly decreased throughout the entire right lung field, some areas more than others. Segmental-appearing perfusion defects are seen in the right lung, particularly the lower lobe basal segments. Ventilation is nearly normal except for truncation of the costophrenic angle on the left, likely due to a small effusion. Thus, there are innumerable perfusion-ventilation mismatches. The chest x-ray is clear.

3. High probability for pulmonary embolus, greater than 80% probability of pulmonary embolus by PIOPED data.

4. Chest x-ray findings in pulmonary embolus are uncommon without infarction. The most common findings are a normal chest x-ray or discoid atelectasis. These are also the most common chest x-ray findings in patients determined not to have emboli.

References

Freeman LM, Stein EG, Sprayregen S, et al: The current and continuing role of ventilation perfusion scintigraphy in evaluating patients with suspected pulmonary embolism, *Semin Nucl Med* 38:432–430, 2008.

Gottschalk A, Stein P, Coleman RE, et al: Ventilation-perfusion scintigraphy in the PIOPED study. Part II, *J Nucl Med* 34:1119–1126, 1993.

Cross-Reference

Nuclear Medicine: THE REQUISITES, 3rd ed, pp 508–534.

Comment

In this case, segmental perfusion defects are seen bilaterally even though there is severely decreased perfusion of the right lung. With this degree of hypoperfusion, a characteristic segmental pattern is not always seen. Reduced perfusion has the same significance as no perfusion when it comes to interpretation of perfusion scans.

Although a high-probability lung scan is strongly suggestive of pulmonary embolus (80% probability), 20% of patients have other diagnoses (e.g., vasculitis, malignancy). Mediastinal tumors can occlude the pulmonary artery, which is compressible in contrast to the more rigid bronchi.

Although the lung scan has high specificity, less than half of patients ultimately determined to have pulmonary embolus have a high-probability scan. The majority have an intermediate-probability scan. An intermediate-probability scan (35% probability) is not the same as a low-probability scan (<20%). Whether to do further workup is a clinical decision. Often, lower extremity Doppler is performed for possible thrombophlebitis.

Ventilation-perfusion scan interpretation requires incorporation of the chest x-ray findings. Acute findings of infiltrate, atelectasis, and effusion make those regions abnormal. Chronic changes (e.g., scarring and fibrosis, previous surgery, cardiomegaly, other anatomic findings) are not considered abnormal for PIOPED interpretation. A region of acute infiltrate in the same region as a perfusion and ventilation defect is considered "triple matched" and thus intermediate probability. Upper lobe triple match is considered low probability.

Notes

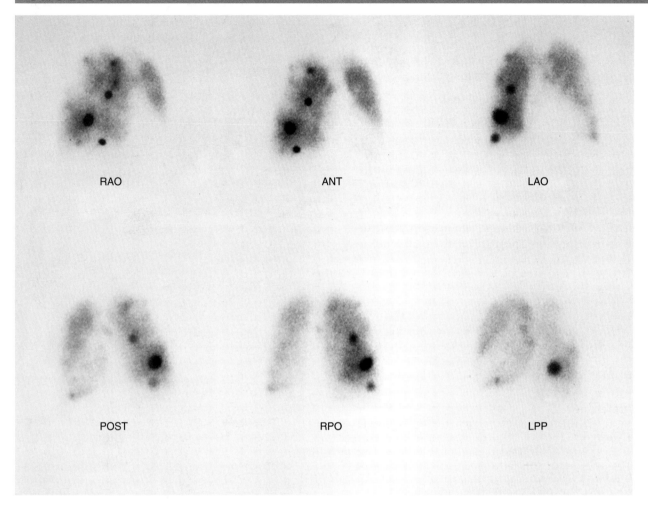

RAO   ANT   LAO

POST   RPO   LPP

A 45-year-old woman was referred for a ventilation-perfusion study. Only the perfusion scan is shown.

1. Describe the abnormal scintigraphic findings.

2. What is the likely cause of the findings?

3. What could have been done to prevent this from happening?

4. What are relative contraindications to injection of the radiopharmaceutical?

Pulmonary System: "Hot Spots" on a Lung Scan

1. Multiple "hot spots" are present in the upper and lower lobes, mostly in the right lung field.

2. MAA accelerates blood clotting, and the clots (hot spots) adhere to MAA.

3. The radioactive emboli are the result of poor technique caused by drawing back blood into the syringe containing the ^{99m}Tc-MAA before injection. Technologists are taught not to draw blood back into the ^{99m}Tc-MAA syringe. However, sometimes this happens.

4. Patients with known right-to-left shunts or severe pulmonary hypertension. These are relative contraindications, and MAA dose reduction is recommended.

References

Conca DM, Brill DR, Shoop JD: Pulmonary radioactive microemboli following radionuclide venography, *J Nucl Med* 18:1140–1141, 1977.

Preston DF, Greenlaw RH: "Hot spots" on lung scans, *J Nucl Med* 11:422–425, 1970.

Cross-Reference

Nuclear Medicine: THE REQUISITES, 3rd ed, pp 510–516.

Comment

Approximately 200,000 to 400,000 radiolabeled MAA particles are normally administered. Side effects are extremely rare. The particles do not totally occlude vessels, are quite malleable, and begin breaking down rapidly with a half-life of 4 hours. Reducing the number of particles in patients with severe pulmonary hypertension or a large right-to-left shunt is generally recommended, but the likelihood of side effects is very low.

The cause of this abnormal hot spot scan pattern is poor technique. In contrast to other radiopharmaceuticals, blood should not be drawn back into the syringe to prove that it is in the vein. ^{99m}Tc-MAA particles should be agitated before injection to avoid settling and aggregation of the particles, which also can cause hot spots. This hot spot pattern has also been reported in patients injected distally in an extremity with proximal thrombophlebitis. Injection of the radiopharmaceutical can dislodge part of the labeled thrombus.

Other important technical aspects of MAA injection include ensuring that the patient breathes deeply and is in the supine position to ensure uniform particle distribution. Gravity produces lower lobe predominance if the patient is upright. The MAA should be injected through a 23-gauge or larger needle to prevent particle fragmentation. Six to eight views are recommended. The anterior, posterior, and posterior oblique views are the most important. Lateral views should be interpreted cautiously because of shine-through from the opposite side. Anterior oblique views sometimes are helpful.

Notes

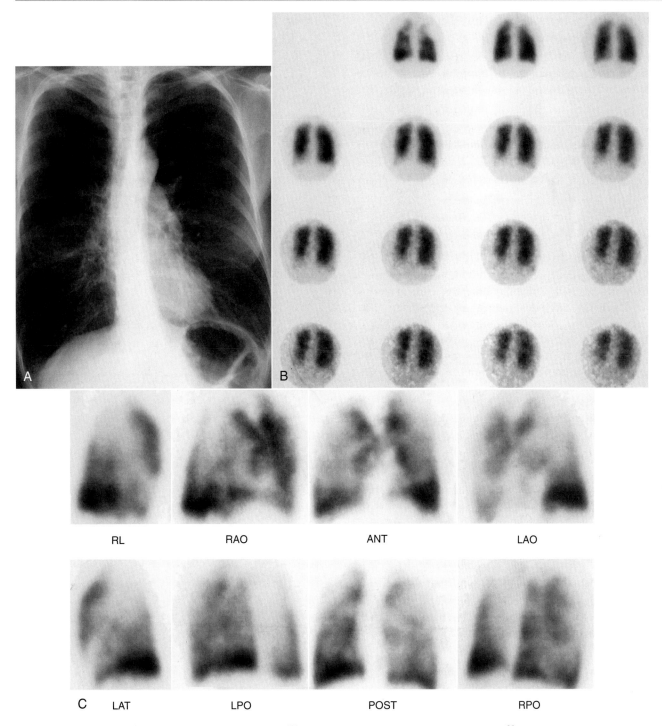

RL   RAO   ANT   LAO

C   LAT   LPO   POST   RPO

Chest radiography (A), posterior xenon-133 (^{133}Xe) ventilation (B), and eight-view ^{99m}Tc-MAA perfusion study (C) were performed for shortness of breath.

1. Describe the findings on the ventilation study.

2. Describe the findings on the perfusion study.

3. Provide an interpretation regarding the presence or absence of pulmonary embolism.

4. What term could be applied to this perfusion pattern?

CASE 26

Pulmonary System: Ventilation-Perfusion-Stripe Sign, Emphysema

1. Decreased upper lobe ventilation is seen on the initial single-breath image with air trapping in both upper lobes and the right lower lobe on washout images (B).

2. Decreased perfusion to the majority of both lungs, with preserved perfusion in the subpleural lung, most evident at the lung bases and medial aspect of both upper lobes (C).

3. Low probability.

4. Stripe sign.

References

Gottschalk A, Stein PD, Sostman HD, et al: Very low probability of interpretation of V/Q lung scans in combination with low probability objective clinical assessment reliably excludes pulmonary embolism: data from PIOPED II, *J Nucl Med* 48:1411–1415, 2007.

Sostman HD, Gottschalk A: The stripe sign: a new sign for diagnosis of nonembolic defects on pulmonary perfusion scintigraphy, *Radiology* 142:737–741, 1982.

Cross-Reference

Nuclear Medicine: THE REQUISITES, 3rd ed, pp 512–519, 527.

Comment

The stripe sign refers to subpleural ^{99m}Tc-MAA lung uptake peripheral to decreased perfusion proximal or more central. The perfusion defect is not pleural based because a rim or stripe of activity at the pleura is greater than the activity seen in the defect. This assessment should be made from the best tangential view of the area in question. The stripe sign is useful and reliable for discounting pulmonary embolus as the cause of the perfusion defect. It is approximately 90% reliable as an indication of nonembolic disease and thus low probability of pulmonary embolus. However, the remainder of the lungs should be inspected because the sign is only a predictor for the area where it appears and not for the remaining lung fields overall.

^{133}Xe is an inert radioactive gas that is very sensitive for chronic obstructive lung disease, usually with a pattern of regional delayed washin and washout. Because of rapid gas inhalation/exhalation imaging, imaging can only be done in two views (with a two-headed camera). ^{133}Xe is also not an ideal imaging agent. It has an 81-keV photopeak, lower than optimal for the gamma camera. The rapid dynamics result in low count images. ^{133}Xe also has some radiation safety issues. This heavy gas can layer out on the floor of the imaging room if there is inadequate negative-pressure air flow. This is required by the Nuclear Regulatory Commission (NRC). Furthermore, ^{133}Xe has a long half-life; when exhaled, it is "trapped" in charcoal until it decays.

Emphysema or chronic obstructive lung disease is a major cause of chronic airflow obstruction, a diagnosis indicating pathologic permanent abnormal enlargement of air spaces distal to the terminal bronchiole. The best radiographic indicator is hyperinflation, but vascular change, bullae, and increased lung markings also may be demonstrated. The ^{133}Xe study is a sensitive indicator of obstructive lung disease, as shown in this case. While regional patterns of delayed washout are more diagnostically specific, globally delayed washout can be caused by poor patient cooperation and hypoventilation.

Notes

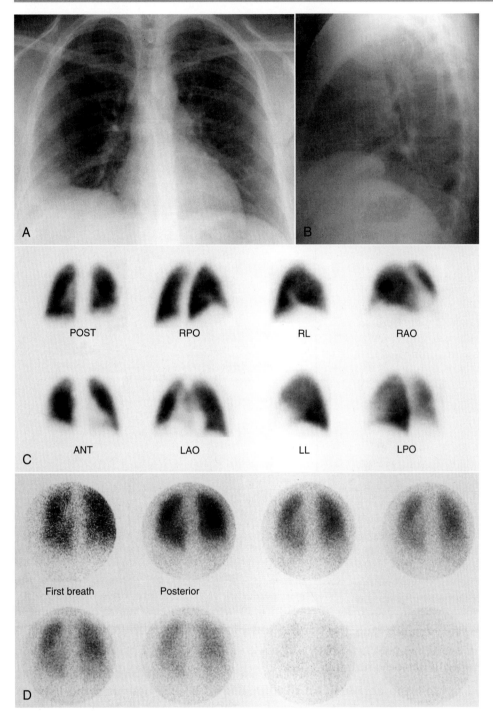

A young female patient presents to the emergency department with chest pain. Posteroanterior (A) and lateral chest radiographs (B), perfusion scan (C), and ventilation study (D) are shown.

1. Describe the findings on the chest radiographs.

2. Describe the perfusion and ventilation scans.

3. Does the single-view ventilation study limit interpretation of this study?

4. Categorize the study regarding the presence or absence of pulmonary embolism using PIOPED criteria.

Pulmonary System: Hampton's Hump— Intermediate Probability

1. Radiographs: a pleural-based opacity in the lateral right lung base.

2. Perfusion study: a single wedge-shaped, pleural-based defect in the same location as the radiographic abnormality, probably the anterobasal segment of the right lower lobe. Normal ^{133}Xe ventilation study.

3. Yes, the single posterior view makes it impossible to see the anterior basal segment where the perfusion defect is located.

4. Intermediate probability for pulmonary embolism.

References

Armstrong P, Wilson AG, Dee P, et al: *Images of Diseases of the Chest*, 3rd ed. St. Louis: Mosby, 2000, pp 75, 407–408.

Lu P, Chin BB: Simultaneous chest radiographic findings of Hampton's hump, Westermark's sign, and vascular redistribution in pulmonary embolism, *Clin Nucl Med* 23:701–702, 1998.

Cross-Reference

Nuclear Medicine: THE REQUISITES, 3rd ed, pp 515–522.

Comment

The radiographic signs of acute pulmonary embolism without infarction or hemorrhage include oligemia of the lung (Westermark's sign), increase in size of the main pulmonary artery, and elevation of the hemidiaphragm. All are nonspecific. Most emboli do not cause infarction. However, when present, infarction appears as lung consolidation and occurs predominantly in the lower lung fields. The radiographic finding described by Hampton and Castleman (1940) is known as Hampton's hump: "infarcts are always in contact with pleural surfaces and the shadows are rarely, if ever, triangular in shape." When pulmonary embolism is associated with consolidation because of hemorrhage and not true infarction, the infiltrate clears quickly, often within a week. In contrast, true infarction resolves over several months and may be associated with permanent linear scarring. Because cavitation is rare, it suggests secondary infection.

Because there is a single segmental mismatch, the study cannot be categorized as low probability (<20% probability). Even a single, moderately sized (25–75%) subsegmental perfusion defect should be classified as intermediate probability (35%). Two or more mismatched segmental defects are not present, so the study cannot be categorized as high probability (>80% probability). Therefore, by default and definition, the study indicates intermediate probability of pulmonary embolism. Whether the perfusion and ventilation defects are matched or mismatched with the chest x-ray (infiltrate, effusion, atelectasis) does not alter the intermediate probability interpretation according to PIOPED criteria. However, they usually are matched.

Notes

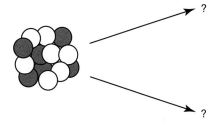

1. What is a positron?

2. Describe positron decay and how gamma rays are generated and detected (see figure above).

3. List five positron radionuclides used clinically, their half-lives, and detected photopeaks.

4. How are PET radiotracers most commonly used in medicine?

PET: Positron Decay/Gamma Ray Emissions

1. A positron is the antimatter counterpart of an electron (i.e., a positive electron, or beta plus [beta⁺] particle). It has an electric charge of +1 and the same mass as an electron.

2. Positron or beta⁺ decay is shown: $p \rightarrow n + beta^+ + v$

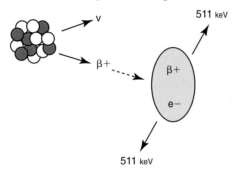

Beta⁺ decay occurs in proton-rich radionuclides. A proton (p) is converted into a neutron (n), emitted positron (beta⁺), and neutrino (*v*). After the positron is ejected from the nucleus, it loses kinetic energy and collides with an electron, causing annihilation of both particles. Two 511-keV photons (gamma rays) are produced, which travel 180 degrees apart. PET coincidence detectors register an event if the emitted photons are detected simultaneously.

3. The photopeak of all positron emitters is 511 keV.

Positron Emitter	Half-life ($T_{1/2}$)
R-82	75 sec
O-15	2 min
N-13	10 min
C-11	20 min
F-18	110 min

4. The radioinuclide binds to a biological marker (chemical, molecule, cell type) that acts as a probe for a specific physiologic process. Some PET clinical radiopharmaceuticals are listed below.

Positron Radiopharmaceutical	Physiologic Probe
O-15 water	Blood flow
N-13 ammonia	Myocardial perfusion
C-11 methionine, acetate	Protein synthesis, tumor metabolism
¹⁸F-FDG, fluoride, fluorothymidine	Metabolism, bone uptake, tumor proliferation
R-82 chloride	Myocardial perfusion

References

Karp JS, Surti S, Daube-Witherspoon ME, Muehllehner G: Benefit of time-of-flight in PET: experimental and clinical results, *J Nucl Med* 49:462–470, 2008.

Wahl RL: *Principles and Practice of PET and PET/CT*, 2nd ed. Philadelphia: Lippincott Williams & Williams, 2009.

Cross-Reference

Nuclear Medicine: THE REQUISITES, 3rd ed, pp 5, 63–67, 302–304.

Comment

The positron emitters with shorter half-lives, such as O-15 and N-13, require an on-site cyclotron, because the radiotracer must be administered to the patient promptly after production. ⁸²Rb also has a very short half-life; however, it is obtained from a portable Sr-82/Rb-82 generator on-site, similar to the molybdenum/⁹⁹ᵐTc generator.

For the typical or conventional PET scanner, the patient is surrounded by a ring of detectors allowing the registration of two 511-keV annihilation photons simultaneously (coincidence detection). This then generates electrical pulses permitting the system to count each coincidence event. A list of counts along each line of response (anywhere within the column between paired detectors) is determined for the PET raw data.

Time-of-flight PET scanners are now commercially available. The exact time that a photon is detected can be determined (i.e., the position at the time of detection along the line of response). This improves the signal-to-noise ratio without compromising spatial resolution; this may have greatest impact in the imaging of larger patients.

Notes

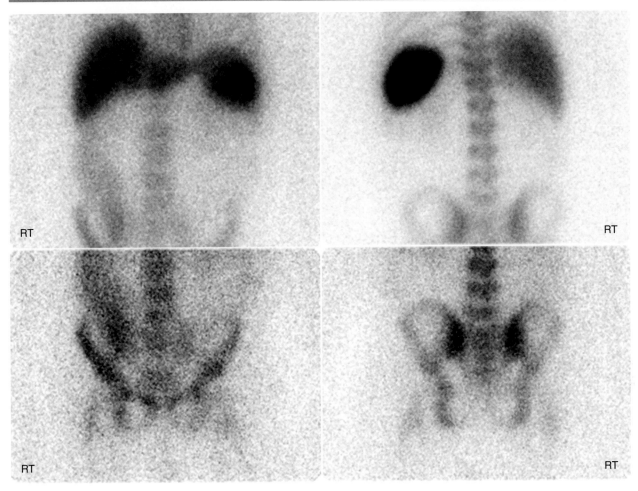

A 65-year-old woman has a complicated postoperative course after surgery for biliary obstruction requiring intensive antibiotic treatment, with persistent fever and diarrhea.

1. What is the radiopharmaceutical?

2. What is this radiopharmaceutical's normal distribution and pattern of clearance?

3. Describe the findings on this study.

4. Provide a differential diagnosis and the most likely diagnosis.

Inflammatory Disease: Inflammatory Bowel Disease

1. ^{111}In-oxine–labeled leukocytes.

2. Normal uptake is highest in the spleen, next highest in the liver, then the bone marrow. There is no genitourinary or hepatobiliary clearance normally.

3. Increased uptake along the right side of the abdomen. There is also some uptake in the rectosigmoid region.

4. Intraperitoneal infection, inflammatory bowel disease (e.g., ulcerative colitis, antibiotic-induced colitis). Flexible colonoscopy diagnosed pseudomembranous colitis.

References

Lantto E, Jarvi K, Krekela I, et al: Tc-99m hexamethyl propylene amine oxime leucocytes in the assessment of disease activity in inflammatory bowel disease, *Eur J Nucl Med* 18:14–18, 1992.

Stathaki MI, Koukouraki SI, Karkavitsas NS, Koutroubakis IE: Role of scintigraphy in inflammatory bowel disease, *World J Gastroenterol* 15:2693–2700, 2009.

Cross-Reference

Nuclear Medicine: THE REQUISITES, 3rd ed, pp 388–394.

Comment

Radiolabeled leukocytes can be used to localize active ulcerative colitis, Crohn's disease (regional enteritis), and pseudomembranous colitis. Although the initial diagnosis is often made by endoscopic biopsy, scintigraphy is valuable for determining the effectiveness of treatment and detecting and localizing recurrent disease. Both ^{111}In-oxine leukocytes and ^{99m}Tc-HMPAO leukocytes have been used for this purpose. The advantage of ^{111}In leukocytes is that there is no intra-abdominal clearance of the radiopharmaceutical. ^{99m}Tc-HMPAO is cleared through both the kidneys and hepatobiliary system, so this can be a problem diagnostically. Despite these limitations, ^{99m}Tc-HMPAO–labeled leukocytes have been successfully used for this purpose, and some reports suggest that they are superior because of their better imaging characteristics and better differentiation of abscess from inflammation. The addition of SPECT/CT improves the diagnostic accuracy. ^{111}In-labeled leukocytes are normally imaged at 24 hours. Inflammatory bowel disease is an exception. This is an exception because there is shedding of the inflamed mucosa and leukocytes into the bowel lumen. This sloughing occurs rapidly, and 24-hour imaging may not correctly localize the inflamed bowel. Thus, imaging is usually performed at 4 hours. With ^{99m}Tc-HMPAO–labeled leukocytes, imaging is usually performed 2 hours after injection when inflammatory bowel disease is suspected, before urinary and hepatobiliary clearance is likely to occur. Pseudomembranous colitis is acquired almost exclusively in association with antimicrobial use and is caused by *Clostridium difficile*.

Notes

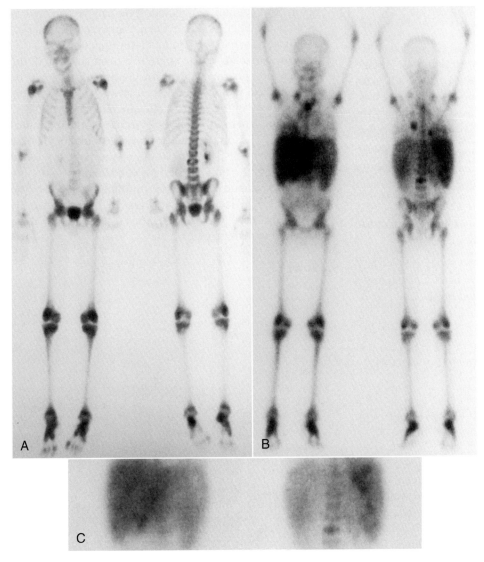

A 9-year-old patient had back pain and fever for 4 weeks. Bone scan (A), gallium-67 (^{67}Ga) citrate whole-body scan (B) with abdominal spot views (C) are shown.

1. Describe the scintigraphic findings on the bone and gallium scans.

2. When both studies are ordered at the same time, which should be performed first?

3. Provide the differential diagnosis and the most likely diagnosis.

4. List the ^{67}Ga photopeaks. Which are used for imaging? Which collimator should be used to perform the study?

Inflammatory Disease: ^{67}Ga—Fever of Unknown Origin

1. The bone scan shows mild increased L3 uptake. The ^{67}Ga scan shows abnormal L3 vertebral body uptake, as well as neck uptake bilaterally (right > left side), mediastinal, right paratracheal nodes, right lung base, posterior thorax, and multifocal uptake in the liver. The lower intensity camera setting optimizes liver visualization (C).

2. Bone scan. The ^{67}Ga has high-energy photopeaks that would downscatter into the bone scan if performed first.

3. Hodgkin's disease, tuberculosis, or atypical mycobacteria; Hodgkin's disease is likely.

4. Photopeaks occur at 91 to 93, 185, 300, and 394 keV. The lower three photopeaks are used for imaging. A medium-energy collimator should be used.

Reference

Rehm PK: Radionuclide evaluation of patients with lymphoma, *Radiol Clin North Am* 39:957–978, 2001.

Cross-Reference

Nuclear Medicine: THE REQUISITES, 3rd ed, pp 263–271.

Comment

^{67}Ga has been used for infection imaging since the early 1970s. Today, its role is limited because of the availability of radiolabeled leukocytes. ^{67}Ga occasionally is useful in patients with persistent fever but without localizing signs on examination and negative CT findings. In the setting of a fever of unknown origin (FUO), ^{67}Ga may localize to the site of infection, tumor, or both. While tumor may occasionally present as FUO, if an intra-abdominal source of infection is being sought, ^{67}Ga scanning is disadvantageous because of normal bowel clearance that may obscure pathologic uptake.

^{67}Ga is normally taken up by both the marrow and bone. The findings in this patient, however, indicate soft-tissue and focal bone involvement; thus, gallium-avid tumors and inflammatory and infectious conditions form the primary differential diagnosis. Given the distribution and age group, the gallium-avid tumor for primary consideration would be Hodgkin's disease. The involvement of a single vertebra on the bone scan, rather than two adjacent vertebral levels, would be atypical for vertebral osteomyelitis. The presence of skeletal (independent of marrow) involvement indicates stage IV disease.

To avoid downscatter of higher-energy photons of ^{67}Ga (393, 300, and 185 keV) into the ^{99m}Tc window centered at 140 KeV, the bone scan must be completed before the gallium is injected. ^{67}Ga can be injected as soon as the bone scan has been completed. Imaging of ^{67}Ga is initiated 48 to 72 hours after injection.

If osteomyelitis of the spine had been suspected, the proper radiopharmaceutical for confirmation would be ^{67}Ga because radiolabeled leukocytes have a high false-negative rate in the spine. Radiolabeled leukocytes (e.g., ^{111}In-oxine) are more commonly used for intra-abdominal infection. The disadvantages of labeled leukocytes are the requirement of up to 50 mL of the patient's blood for labeling, the time needed for cell labeling (minimum of 2 hours), and the serious problem of blood-borne diseases. ^{99m}Tc-labeled leukocytes are cleared via the biliary and urinary tract, and, thus, are not optimal for intra-abdominal imaging.

Notes

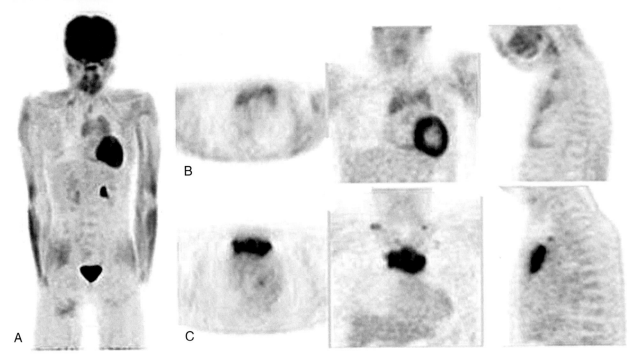

A and B, A 32-year-old man who has undergone chemotherapy for malignant lymphoma. C, A 45-year-old man with an anterior mediastinal mass without previous treatment.

1. Describe the abnormal FDG chest uptake in the first patient (A and B). What is the likely cause?

2. Describe the FDG uptake in the patient in figure C. What is its likely etiology?

3. Provide a differential diagnosis for a mass in the anterior mediastinum.

4. Give the likely cause of increased uptake in the lateral pelvis and upper extremities in the patient in figure A.

Oncology: FDG-PET—Lymphoma, Thymus Uptake

1. Low-grade homogeneous FDG uptake in a structure that has a smooth inverted Y configuration of normal thymus in a patient who has recently undergone chemotherapy. Thymic rebound is commonly seen in this setting.

2. Intense FDG uptake in a heterogeneous lobular pattern. Malignancy would be at the top of differential diagnosis.

3. Goiter, thymoma, lymphoma, teratoma, germ cell tumor, metastatic adenopathy.

4. Physiologic muscle uptake related to muscular activity during or immediately before the FDG uptake period.

References

Brink I, Reinhardt MJ, Hoegerle S, et al: Increased metabolic activity in the thymus gland studied with 18F-FDG PET: age dependency and frequency after chemotherapy, *J Nucl Med* 42:591–595, 2001.

Ferdinand B, Gupta P, Kramer EL: The spectrum of thymic uptake at ^{18}F-FDG PET, *Radiographics* 24:1611–1616, 2004.

Suster S, Moran CA: Thymoma classification: current status and future trends, *Am J Clin Pathol* 125:542–544, 2006.

Cross-Reference

Nuclear Medicine: THE REQUISITES, 3rd ed, p 311.

Comment

Thymic rebound is a common finding in patients after chemotherapy, particularly younger patients even into their late 30s. Normal thymic tissue is suppressed during chemotherapy but rebounds or redevelops afterward. This phenomenon was also described with ^{67}Ga imaging. The thymic uptake is usually mild to moderate, diffuse in a "butterfly-" or "triangle-shaped" pattern. It is commonly seen in the adult patient who has recently received chemotherapy and marrow-stimulating drugs. This uptake may last for up to a year after therapy. The enlarged thymus demonstrates normal cell morphology on histopathology. Serial repeat PET scans typically demonstrate decreasing uptake with time. In children, thymic rebound is commonly seen after illness, burns, surgery, and steroid use.

The four most common causes of anterior mediastinal masses are known as the "terrible Ts": thyroid extension/goiter, terrible lymphoma, thymoma (benign, atypical, or malignant carcinoma), and teratoma. Other causes include metastatic lymphadenopathy and germ cell tumor. All these causes can have varying degrees of FDG uptake.

Notes

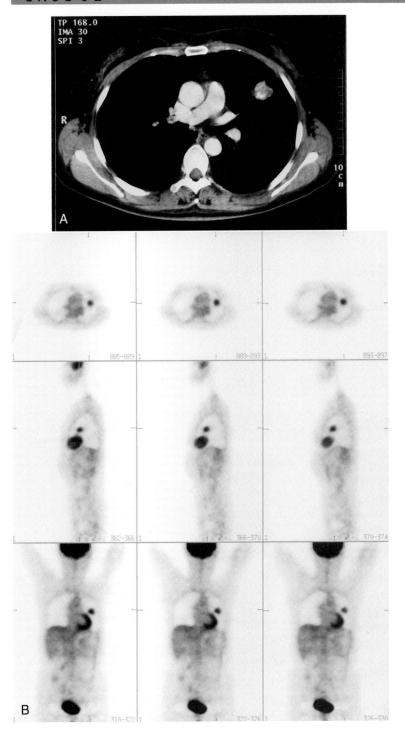

A 67-year-old man has a 2.5-cm left upper lobe lung lesion detected on chest radiographs and confirmed by CT (A). An FDG-PET scan is shown (B).

1. What percentage of all newly discovered pulmonary nodules is malignant?

2. What percentage of single pulmonary nodules is indeterminate in etiology after chest radiography and CT? What percentage is ultimately benign?

3. What is the likelihood of lung cancer in this case?

4. What are causes for false-negative/false-positive results on ^{18}F-FDG-PET studies?

Oncology: FDG-PET—Single Pulmonary Nodule

1. Only 20% to 30% are malignant overall. However, the incidence is as high as 50% in smokers.

2. By radiographic/CT criteria, 30% to 40% are indeterminate; 50% of these are benign.

3. High.

4. False-negative findings: small lesion size (<1 cm), bronchoalveolar carcinoma, and carcinoid tumors. False-positive findings: can be caused by benign tumor and inflammatory or infectious disease (e.g., histoplasmosis, tuberculosis). Inflammatory lesions typically have less FDG uptake than malignant tumors, but overlap exists.

Reference

Gould MK, Maclean CC, Kuschner WG, et al: Accuracy PET for diagnosis of pulmonary nodules and mass lesions: a meta-analysis, *JAMA* 285;936–937, 2001.

Cross-Reference

Nuclear Medicine: THE REQUISITES, 3rd ed, pp 317–319.

Comment

Of approximately 130,000 pulmonary lung nodules diagnosed annually, one third are malignant. CT scans can further characterize the lesion. However, after CT, 30% to 40% remain indeterminate; 50% of these ultimately are malignant. If characteristic benign changes are not seen in a low-risk patient, multiple follow-up CT scans are performed over 2 years to confirm that the lesion is benign. Various invasive procedures are used to make the diagnosis, including bronchoscopy, percutaneous biopsy, and video-assisted thoracoscopy and thoracotomy. Resection of pulmonary nodules has associated risk. A noninvasive method to preoperatively determine which patients require a more invasive diagnostic procedure could avoid unnecessary surgery, morbidity, and even death for many patients. ^{18}F-FDG-PET can help differentiate benign from malignant lesions. Data from 17 investigations and 588 patients show 96% sensitivity for the diagnosis of malignancy in single pulmonary nodules, 88% specificity, and 94% overall accuracy. A negative FDG-PET study result lessens the urgency of diagnostic surgery in patients at high risk for surgical complications who have chronic obstructive pulmonary disease or other serious medical problems and young patients at low risk of malignancy.

Notes

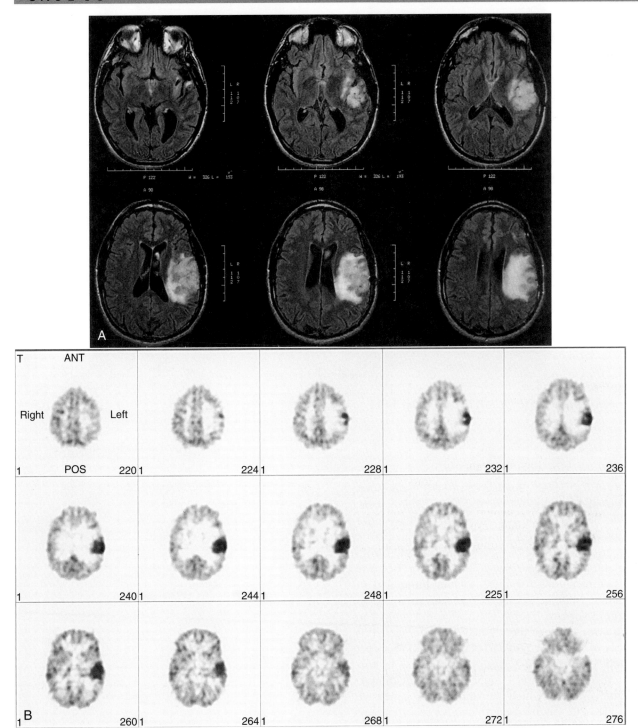

A 38-year-old man had a diagnosis of grade I–II astrocytoma 9 years previously. He has had a recent onset of seizures. MRI (A) showed no definite change from the previous studies. An FDG-PET brain scan was performed (B).

1. What FDG-PET scan findings are expected with a low-grade glioma?

2. What is the finding on this FDG-PET scan (B)?

3. Interpret this study.

4. Would SPECT perfusion agents (^{99m}Tc-HMPAO or ^{99m}Tc-ethylcysteinate dimer [ECD]) have a similar appearance?

C A S E   3 3

FDG-PET: Primary Brain Tumor

1. Low-grade gliomas typically have low levels of uptake or no uptake.

2. Intense uptake in a large left temporoparietal mass that corresponds to that seen on MRI.

3. Transformation of a low-grade to a high-grade glioma.

4. No. Malignant tumors usually do not have receptors for binding of the radiopharmaceutical, which is necessary before intracellular incorporation.

References

Delbeke D, Myerowitz C, Lapidus RL, et al: Optimal cutoff levels of F-18 FDG uptake in the differentiation of low-grade from high-grade brain tumors with PET, *Radiology* 195:47–52, 1995.

Langleben DB, Segall GM: PET in differentiation of recurrent brain tumor from radiation injury, *J Nucl Med* 41:1861–1867, 2000.

Cross-Reference

Nuclear Medicine: THE REQUISITES, 3rd ed, p 440.

Comment

Primary brain tumors were among the first to be imaged with FDG-PET in 1982. The degree of FDG uptake correlates with the tumor grade and the patient's prognosis. Low-grade tumors (grade I–II astrocytomas) have poor or no uptake. High-grade tumors (grade III anaplastic astrocytomas and grade IV glioblastoma multiforme) have uptake greater than that of gray matter. Because gray matter metabolism is three to four times that of white matter, white matter typically is seen as having no uptake on FDG scans. Biopsy is invasive and subject to sampling error because the gliomas are heterogeneous with areas of necrosis. FDG-PET can be used to direct stereotactic biopsy in heterogeneous tumors. In this case, the high uptake of FDG signifies transformation to a high-grade tumor, which demands more aggressive therapy. FDG-PET can be used to look for recurrence of tumor after therapy. MRI is often not able to differentiate tumor recurrence and radiation necrosis. Usually the recurrence is at the periphery of the lesion seen on MRI. FDG-PET also may be important in the evaluation of the effectiveness of therapy. The presence or absence of uptake of FDG after therapy can determine whether the tumor has responded to radiation therapy. Areas of radiation necrosis have very low glucose metabolism, whereas ineffective therapy is indicated by persistent FDG uptake.

FDG-PET can be helpful in the differential diagnosis of intracranial masses in patients with AIDS. Tumors, such as lymphoma, take up the FDG, whereas infection (e.g., toxoplasmosis) usually does not have increased uptake. This evaluation can also be done with SPECT ^{201}Tl chloride.

Notes

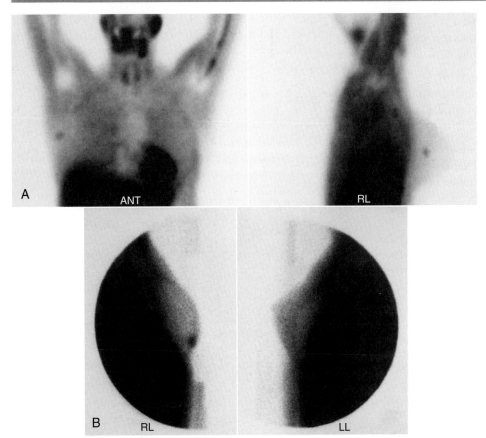

Scintimammography is performed in two different patients: A, a mammographically detected right breast mass; B, a palpable mass adjacent to a right breast prosthesis.

1. What is the radiopharmaceutical? What is its mechanism of uptake?

2. Describe the imaging findings and give an interpretation.

3. What is the accuracy of conventional mammography versus scintimammography for breast cancer?

4. What are causes of false-negative and false-positive findings on scintimammography?

CASE 34

Oncology: Scintimammography

1. ^{99m}Tc-sestamibi lipophilicity allows it to enter the cell where it is then concentrated in mitochondria as a function of charge.

2. Patient A has prominent focal uptake in a right breast mass. Patient B has definite focal uptake at the periphery of the breast prosthesis.

3. Accuracy of conventional mammography: sensitivity, 70% to 95%; positive predictive value for cancer, 20% to 30%. Scintimammography multicenter trial: sensitivity/specificity, 75%/83%. Palpable lesion sensitivity, 87%; nonpalpable lesion sensitivity, 71%.

4. Most false-negative findings are in lesions less than 1 cm. False-positive findings occur in fibroadenomas and benign and malignant tumors other than breast cancer.

References

Khalkali I, Villaneuva-Meyer J, Edell SL, et al: Diagnostic accuracy of ^{99m}Tc-sestamibi breast imaging: multicenter trial results, *J Nucl Med* 41:1973–1979, 2000.

Taillefer R: The role of ^{99m}Tc-sestamibi and other conventional radiopharmaceuticals in breast cancer diagnosis, *Semin Nucl Med* 29:16–40, 1999.

Cross-Reference

Nuclear Medicine: THE REQUISITES, 3rd ed, pp 277–278.

Comment

Mammography has good sensitivity for detection of malignancy. Its sensitivity is lower in patients with dense breasts, implants, or after breast surgery or radiotherapy. Of greater concern is its poor positive predictive value. Many women require biopsy because of the limitations of mammographic diagnosis. Cancer is ultimately diagnosed in only one third to one fourth of patients who have breast biopsies for suspected cancer. Ultrasonography can differentiate a cyst from a solid tumor but has limitations for solid masses. MRI is quite sensitive, but its specificity is low. The role of scintimammography is evolving. Because its negative predictive value (10–15%) is not adequate to exclude malignancy with confidence, biopsy is still needed. Scintimammography is clinically useful for patients with nondiagnostic mammograms, those with dense breasts, those with breast implants, those who have had previous surgery, those with nodular breasts, and those with fibrocystic disease. ^{99m}Tc-tetrofosmin, a cardiac imaging agent similar to ^{99m}Tc-sestamibi, has been used for scintimammography, and the two have similar accuracy. Better imaging devices, including dedicated breast scanners, are being developed with the goal of improved sensitivity for small lesions and the potential to perform concurrent imaging and biopsy at the same setting. Similar instruments are being developed for FDG-PET.

Notes

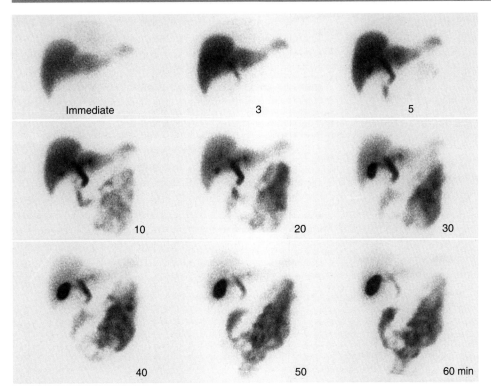

Immediate 3 5

10 20 30

40 50 60 min

A 39-year-old woman had acute upper abdominal pain. Ultrasonography showed gallstones and gallbladder wall thickening. Cholescintigraphy was requested to confirm or exclude acute cholecystitis.

1. What is the radiopharmaceutical? What is its mechanism of uptake and clearance?

2. What patient preparation is required before the study?

3. What is your interpretation of the study?

4. What are the sensitivity and specificity of cholescintigraphy for acute cholecystitis?

Hepatobiliary System: Cholescintigraphy— Normal Study

1. ^{99m}Tc-disofenin (disofenin, DISIDA, Hepatolite) or ^{99m}Tc-mebrofenin (BrIDA, Choletec), the two approved radiopharmaceuticals for this purpose. Hepatoiminodiacetic acid (HIDA) radiopharmaceuticals are extracted by hepatocytes and secreted into biliary ducts in a manner similar to that of bilirubin, except unconjugated.

2. No oral intake for 3 to 4 hours before radiopharmaceutical injection. No opiate drugs for 6 hours.

3. Normal study. Negative for acute cholecystitis or biliary obstruction.

4. Sensitivity (percentage of patients with a positive test result for the disease who have the disease) is 95% to 98%; specificity is 90%.

Reference

Ziessman HA: Acute cholecystitis, biliary obstruction, biliary extravasation, *Semin Nucl Med*, 33:279–295, 2003.

Cross-Reference

Nuclear Medicine: THE REQUISITES, 3rd ed, pp 159–174.

Comment

The patient should fast for 3 to 4 hours before initiating cholescintigraphy because if the patient has recently eaten, endogenously stimulated cholecystokinin will cause the gallbladder to contract, preventing radiotracer entry. Conversely, if the patient has not eaten for 24 hours and the gallbladder has had no stimulus for contraction, it is likely to be full of viscous concentrated bile that may prevent radiotracer entry. In either case, this could result in a false-positive study result (nonfilling of the gallbladder in a patient without cholecystitis). For patients fasting longer than 24 hours, sincalide (Kinevac), a cholecystokinin analogue, is infused to contract and empty the gallbladder. ^{99m}Tc-iminodiacetic acid is injected 30 minutes after completion of the sincalide infusion to allow time for gallbladder contraction and relaxation.

Ultrasonography is a standard part of the workup of upper abdominal pain and hepatobiliary disease. However, for the diagnosis of acute cholecystitis, cholescintigraphy has superior accuracy. The reason is that cholescintigraphy demonstrates the primary physiology of acute cholecystitis, obstruction of the cystic duct, whereas ultrasonographic findings are secondary (thickened gallbladder wall) and nonspecific (stones, pericholecystic fluid).

The hepatic function in this patient is good, confirmed by the prompt background (heart blood pool) clearance by 5 minutes. The common duct is visualized by 5 minutes. The gallbladder begins filling at 5 to 10 minutes and is filled by 60 minutes, at which time the liver has mostly washed out. Normal biliary-to-bowel clearance is seen by 10 minutes, and the common duct is substantially cleared by 50 to 60 minutes. Gallbladder filling and common duct visualization by 60 minutes is defined as normal. The false-negative rate for cholescintigraphy (filling of gallbladder in the presence of acute cholecystitis) is extremely low, and the study excludes the diagnosis with a high degree of certainty. The study should be interpreted not only for the presence or absence of gallbladder filling but also for the adequacy of common duct clearance and biliary-to-bowel transit. Poor ductal clearance (<50%) and transit to the small bowel would suggest partial biliary obstruction.

Notes

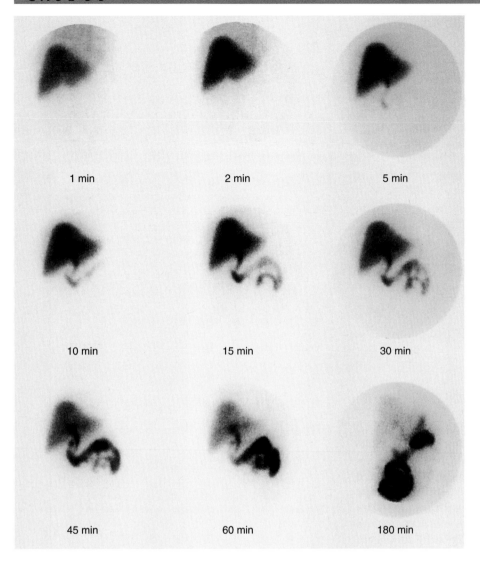

1 min 2 min 5 min

10 min 15 min 30 min

45 min 60 min 180 min

A 45-year-old woman has acute biliary colic with suspected acute cholecystitis.

1. Is the study normal or abnormal at 60 minutes?

2. Is the study normal or abnormal at 180 minutes?

3. If the gallbladder had filled at 180 minutes, what would be the diagnosis?

4. What are the most common causes of false-positive cholescintigraphy results (nonfilling of the gallbladder in a patient without cholecystitis) in the evaluation of acute cholecystitis?

Hepatobiliary System: Acute Cholecystitis

1. Abnormal. Nonfilling of the gallbladder.

2. Abnormal. Nonfilling of the gallbladder.

3. Negative for acute cholecystitis. Most likely chronic cholecystitis.

4. Prolonged fasting, hyperalimentation, serious concurrent illness, chronic cholecystitis, and hepatic insufficiency.

References

Swayne LC: Acute acalculous cholecystitis: sensitivity in detection using technetium-99m iminodiacetic acid cholescintigraphy, *Radiology* 160:33–38, 1986.

Weissman HS, Badia J, Sugarman LA, et al: Spectrum of 99m-Tc-LIDA cholescintigraphic patterns in acute cholecystitis, *Radiology* 138:167–175, 1981.

Cross-Reference

Nuclear Medicine: THE REQUISITES, 3rd ed, pp 159–174.

Comment

In the setting of acute upper abdominal pain, nonvisualization of the gallbladder is diagnostic of acute cholecystitis. Although nonvisualization of the gallbladder at 60 minutes is abnormal, it is not diagnostic of acute cholecystitis. Delayed images for up to 3 to 4 hours are acquired to make or exclude the diagnosis. With delayed imaging, the specificity for acute cholecystitis is increased and the false-positive rate reduced, with no significant change in sensitivity and improved overall accuracy. An alternative to delayed imaging would be to administer morphine sulfate and image for an additional 30 minutes.

Acute *acalculous* cholecystitis typically occurs in sick hospitalized patients (e.g., those with severe trauma, sepsis, shock). It has a high morbidity and mortality. In many of these patients, the cystic duct is obstructed by inspissated bile and inflammatory debris; however, sometimes the gallbladder is inflamed directly from sepsis, toxins, or ischemia, without obstruction. Because the cystic duct is patent, the sensitivity for detection with cholescintigraphy might be expected to be less than with acute *calculous* cholecystitis. It is probably in the range of 75% to 80%. If the gallbladder fills in a patient with a high clinical suspicion for cholecystitis and a false-negative study result is suspected, cholecystokinin can be administered. Good gallbladder contraction would exclude the disease. However, poor gallbladder contraction would not distinguish between acute or chronic cholecystitis. A radiolabeled leukocyte study may be helpful to confirm or exclude the diagnosis.

Notes

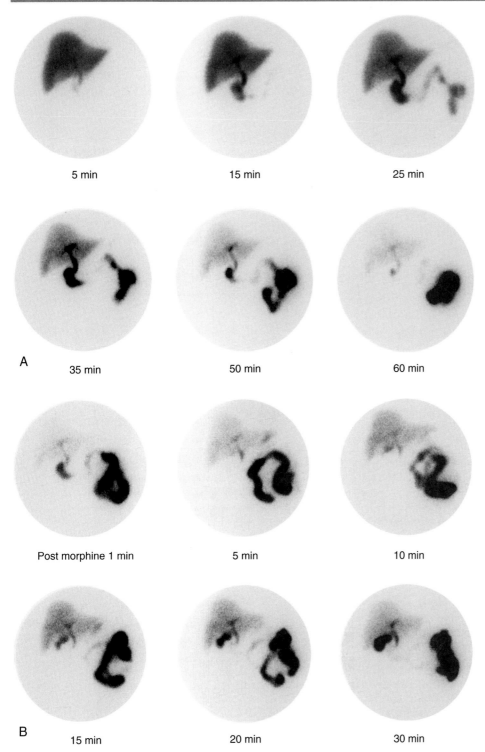

A 5 min   15 min   25 min

35 min   50 min   60 min

B Post morphine 1 min   5 min   10 min

15 min   20 min   30 min

A 53-year-old woman has recent onset of right upper quadrant pain and suspected acute cholecystitis. A, 60-minute cholescintigraphy. B, 30-minute post-morphine sulfate injection and acquisition.

1. What is the mechanism of morphine sulfate when used to diagnose acute cholecystitis? What is its advantage over the delayed imaging method?

2. In a patient with nonvisualization of the gallbladder at 60 minutes, what must be determined before morphine is administered?

3. What is the accuracy of morphine cholescintigraphy compared with the delayed imaging method?

4. What dose of morphine is used in hepatobiliary imaging to confirm the diagnosis of acute cholecystitis?

Hepatobiliary System: Morphine-Augmented Cholescintigraphy

1. Morphine causes contraction of the sphincter of Oddi, which increases intraluminal common bile duct pressure. Thus, bile flow is directed to the cystic duct and gallbladder if it is patent. The morphine portion of the study requires 30 minutes compared with delayed imaging up to 3 to 4 hours.

2. Besides a drug allergy, morphine should not be given if there is any evidence of common duct obstruction (e.g., delayed clearance of the common duct or delayed transit into the bowel).

3. The accuracy is at least as good, if not better, than the delayed imaging method.

4. Intravenous administration of 0.04 mg/kg morphine (e.g., 2.4 mg for a 60-kg patient).

References

Choy D, Shi EC, McLean RG, et al: Cholescintigraphy in acute cholecystitis: use of intravenous morphine, *Radiology* 151:203–207, 1984.

Fink-Bennett LM, Balon H, Robbins T, Tsai D: Morphine-augmented cholescintigraphy: its efficacy in detecting acute cholecystitis, *J Nucl Med* 32:1231–1233, 1991.

Cross-Reference

Nuclear Medicine: THE REQUISITES, 3rd ed, pp 172–174.

Comment

The 60-minute study (A) shows nonfilling of the gallbladder, near-complete washout of the liver, and normal biliary-to-bowel transit. Note that a repeat half-dose of ^{99m}Tc-HIDA was administered at the same time as morphine infusion (B), thus increasing hepatic uptake at 5 to 10 minutes. The gallbladder is promptly visualized, ruling out acute cholecystitis. With rapid hepatic washout, delayed imaging can be problematic and, thus, sometimes a smaller second dose of HIDA is given.

A 3- to 4-hour test is not optimal in a seriously ill patient. Reducing the length of the study from 3 to 4 hours to 90 minutes is a major advantage of morphine scintigraphy. However, the handling of narcotics requires accountability and can be a logistical problem on weekends and nights at some hospitals. Because morphine causes a functional partial common duct obstruction, the diagnosis of common duct obstruction cannot be made once it is given. Thus, common duct obstruction must be excluded before morphine administration. If this cannot be done, then the delayed imaging method should be used. Notice the irregular filling of the gallbladder due to gallstones.

Notes

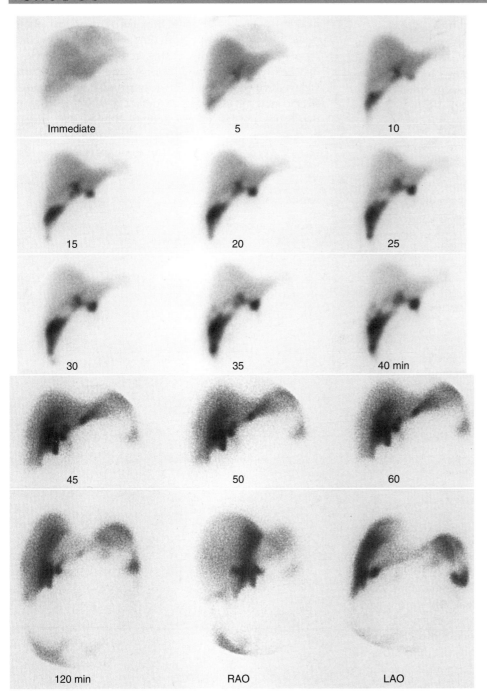

Immediate   5   10

15   20   25

30   35   40 min

45   50   60

120 min   RAO   LAO

A 43-year-old woman has a low-grade fever and abdominal discomfort, which began 2 days after cholecystectomy.

1. Describe the cholescintigraphic findings. What is your interpretation?

2. What other information does this study provide to the referring physician?

3. What are possible causes of this problem?

4. What unique information does cholescintigraphy provide that is not obtainable from other diagnostic imaging procedures?

Hepatobiliary System: Biliary Leak

1. Rapid bile intraperitoneal leakage probably originating from the region of the ligated cystic duct, extending toward the right paracolic gutter and, with time, over the dome of the liver and into the lower pelvis. This is diagnostic of a biliary leak.

2. This is a rapid leak, which is likely to be treated aggressively (e.g., reoperation). A slow leak often resolves spontaneously with time.

3. The most common cause is disruption of the cystic duct ligature after cholecystectomy. Other causes for leak include disruption of a surgical anastomosis or duct perforation, as may be seen in blunt or penetrating trauma, interventional radiographic procedures, tumor, or inflammatory processes.

4. Confirms that fluid collections seen by anatomic imaging modalities are biliary in nature.

References

Rosenberg DJ, Brugge WR, Alavi A: Bile leak following an elective laparoscopic cholecystectomy: the role of hepatobiliary imaging in the diagnosis and management of bile leaks, *J Nucl Med* 32:1777–1781, 1991.

Ziessman HA. Acute cholecystitis, biliary obstruction, biliary extravasation, *Semin Nucl Med* 33:279–295, 2003.

Cross-Reference

Nuclear Medicine: THE REQUISITES, 3rd ed, pp 185–187.

Comment

Biliary tract injury resulting in bile leakage has been said to occur in less than 1% of patients undergoing cholecystectomy. However, there is definitely an increased incidence with laparoscopic cholecystectomy. The complication can have dire consequences. Bile leakage can result in peritonitis, subhepatic fluid collection, abscess, and fistula formation. A reduction in morbidity and mortality is achieved by early detection. Sterile slow biliary leaks often seal themselves off spontaneously, whereas larger and more rapid leaks often require surgical intervention. Cholescintigraphy is a very sensitive and specific noninvasive method for detection of a bile leak and the rate of bile leakage can be qualitatively estimated.

Ultrasonography and CT can reliably detect fluid collections but often cannot determine whether they freely communicate with the biliary tree. Cholescintigraphy can answer that question. Because a frequent cause of postoperative bile leakage is incomplete cystic duct ligation, the most common site of bile collection is in the gallbladder fossa, although subcapsular and intraperitoneal locations may be seen. Bilomas often appear photopenic initially; however, with time they fill in and become more obvious with increasing activity. Multiple views may be helpful to accurately locate and confirm the leak. Delayed views beyond the routine 60-minute imaging period may be required to detect a slow leak or one that is obscured by enteric activity. If immediate surgery is not clinically indicated, cholescintigraphy may be repeated on a later day to confirm improvement or resolution of the biliary leak.

Notes

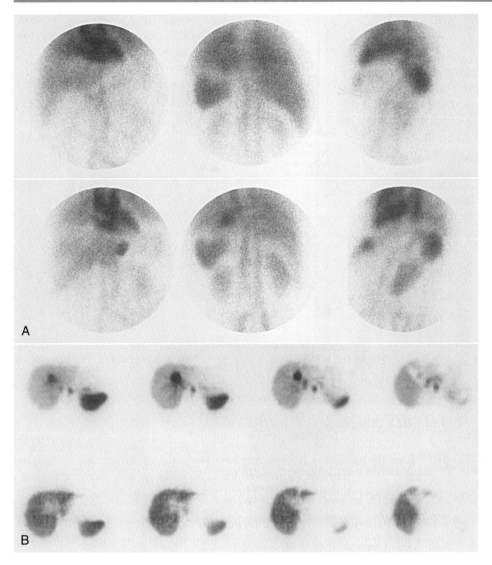

Two patients: A, A 59-year-old man had an abnormal CT reported to show a lesion of uncertain etiology in the left lobe of the liver (immediate, delayed images). B, A 46-year-old woman with colon cancer who underwent resection 1 year ago had two different SPECT radionuclide liver studies. Comparable transaxial slices are shown for the two studies.

1. What is the radiopharmaceutical used in study A? Describe the findings. What is the diagnosis?

2. What are the two radiopharmaceuticals used for study B and what is their mechanism of uptake/ distribution?

3. Describe the findings and give the likely diagnosis for the second study (B).

4. What are the advantages/disadvantages and accuracy of the radionuclide planar and SPECT studies?

Gastrointestinal System: Cavernous Hemangioma of the Liver

1. [99mTc]-labeled red blood cells (RBCs). Immediate images show no definite abnormality. Delayed images show increased focal uptake in the left lobe, seen in the anterior and left lateral views. Diagnosis: cavernous hemangioma of the liver.

2. [99mTc]-RBCs (*above*) and [99mTc]-sulfur colloid (*below*). [99mTc]-sulfur colloid is taken up by the liver Kupffer cells.

3. The cold defect seen on the [99mTc]-sulfur colloid study corresponds to the increased (hot) uptake on the [99mTc]-RBCs. This is also a cavernous hemangioma.

4. Very specific (>99%) for diagnosis of cavernous hemangioma. Poor sensitivity for small lesions.

References

Birnbaum BA, Weignreb JC, Meigibow AJ, et al: Definitive diagnosis of hepatic hamartomas: MR versus [99mTc] labeled RBC SPECT, *Radiology* 176:95–101, 1990.

Ziessman HA, Silverman PM, Patterson J, et al: Improved detection of small cavernous hemangiomas of the liver with high-resolution three-headed SPECT, *J Nucl Med* 32:2086–2091, 1991.

Cross-Reference

Nuclear Medicine: THE REQUISITES, 3rd ed, pp 190–198.

Comment

Cavernous hemangiomas are the most common benign liver tumor, second in occurrence only to hepatic metastases. They are composed of abnormally dilated endothelium-lined vascular channels of varying size separated by fibrous septae. They are not hypervascular but have increased vascular space (blood pool) compared with normal tissue. The explanation for the characteristic change in appearance from early to delayed images is the time required for the labeled RBCs to exchange and equilibrate with the large, relatively stagnant, nonlabeled blood pool of the hemangioma. Blood flow usually is normal.

Ultrasonography has poor specificity for the diagnosis of hemangiomas. CT with contrast and delayed imaging often can make the diagnosis; however, its sensitivity and specificity are inferior to MRI. MRI accuracy is probably greater than 90%; however, false-positive results occur because of a variety of benign and malignant tumors. Direct comparison studies of MRI and SPECT have shown similar accuracy down to a size of 2 cm; MRI is superior for small hemangiomas and those adjacent to major vessels. The specificity and positive predictive value of the RBC study is very high.

SPECT has superior sensitivity compared with planar imaging. Multiheaded SPECT cameras allow detection of most hemangiomas 1.4 cm or larger in size. [99mTc]-sulfur colloid was used in this case for anatomic correlation, but is not commonly used today. Hybrid RBC SPECT/CT would be the ideal methodology.

Notes

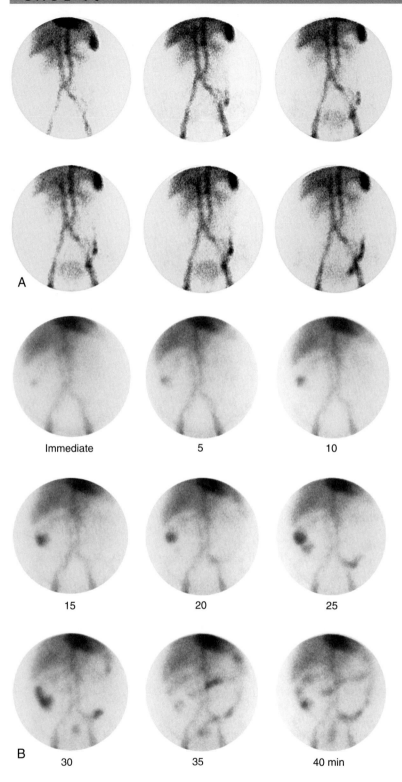

A

Immediate 5 10

15 20 25

B 30 35 40 min

1. What type of studies are these and which radiopharmaceutical is used?

2. What is the diagnosis in study A?

3. What is the diagnosis in study B?

4. What is the sensitivity of contrast angiography for these diagnoses?

Gastrointestinal System: ^{99m}Tc-RBC Colonic Bleeding

1. Gastrointestinal bleeding studies. ^{99m}Tc-RBCs.

2. Bleeding originating from the descending colon, rectosigmoid region.

3. Bleeding originating from the right colon, hepatic flexure. It moves rapidly to the left colon.

4. Contrast angiography can detect bleeding rates of 1 mL/min compared with 0.1 mL/min for the radionuclide gastrointestinal bleeding study. The radionuclide study is 10 times more sensitive for detection.

References

Howarth DM: The role of nuclear medicine in the detection of acute gastrointestinal bleeding, *Semin Nucl Med* 36:133–146; 2006.
Maurer AH: Gastrointestinal bleeding and cine-scintigraphy, *Semin Nucl Med* 26:43–50, 1996.

Cross-Reference

Nuclear Medicine: THE REQUISITES, 3rd ed, pp 365–373.

Comment

The purpose of the radionuclide gastrointestinal bleeding study is twofold: (1) to determine whether the patient is actively bleeding and (2) to diagnose the approximate site of bleeding. Gastrointestinal bleeding is intermittent, and symptoms often manifest after the bleeding has ceased. If the radionuclide study results are negative, it is very unlikely that angiography will be positive. If the radionuclide study results are positive, angiography should promptly follow. Localizing the approximate site of bleeding on the radionuclide study, particularly whether the bleed originates from the celiac, superior, or inferior mesenteric arteries can save the angiographer time and contrast media.

To accurately diagnose the site of active bleeding requires the application of specific scintigraphic criteria. The radionuclide study will initially show no intra-abdominal activity; with active bleeding, activity will be detected and seen to increase in intensity, and then move in a pattern consistent with intestinal anatomy. Imaging should not be discontinued until the imager is certain of the approximate site of bleeding. Small and large bowel can sometimes be misinterpreted if imaging is discontinued too soon. Fixed regions of uptake should not be diagnosed as bleeding, but are often due to hemangiomas, aneurysms, renal transplants, etc., which have an increased blood pool.

Notes

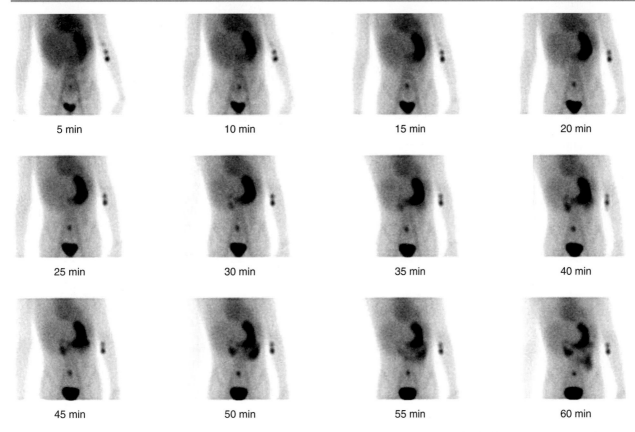

5 min	10 min	15 min	20 min
25 min	30 min	35 min	40 min
45 min	50 min	55 min	60 min

A 3-year-old girl is referred because of two episodes of rectal bleeding, which has now stopped.

1. What is the radiopharmaceutical, its mechanism of uptake, and study type?

2. Which pharmacologic drug is used to enhance detectability? What is its mechanism?

3. Provide an interpretation of the study.

4. Why is bleeding a common complication of this disease entity?

Gastrointestinal System:
Meckel's Diverticulum

1. ^{99m}Tc-pertechnetate. It is taken up from the bloodstream and secreted into the gastric lumen by gastric mucosa. Meckel's scan.

2. Cimetidine, a histamine H_2-receptor antagonist. It increases and prolongs uptake of the radiopharmaceutical by inhibiting ^{99m}Tc-pertechnetate secretion from gastric mucosal cells.

3. Increasing focal accumulation of radiotracer in the mid-lower abdomen is suspicious for Meckel's diverticulum.

4. Acid and pepsin secretion by the ectopic gastric mucosa causes inflammation and ulceration of adjacent bowel mucosa.

References

Sfakianakis GN, Conway JJ: Detection of ectopic gastric mucosa in Meckel's diverticulum and in other aberrations by scintigraphy: pathophysiology and 10-year clinical experience, *J Nucl Med* 22:647–654, 1981.

Treves ST, Grand RJ: Gastrointestinal bleeding. In: Traves ST (ed): *Pediatric Nuclear Medicine*, 3rd ed. New York: Springer-Verlag, 2007, pp 192–200.

Cross-Reference

Nuclear Medicine: THE REQUISITES, 3rd ed, pp 375–379.

Comment

Meckel's diverticulum is the most common gastrointestinal congenital anomaly. It is caused by failed closure of the omphalomesenteric (vitelline) duct in the embryo. It is a true diverticulum and arises on the antimesenteric side of the small bowel, usually 80 to 90 cm proximal to the ileocecal valve. Gastric mucosa occurs in 10% to 30% of all cases, in 60% of symptomatic patients, and in 98% of patients who bleed.

The Meckel's scan has been used since the 1970s and remains the standard diagnostic imaging study. Pharmacologic augmentation with cimetidine is used at many centers. Radiopharmaceutical uptake typically occurs simultaneously with stomach uptake. In this case, the uptake appears to be delayed relative to gastric uptake, probably because of the small size of the diverticulum. The most common reason for false-positive studies is accumulation of radiotracer in the urinary tract (e.g., extrarenal pelvis, hydronephrosis, reflux, bladder diverticulum). Other reported causes of false-positive uptake include local inflammatory bowel disease, abscess, appendicitis, tumors, and gastrointestinal duplications.

False-negative results occasionally occur because of the rapid ^{99m}Tc washout or lack of sufficient gastric mucosa (e.g., <2 cm). However, the overall accuracy is very good: 85% sensitivity and 95% specificity.

Notes

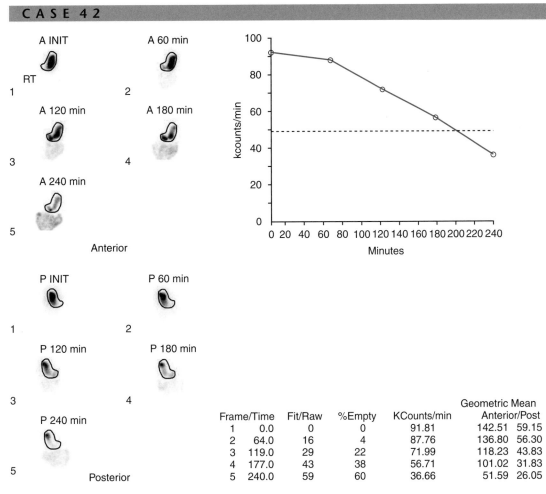

Frame/Time		Fit/Raw	%Empty	KCounts/min	Geometric Mean Anterior/Post	
1	0.0	0	0	91.81	142.51	59.15
2	64.0	16	4	87.76	136.80	56.30
3	119.0	29	22	71.99	118.23	43.83
4	177.0	43	38	56.71	101.02	31.83
5	240.0	59	60	36.66	51.59	26.05

This insulin-dependent diabetic patient had symptoms suggestive of gastroparesis, including early satiety, postprandial bloating, and abdominal discomfort. The patient ingested a radiolabeled egg meal.

1. What is the radiopharmaceutical used for an egg meal? What is its mechanism of binding to the egg?

2. What is normal solid gastric emptying?

3. Why is attenuation correction necessary for accurate quantification of solid gastric emptying? What is the standard method used for this correction?

4. What factors can affect the amount of gastric emptying in addition to patient pathophysiology?

Gastrointestinal System: Gastric Emptying

1. Tc-99m-sulfur colloid is used for radiolabeling egg. The radiotracer binds to albumin in the egg white.

2. Normal values depend on the meal and the acquisition and processing methodology used. According to this meal and methodology, normal is greater than 90% emptying at 4 hours (frame 5, 240 minutes).

3. The anterior view alone underestimates and the posterior view overestimates emptying because of variable attenuation as the meal moves through the stomach. The geometric mean (square root of the product of the anterior and posterior image counts at each time point) is the standard method of correction.

4. Delayed emptying may be caused by hyperglycemia per se without diabetic gastroenteropathy. Many drugs may delay emptying (e.g., opiates, progesterone, nifedipine, theophylline, anticholinergics, diazepam).

References

Abell TL, Camilleri M, Donohoe K, et al: Consensus recommendations for gastric emptying scintigraphy. A Joint Report of the Society of Nuclear Medicine and the American Neurogastroenterology and Motility Society, *Am J Gastroenterol* 103:753–763, 2008; *J Nucl Med Technol* 36:44–54, 2008.

Ziessman HA, Goetze S, Bonta D, Ravich W: Experience with a new standardized 4-hr gastric emptying protocol, *J Nucl Med* 48:568–572, 2007.

Cross-Reference

Nuclear Medicine: THE REQUISITES, 3rd ed, pp 354–364.

Comment

Consensus recommendations have now been published in the gastroenterology and nuclear medicine literature. The purpose of these recommendations is to standardize methodology and normal values among imaging centers. Normal values depend very much on the meal ingested. Solids empty faster than semisolids and semisolids empty more rapidly than full liquids, which empty faster than clear liquids. Increased calories, meal size, meal particle size, and so on all delay emptying. Thus, normal values must be established for the meal used. The consensus guidelines recommend a simplified protocol (1-minute images at time 0 and 1, 2, and 4 hours), a standardized protocol (meal, methodology specified in the consensus recommendations), and established normal values. A major strength of the recommended protocol is that normal values are based on 123 normal subjects from multiple countries. The meal is primarily an egg substitute sandwich. Using this meal and protocol, solid emp-

tying is delayed if there is more than 10% retention (<90% emptying) at 4 hours.

The stomach consists of two compartments from a functional standpoint. The antrum has phasic contractions and is responsible for solid emptying, grinding up food into small enough particles that can pass through the pylorus. The delay before emptying begins (see time activity curve in case study) is called the lag phase. Emptying is usually linear in character after that. The fundus is responsible for relaxation and accommodation of the meal and liquid emptying as a result of tonic continuous contraction. Liquids empty continuously in a single exponential pattern. Clear liquids (water) empty with a half-time of less than 20 minutes. Liquids are sometimes used when the patient is allergic to eggs and cannot tolerate the volume of the solid meal.

Notes

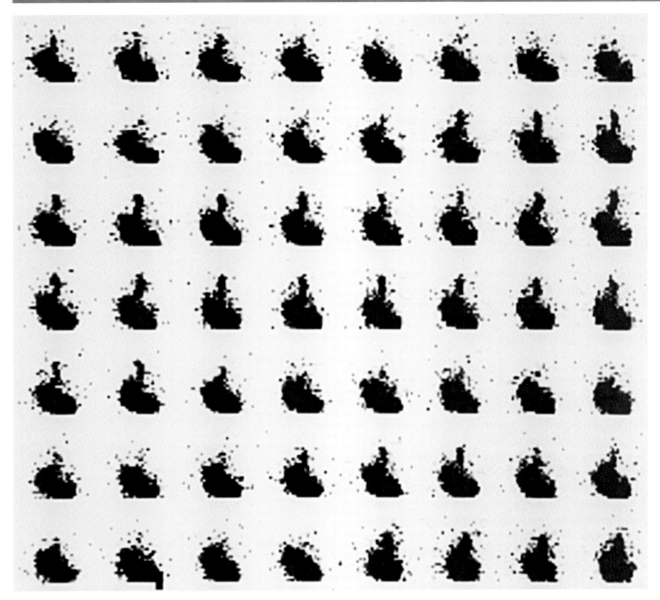

A 3-month-old infant was referred with symptoms of gastroesophageal reflux. A radionuclide gastroesophageal reflux study (milk study) was performed (posterior view). The intensity setting is set high for best visualization of the abnormality.

1. What are common symptoms and problems in children associated with reflux?

2. What other method is used by pediatricians for detection of reflux?

3. What radiolabel and meal are commonly used for this study?

4. How frequently should images be acquired to maximize sensitivity of this test?

Gastrointestinal System: "Milk" Study—Gastroesophageal Reflux

1. Vomiting, pulmonary symptoms, asthma, pneumonia, sudden death, failure to thrive, anemia.

2. 24-hour pH monitoring.

3. ^{99m}Tc-sulfur colloid (1 mCi) mixed with the child's usual feeding, formula, or milk.

4. 5 to 10 seconds per frame.

References

Heyman S, Kirkpatrick JA, Winter HS, Treves S: An improved radionuclide method for the diagnosis of gastroesophageal reflux and aspiration in children (milk scan), *Radiology* 131:474–482, 1979.

Piepsz A: Recent advances in pediatric nuclear medicine, *Semin Nucl Med* 25:165–182, 1995.

Cross-Reference

Nuclear Medicine: THE REQUISITES, 3rd ed, pp 350–354.

Comment

Gastroesophageal reflux is a common clinical pediatric problem. Although this occurs in healthy infants, it usually resolves by approximately 8 months and rarely causes serious medical problems. However, some children have symptomatic reflux that can persist into adulthood. Symptoms associated with reflux can be serious, including failure to thrive, esophagitis with stricture, anemia, aspiration, recurrent respiratory infections, asthma, and sudden death syndrome.

The 24-hour pH probe monitoring technique often is considered the gold standard. However, comparative studies of the two techniques have shown similar sensitivity for detection of gastroesophageal reflux by scintigraphy (milk study) and pH probe. The disadvantages of the pH probe are that children younger than 5 years must be hospitalized and there is a possible underestimation of reflux because a small volume of acid reflux may adhere to the probe, preventing subsequent events from being recorded. Conversely, the milk study is most sensitive when the stomach is full. As it empties, the detected reflux events decline. The milk study is a simple study to perform. Frequent image acquisition (every 5–10 seconds) is necessary to detect short recurrent reflux events. After ingesting the milk or formula feeding, the study is acquired for an hour with the child supine on the gamma camera. Reflux events can be detected easily on computer review of the study. Various quantitative methods have been used; the most simple and straightforward is counting the number of reflux events and categorizing them as high (greater than half the distance to the mouth) or low and short (<10 seconds) or long events. This case study has frequent short and long and many high and long recurrent reflux events.

Notes

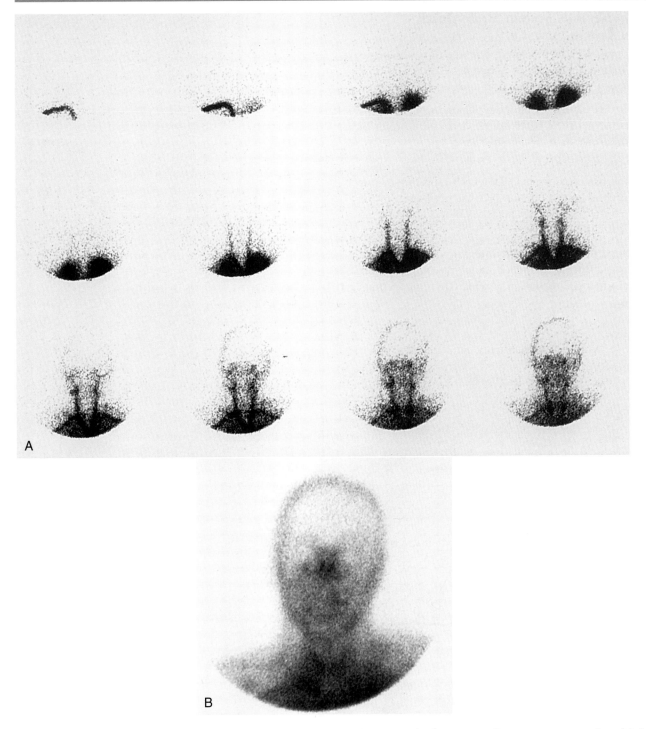

A

B

A 30-year-old potential organ donor has been comatose for 2 weeks because of a recent severe head injury. The patient is being treated with hypothermia and barbiturates. Brain death is suspected clinically. The electroencephalogram is flat.

1. How is the diagnosis of brain death made clinically?

2. If the electroencephalogram in this patient is a flat line, why is another study indicated?

3. List the radiopharmaceuticals and their physiologic mechanisms that are useful for this purpose.

4. What are the scintigraphic findings and diagnosis?

Central Nervous System: Brain Death

1. Brain death is a clinical diagnosis. The clinical criteria are coma, lack of brainstem reflexes or spontaneous respiration, and exclusion of reversible causes, and the cause of the brain dysfunction must be diagnosed.

2. An isoelectric flat electroencephalogram can be due to the presence of barbiturates, depressive drugs, or hypothermia, as well as brain death.

3. ^{99m}Tc-HMPAO (Ceretec) and ^{99m}Tc-ECD (Neurolite) are the preferred agents. They both bind irreversibly to cerebral cortex. ^{99m}Tc-DTPA has been used in the past, but provides only first-pass blood flow and no cortical binding.

4. A, Blood flow through the internal carotids is seen, but no intracerebral blood flow. B, Only external carotid blood distribution is seen. There is no brain uptake.

Reference

Zuckier LS, Kolano J: Radionuclide studies in the determination of brain death: criteria, concepts, and controversies, *Semin Nucl Med* 38:262–273, 2008.

Cross-Reference

Nuclear Medicine: THE REQUISITES, 3rd ed, pp 434–437.

Comment

The diagnosis of brain death is clinical. Ancillary tests are used to increase the diagnostic certainty when conventional clinical testing and electroencephalography are not diagnostic or are unreliable (e.g., when the patient is being treated with barbiturates or hypothermia). The radionuclide brain death study shows the physiology of brain death (i.e., no intracerebral blood flow). The study is diagnostic.

Although ^{99m}Tc-DTPA has been used successfully for many years to evaluate cerebral blood flow for brain death, it has limitations. Technical problems (e.g., a bad bolus or camera or computer malfunction during acquisition) can complicate interpretation. The cerebral perfusion agents ^{99m}Tc-HMPAO and ^{99m}Tc-ECD have the advantage that they fix intracellularly in brain cells. A flow study is not even mandatory. Static images within 10 minutes after the flow show whether the radiopharmaceutical is taken up by the cerebral cortex. If cortical uptake does not occur, the diagnosis of brain death is confirmed. This is the only indication for ^{99m}Tc-labeled brain perfusion agents for which SPECT is not required.

Notes

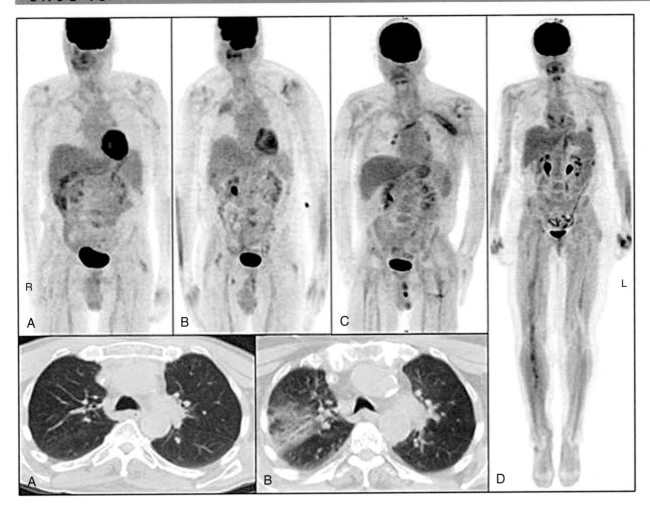

Three patients with malignant lymphoma are shown. The first study (A) and second study (B) are from the same patient, who is clinically in remission. Patient C has an unknown source of infection. Image D is another patient in remission.

1. What is the major change between the FDG-PET studies A and B? What is the likely cause?

2. Describe the abnormality in patient C. What is the likely source of infection?

3. Describe the abnormality and provide a differential diagnosis for patient D.

4. For which clinical settings has FDG-PET/CT proven most useful for infection detection?

C A S E 4 5

Inflammatory Disease: Infection and Inflammation

1. PET B shows FDG uptake in the right upper lung, which correlates with pneumonic infiltrate seen on CT B.

2. Abnormal linear uptake in the left upper chest and superior mediastinum most consistent with inflammation/infection of a central line.

3. FDG vertical linear uptake in the right lower extremity as well as increased soft-tissue activity. Differential diagnosis includes cellulitis and deep venous thrombosis or phlebitis. The linear activity suggests phlebitis. Atherosclerosis is unlikely because it is usually bilateral and symmetrical.

4. Immunocompromised patients and those with fever of unknown origin, particularly when results of other imaging modalities and laboratory tests are negative. FDG-PET has a high negative predictive value.

References

Love C, Tomas MB, Tronco GG, Palestro CJ: FDG PET of infection and inflammation, *Radiographics* 25:1357–1368, 2005.

Mahfouz T, Miceli MH, Saghafifar F, et al: F-18-FDG PET contributes to the diagnosis and management of infections in patients with multiple myeloma, *J Clin Oncol* 23:7857–7863, 2005.

Miceli M, Atoui R, Walker R, et al: Diagnosis of deep septic thrombophlebitis in cancer patients by fluorine-18 FDG positron emission tomography scanning: a preliminary report, *J Clin Oncol* 22:1949–1956, 2004.

Cross-Reference

Nuclear Medicine: THE REQUISITES, 3rd ed, pp 384–418.

Comment

The role of FDG for infection imaging is evolving. Compared with other scintigraphic methods for imaging infection or unknown sources of fever, FDG-PET/CT has advantages. It does not require handling and radiolabeling of patient blood products. Patient preparation and image acquisition require considerably less total time than leukocyte imaging. FDG produces better image quality and is cross-sectional. Sensitivity for detecting infection is similar to ^{111}In leukocyte scintigraphy and more sensitive than ^{67}Ga for localizing a source of fever. FDG has a particularly high negative predictive value. Like ^{67}Ga, FDG detects tumors as well as infection. This can be helpful in patients with a fever of unknown origin because tumors may be the fever cause.

FDG-PET has an important role in the evaluation of the immunocompromised patient. In multiple myeloma patients, FDG-PET/CT has been shown to detect infections not seen with other imaging modalities (often in the respiratory tract), contributing to better patient management in 46% of the cases.

Atherosclerosis is a dynamic inflammatory process. FDG accumulates in plaque macrophages in large arteries. Uptake is commonly seen in major vessels on routine oncologic imaging. The amount of uptake correlates with the macrophage density. In general, vulnerable plaques have inflamed intima with macrophage infiltration and thus increased FDG uptake, whereas stable plaques typically do not.

Notes

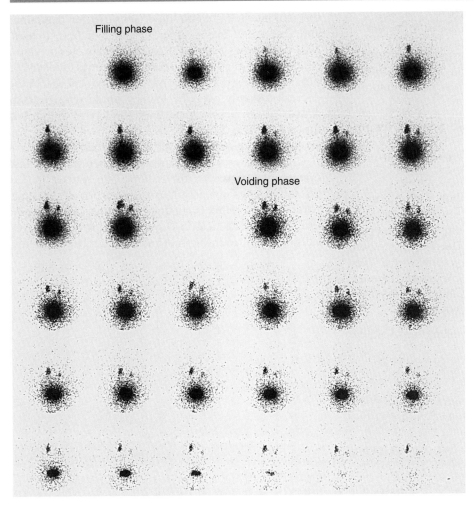

Filling phase

Voiding phase

A 5-year-old girl has had two urinary tract infections in the past 6 months.

1. Which radiopharmaceuticals can be used for cystography?

2. What are the advantages of radionuclide cystography over the contrast study?

3. What is the difference between indirect and direct radionuclide cystography?

4. What is your interpretation of this study?

Genitourinary System:
Radionuclide Cystography

1. ^{99m}Tc-DTPA, Tc-99m-pertechnetate, and ^{99m}Tc-sulfur colloid are most commonly used. They are mixed with saline solution and infused via a catheter into the bladder.

2. Radionuclide cystography is more sensitive for the detection of vesicoureteral reflux (VUR) than the contrast study and results in 50 to 200 times less radiation exposure to the gonads.

3. The direct method is most commonly used and most sensitive; it requires urinary catheterization and instillation of radiotracer with saline solution volume into the bladder via a urinary catheter. The indirect method is performed after routine renography with ^{99m}Tc-mercaptylacetyltriglycine (MAG3). When the bladder is full, a prevoiding image is obtained, followed by dynamic images during and after voiding.

4. Bilateral VUR seen on both the filling and voiding phases.

References

Eggli DF, Tulchinsky M: Scintigraphic evaluation of pediatric urinary tract infection, *Semin Nucl Med* 23:199–218, 1993.

Treves ST, Willi U: Vesicoureteral reflux, In: Treves ST (ed): *Pediatric Nuclear Medicine/PET*, 3rd ed. New York: Springer, 2007, pp 286–306.

Cross-Reference

Nuclear Medicine: THE REQUISITES, 3rd ed, pp 255–259.

Comment

VUR is caused by failure of physiologic valve function. The ureter normally passes obliquely through the bladder wall and submucosa to its opening at the trigone. As urine fills the bladder, the valves passively close, thus preventing reflux. If the intramural ureteral length is too short compared with its diameter, the valve does not close and reflux results. In more than 80% of cases, the abnormality resolves as the child grows. Untreated reflux and pyelonephritis may result in renal scarring, hypertension, and renal failure. The combination of VUR and infected urine are required to produce injury to the kidneys. The goal of therapy is to prevent renal damage until the reflux resolves spontaneously or is surgically corrected.

In many centers, contrast cystography is used for the initial evaluation of children suspected of reflux because of better anatomic detail, particularly for male patients, to detect posterior urethral valves. The voiding phase of the radionuclide study is more sensitive for detection, although reflux may be seen in either or both phases. This case shows early VUR on the left (posterior view) reaching the renal pelvis during the later bladder filling phase and lesser reflux into the right pelvis. VUR decreases slowly over the voiding phase with residual activity in the pelvis, particularly the left, at the end of the study. The 10-second per frame acquisition rate allows for high sensitivity for VUR detection.

Grading criteria are similar to those used with contrast cystography; however, the radionuclide study's limited resolution does not permit assessment of calyceal morphology. Mild reflux is confined to the ureter, moderate reaches the pelvicocalyceal system, and severe involves a distorted collecting system and dilated tortuous ureter.

Notes

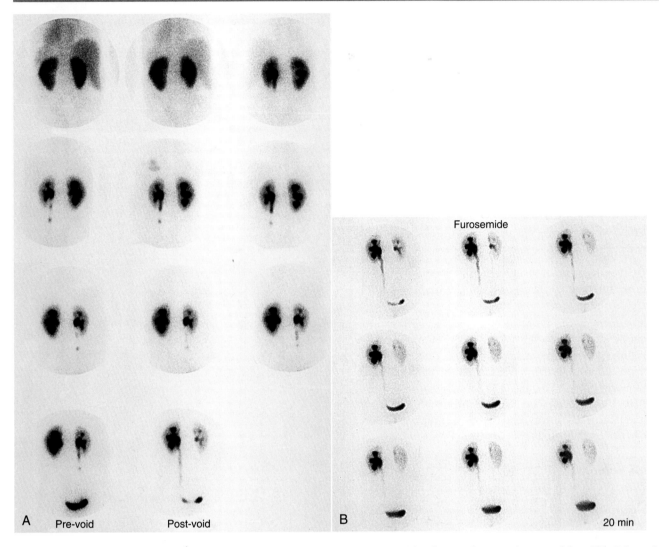

A
Pre-void   Post-void

B   Furosemide

20 min

A 45-year-old woman with cervical carcinoma has new bilateral hydronephrosis detected by CT. Diuretic renography was performed.

1. Describe the scintigraphic findings before and after furosemide (Lasix) administration.

2. What patient preparation is required before the study?

3. Interpret the study after diuretic administration.

4. List some diagnostic limitations of diuretic renography.

Genitourinary System: Diuretic Renography—Unilateral Obstruction

1. A, Good bilateral cortical renal uptake and prompt excretion into collecting systems bilaterally. Retention of activity in left renal collecting system and upper ureter. B, Very poor left kidney response to furosemide. The right is mostly washed out before furosemide administration and completely by the end of the study.

2. Good hydration. Adults usually receive oral hydration. Children are often administered intravenous hydration and have urinary catheters placed.

3. Clinically significant obstruction of the distal left renal collecting system.

4. Dehydration, renal insufficiency, inadequate diuretic dose, full bladder, large collecting system.

References

Connolly LP, Zurakowski D, Peters CA, et al: Variability of diuresis renography interpretation due to method of post-diuretic renal pelvic clearance half-time determination, *J Urol* 164:467–471, 2000.

Shulkin BL, Mandell GA, Cooper JA, et al: Procedure guideline for diuretic renography in children. *J Nucl Med Technol* 36:162–168, 2008.

Cross-Reference

Nuclear Medicine: THE REQUISITES, 3rd ed, pp 237–241.

Comment

Optimal methodology is important to get reproducible results. Good hydration is mandatory. For adults, oral hydration is usually adequate. The patient must receive a sufficient furosemide dose. A larger dose is needed with renal insufficiency; however, the exact dose is often only an estimate. A common reason for an indeterminate response occurs in patients who have had previous intervention for obstruction but still have a dilated collecting system. These patients may be monitored over time to ensure that no deterioration in renal function or diuretic response occurs. Bladder filling backpressure can be a factor in delayed clearance; in such cases, a urinary catheter should be placed. Intravenous fluids and urinary catheterization are routine in many clinics for young children.

An obstructed kidney shows very poor or no washout, usually with a half-time of emptying of greater than 20 minutes. A nonobstructed kidney shows prompt washout, usually with a half-time of less than 10 minutes. However, some patient studies show partial washout, defined as indeterminate for obstruction. Large collecting systems clear out more slowly than small ones, even if not obstructed, and are often in the indeterminate range. Calculation of a washout half-time can be particularly valuable for serial studies.

Notes

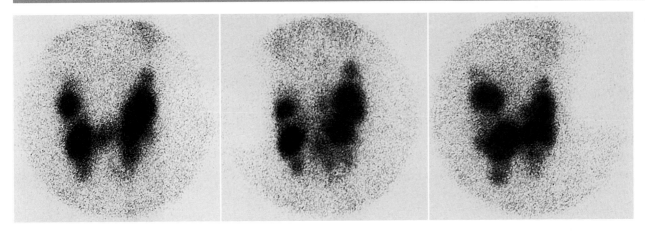

A 53-year-old woman was referred for recent enlargement of the right lower lobe of a known multinodular thyroid gland. Serum thyroid-stimulating hormone (TSH) was suppressed. The patient has a history of radiation therapy for acne as a teenager.

1. Describe the scintigraphic findings of this ^{99m}Tc-pertechnetate scan (*left to right*: anterior, left anterior oblique, right anterior oblique).

2. Give the likely diagnosis.

3. What are the therapeutic options?

4. What is the likelihood of thyroid cancer in this patient?

Endocrine System: Toxic Nodular Goiter

1. Multiple hot and relatively cold regions throughout both lobes with apparent suppression of non-nodular gland.

2. Multinodular toxic goiter.

3. Treat with radioactive ^{131}I.

4. The likelihood of thyroid cancer is less than 5% in patients with a multinodular goiter. A dominant nodule increases the suspicion for cancer. A history of radiation therapy to the head and neck also significantly increases a patient's risk of thyroid cancer.

References

Cases JA, Surks MI: The changing role of scintigraphy in the evaluation of thyroid nodules, *Semin Nucl Med* 30:81–87, 2000.

Sarkar SD: Benign thyroid disease: what is the role of nuclear medicine? *Semin Nucl Med* 36:185–193, 2006.

Cross-Reference

Nuclear Medicine: THE REQUISITES, 3rd ed, pp 88–94.

Comment

This patient not only had a toxic multinodular goiter with a radioactive iodine uptake (RAIU) of 36% but also had papillary follicular thyroid cancer. She subsequently had a near-total thyroidectomy and radioactive iodine therapy. The incidence of thyroid cancer approaches 30% in a patient with a history of radiation therapy to the neck and a nodular gland. Patients treated with radiation to the neck for acne, ringworm, and tonsillar enlargement often received a radiation dose of 10 to 50 rads to the thyroid. The scan has the appearance of a multinodular toxic goiter. This is a ^{99m}Tc-pertechnetate scan. Note the salivary glands above the thyroid and the high background, neither of which is seen with ^{123}I. Normally, thyroid uptake and salivary uptake are similar with ^{99m}Tc-pertechnetate. The high thyroid uptake compared with salivary uptake here is consistent with hyperthyroidism. Ten μCi of ^{131}I was administered orally, for the RAIU. The RAIU was 38%. The usual administered dose for therapy of multinodular toxic goiter is 20 to 30 mCi. Toxic nodular goiter is more resistant to ^{131}I therapy than Graves' disease. Once the nodules are effectively treated, which may require 3 to 4 months, the function of the remaining suppressed gland will return. Hypothyroidism as a result of radioactive iodine therapy is uncommon in patients with nodular toxic goiter because the suppressed gland does not take up the radioactive iodine. However, in this case, the patient's biopsy specimen showed cancer, so she received a near-total thyroidectomy followed by thyroid cancer ablation therapy.

Notes

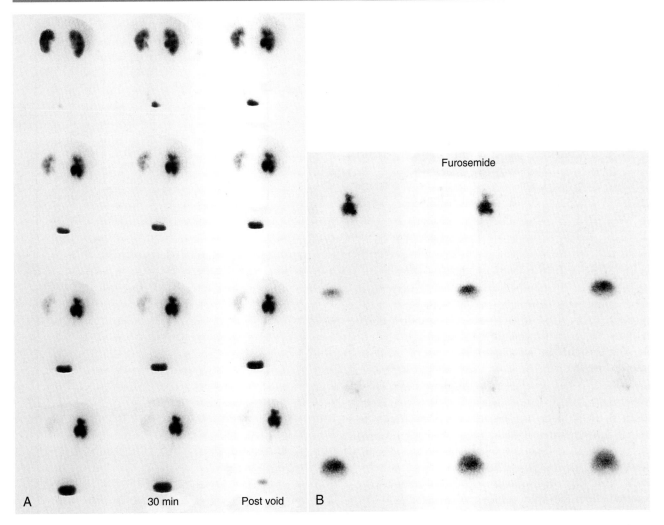

A   30 min   Post void   B

A 31-year-old man with a history of ureteropelvic junction obstruction with surgical correction several years ago. A recent diuretic renogram was interpreted as positive for right renal obstruction. He had a second surgical correction. This present scan was obtained subsequently.

1. Describe the scintigraphic imaging findings before (A) and after (B) administration of furosemide.

2. What is your interpretation of the study?

3. What is the Whittaker test?

4. What is the rationale for furosemide (Lasix) renography?

CASE 49

Genitourinary System: Diuretic Renography—Nonobstructed Hydronephrosis

1. Bilateral prompt cortical uptake and excretion into collecting systems. Retention of activity in the right collecting system at 30 minutes. Good postfurosemide washout.

2. Good response to surgical correction. Negative for obstruction.

3. The Whitaker test measures pressure-flow relationships and requires fluoroscopically guided trocar or spinal needle insertion into the renal pelvis. Basal and pressure measurements are recorded during a constant infusion rate of a contrast solution. Obstruction was defined as greater than 15 cm water and no obstruction as less than 10 to 12 cm water.

4. The rationale is similar to the Whitaker test. Lasix produces increased urinary flow. In a nonobstructed kidney, this results in more rapid washout of the collecting system. In an obstructed one, it will be ineffective.

References

Durand E, Blaufox D, Britton KE, et al: International Scientific Committee of Radionuclides in Nephrourology consensus on renal transit time measurements, *Semin Nucl Med* 38:82–102, 2008.

O'Reilly PH: Consensus Committee of the Society of Radionuclides in Nephrourology, *BJU Int* 91:239–243, 2003.

Cross-Reference

Nuclear Medicine: THE REQUISITES, 3rd ed, pp 237–241.

Comment

Contrast intravenous urography, ultrasonography, and conventional radionuclide renography are not reliable in differentiating obstructive from nonobstructive hydronephrosis. Dilation, delayed opacification, and delayed washout are seen with obstruction on contrast urography but also may be seen with nonobstructive hydronephrosis. Similarly, ultrasonography can depict hydronephrosis but cannot distinguish between obstruction and nonobstruction. The Whittaker test is rarely used today because it is invasive and usually unnecessary; diuretic renography has similar accuracy and is now the standard diagnostic test. The increased urine flow as a result of furosemide diuresis produces prompt washout in a nonobstructed system. With a fixed obstruction, the capacity to augment outflow is limited, resulting in prolonged washout.

Deterioration in renal function or the likelihood of deterioration in the near future is an indication for surgical intervention. Lasix renography is able to predict whether there is a significant obstruction that likely will result in renal deterioration if not corrected. If definite renal dysfunction is demonstrated before Lasix (e.g., a high-grade obstruction with uptake but no urinary clearance), Lasix renography is unnecessary (i.e., the diagnosis of high-grade obstruction is made). Lasix renography is useful with lower grade obstructions that have clearance into the collecting system. Diuretic renography can help determine which patients require surgical correction.

Notes

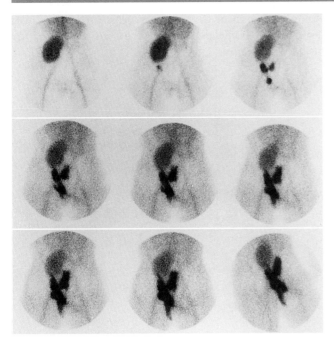

A 30-year-old patient 24 hours after a renal transplant. The patient had decreasing urine output, fullness and tenderness around the graft, and scrotal swelling.

1. Describe the findings on the 25-minute dynamic renal scintigraphy.

2. What is your interpretation?

3. What are causes of postoperative fluid collections adjacent to a renal allograft?

4. What are common complications during the first weeks after transplantation?

Genitourinary System: Transplanted Kidney—Urinary Leak

1. Rapid leakage of urine just inferior to the transplanted kidney extravasating into the scrotal region.

2. Urinary leak caused by disruption of the surgical anastomosis.

3. Hematomas and abscesses occur in the early postoperative course, whereas lymphoceles generally are noted 4 to 8 weeks after surgery.

4. Acute tubular necrosis, acute rejection, obstruction. Cyclosporine toxicity usually occurs months after transplantation.

References

Choyke PL, Becker JA, Ziessman HA: Imaging the transplanted kidney. In: Pollack HM, McLennan BL (eds): *Clinical Urology*, 2nd ed. Philadelphia: WB Saunders, 2000, pp 3091–3118.

Talanow R, Neumann D, Brunken R, et al: Urinary leak after renal transplantation proven by SPECT-CT imaging, *Clin Nucl Med* 32:883–885, 2007.

Cross-Reference

Nuclear Medicine: THE REQUISITES, 3rd ed, pp 239–252.

Comment

Urinary leaks and urinomas usually are diagnosed within the first or second postoperative week. They are typically located between the transplanted kidney and the bladder, although they may descend into the scrotum or thigh. Ureteral breakdown is usually caused by vascular insufficiency leading to ureteral necrosis but also can be caused by increased urinary pressure from distal obstruction. Large urinomas can rupture intraperitoneally to produce urinary ascites, and they can become infected and form abscesses.

Urinary fistulae generally develop in the post-transplantation period. They are managed by reimplantation of the ureter or another reconstructive procedure. Urinomas result from the continued, slow extravasation of urine from the renal pelvis, ureter, or ureteroneocystostomy site. Large urinomas and urinary leaks can be serious complications of renal transplantation. Smaller leaks often result in walled-off collections that may produce symptoms and can resolve spontaneously. Larger and more rapid leaks require prompt intervention. An abrupt halt in urine output from a transplant that was functioning initially after surgery suggests a urinary leak. On ultrasound imaging, urinomas are well-defined, anechoic fluid collections. The radionuclide study can confirm their urinary origin. With a slower leak, delayed images may be required to detect the urinary collection.

Notes

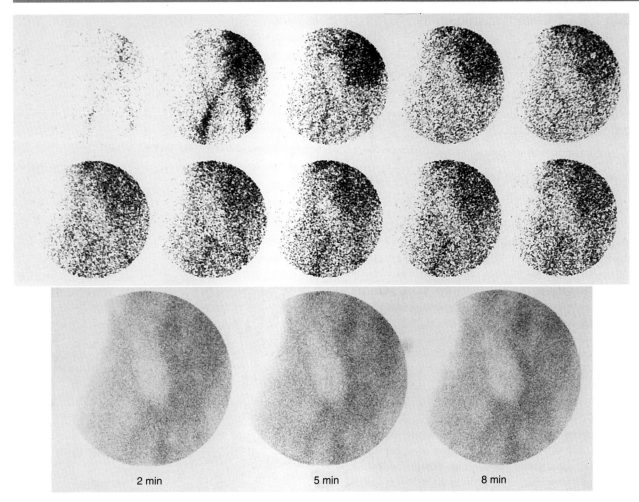

2 min   5 min   8 min

Blood flow (3 s/minute) and early dynamic images (2 minutes per frame) acquired 24 hours after renal transplantation.

1. What are the scintigraphic findings?

2. What is the differential diagnosis?

3. What is your interpretation?

4. What therapy would be appropriate?

Genitourinary System: Transplanted Kidney, Nonviable

1. No blood flow to the transplanted kidney. No renal uptake. A photopenic region in the shape and expected position of the right transplanted kidney.

2. Arterial or venous thrombosis, severe irreversible rejection, acute cortical necrosis.

3. Nonviable kidney.

4. Removal of the nonviable transplanted kidney.

References

Choyke PL, Becker JA, Ziessman HA: Imaging the transplanted kidney. In: Pollack HM, McLennan BL (eds): *Clinical Urology*, 2nd ed. Philadelphia: WB Saunders, 2000, pp 3091–3118.

Russell CD, Yang H, Gastron RS, et al: Prediction of renal transplant survival from early postoperative radioisotope studies, *J Nucl Med* 41:1332–1336, 2000.

Cross-Reference

Nuclear Medicine: THE REQUISITES, 3rd ed, pp 239–252.

Comment

A major benefit of scintigraphy is that radionuclide angiography can demonstrate blood flow at the capillary level. Acute arterial thrombosis is an uncommon complication of renal transplantation. It presents as anuria and is considered an emergency when it occurs. Acute kinking of the transplanted artery may present similarly. Acute venous thrombosis may look identical to arterial thrombosis because of the lack of normal lymphatic drainage after transplantation.

Hyperacute rejection is a rapidly progressive irreversible process first detected immediately after implantation of the kidney transplant. The kidney turns blue in the operating room. The precipitating factor is the presence of preformed antibodies. Immediately after anastomosis an antibody-antigen reaction takes place in the graft, leading to rapid thrombosis of the vascular bed and complete functional destruction within minutes to hours. However, this is uncommon because of the current careful prescreening to determine immunologic compatibility. Renal artery stenosis can occur at any time but usually occurs 3 months or later after transplantation.

Notes

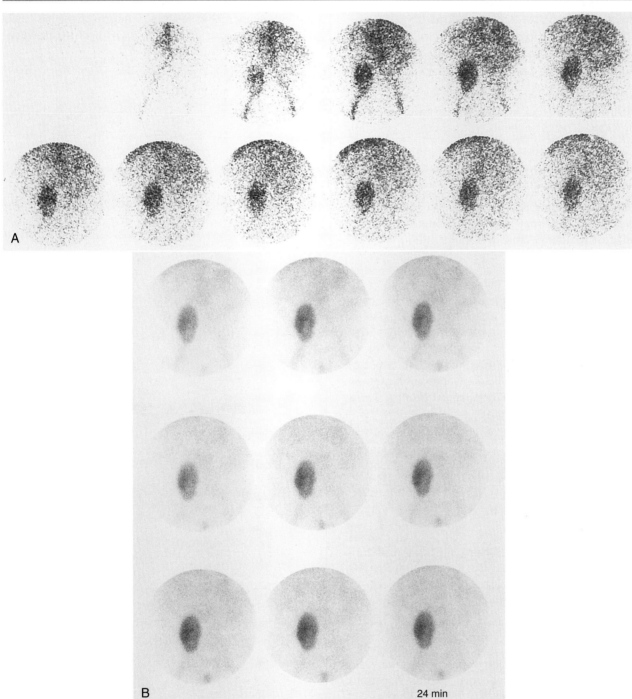

A 25-year-old man is referred for scintigraphy 3 days after renal cadaver transplantation.

1. What postoperative complications occur in the first week after renal transplantation?

2. What post–renal transplantation complications typically occur during the second week?

3. What are the scintigraphic findings in this case?

4. What is the diagnosis?

Genitourinary System: Transplanted Kidney—Acute Tubular Necrosis

1. Acute tubular necrosis (ATN), accelerated acute rejection, urinary leak, urinary obstruction.

2. Acute rejection. Accelerated rejection may occur during the first week in patients who have undergone previous transplantations or received multiple transfusions.

3. Normal blood flow, very poor function manifested by poor uptake and no excretion.

4. The pattern of normal blood flow but poor function during the first week after transplantation is typical of acute tubular necrosis (ATN).

References

Brown ED, Chen MY, Wolfman NT, et al: Complications of renal transplantation: evaluation with ultrasound and radionuclide imaging, *Radiographics* 20:607–622, 2000.

Dubovsky EV, Russell CD, Bischof-Delaloye A, et al: Report of the Radionuclides in Nephrourology Committee for Evaluation of Transplanted Kidney, *Semin Nucl Med* 29:175–188, 1999.

Cross-Reference

Nuclear Medicine: THE REQUISITES, 3rd ed, pp 239–252.

Comment

ATN invariably occurs immediately after transplantation in patients with cadaver allografts; it occurs considerably less frequently with living related donor grafts. An extended time between salvaging the donor kidney and transplantation increases the likelihood and severity of ATN. The scintigraphic findings of ATN are visible within 24 hours of transplantation. ATN usually resolves over 1 to 3 weeks. Thus, it may be superimposed on other postoperative complications (e.g., acute rejection). Acute rejection usually begins 5 to 7 days after transplantation and typically has decreased blood flow compared with the normal flow for ATN.

^{99m}Tc-MAG3 is the radiopharmaceutical of choice for renal transplant evaluation. ^{99m}Tc-DTPA can provide blood flow information but often cannot detect improvement or deterioration in function when the serum creatinine is elevated (e.g., >2.5 mg/dL). ^{99m}Tc-MAG3 allows evaluation of both blood flow at the capillary level and function, even in the setting of poor renal function. The radionuclide study can be particularly valuable when renal function is difficult to determine clinically (e.g., in patients undergoing dialysis). Improvement in renal function often can be detected 24 to 48 hours before changes in the serum creatinine.

Notes

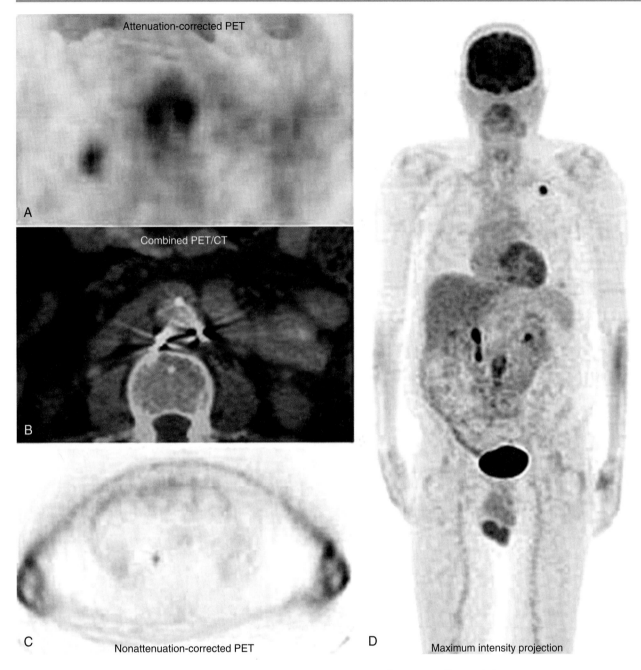

A — Attenuation-corrected PET

B — Combined PET/CT

C — Nonattenuation-corrected PET

D — Maximum intensity projection

1. What is a maximum intensity projection (MIP) image as shown in figure D?

2. Provide a differential diagnosis for the focal uptake in the left upper chest on the MIP image.

3. Name any other areas of abnormal radiotracer uptake in figure D.

4. Figures A, B, and C are the same cross-sectional slice, processed differently as labeled. Describe the diagnostic value of each for this study interpretation.

PET/CT: Attenuation Correction Artifact

1. Volume rendering displays two-dimensional cross-sectional data in a three-dimensional volume display. An MIP image is a type of volume rendering used with PET/CT. It projects in the visualization plane the voxels with the maximum intensity. D, Anterior-facing MIP image. A shaded surface display is another volume-rendering method.

2. Tumor, infection, metallic port artifact, radiotracer contamination.

3. Focal abnormal uptake in the midline abdomen, visualization of renal pelvis bilaterally, and proximal right ureter. Urinary contamination is noted below the scrotum.

4. Two foci of abnormal uptake are seen in the midline on the attenuation-corrected PET (A) and fused PET/CT (B), suggestive of tumor or infection. The PET/CT fused images also show surgical clips from previous surgery, raising the question of possible artifact. The nonattenuation-corrected PET image (C) shows no abnormal uptake, thus confirming artifact as the cause.

References

Kinahan PE, Hasegawa BH, Beyer T: X-ray-based attenuation correction for positron emission tomography/computed tomography scanners, *Semin Nucl Med* 33:166–179, 2003.

Sureshbabu W, Mawlawi O: PET/CT imaging artifacts, *J Nucl Med Technol* 33:156–161, 2005.

Wallis JW, Miller TR, Lerner CA, Keerup EC: Three-dimensional display in nuclear medicine, *IEEE Trans Med Imaging* 8:297–303, 1989.

Cross-Reference

Nuclear Medicine: THE REQUISITES, 3rd ed, p 310.

Comment

MIP images are standard with PET/CT. The rotating images permit quick whole-body analysis that allows rapid detection and localization of increased FDG uptake and possible pathology, whole-body marrow analysis, focal spine uptake, and so on. It is usually reviewed before the cross-sectional slices. While MIP is important and should be reviewed, it should not be relied on exclusively for interpretation.

Nonattenuation-corrected PET images should always be viewed when artifact is suspected. Metallic items that may cause artifactual increased uptake or streak artifact on PET include dental fillings, prostheses, electroencephalographic electrodes, buttons, jewelry, chemotherapy ports, and pacemaker leads. These false-positive artifacts on attenuation-corrected PET images occur when materials are denser than bone, often metal or barium contrast, because of the energy differences between the photons for CT and PET (511 keV). The high CT numbers from metallic implants result in corresponding high PET attenuation coefficients, thus leading to overestimation of the radiotracer activity in that area. On the other hand, some high-density metal implants can produce photopenic (cold) areas on PET images due to the metal attenuating the 511-keV PET photons, which results in no emission data. It is advisable to have patients remove all metallic objects if possible before PET/CT imaging to reduce any potential artifact on images.

Notes

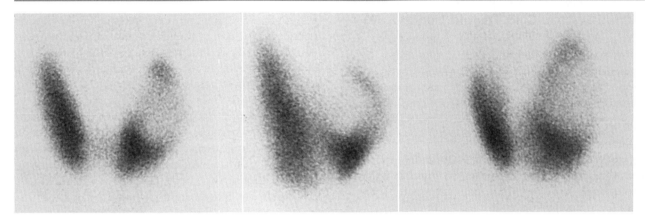

A 55-year-old woman is referred for evaluation of a palpable thyroid nodule. Left to right views are anterior, right anterior oblique, and left anterior oblique.

1. What are the two radiotracers in clinical use for thyroid scintigraphy? How are their mechanisms of uptake in the thyroid gland different?

2. What imaging method is used here? Why?

3. What is the likelihood of thyroid cancer in this patient?

4. What would you recommend as the next diagnostic or therapeutic procedure?

Endocrine System: Cold Thyroid Nodule

1. ^{99m}Tc-pertechnetate is administered intravenously; it is also taken up by thyroid follicular cells, but is not organified. ^{123}I sodium iodide is ingested orally; it is trapped by thyroid follicular cells and organified. Therefore, it remains in the thyroid for a considerably longer time.

2. A pinhole collimator is used because it magnifies and improves resolution. Resolution is dependent on the size of the pinhole insert, usually 3 to 4 mm, and thus resolution is less than 5 mm compared with 1.5 to 2 cm for a parallel-hole collimator.

3. A single cold nodule has a 15% to 20% chance of malignancy.

4. Aspiration needle biopsy.

References

Cases JA, Surks MI: The changing role of scintigraphy in the evaluation of thyroid nodules, *Semin Nucl Med* 30:81-87, 2000.

Sarkar SD: Benign thyroid disease: what is the role of nuclear medicine? *Semin Nucl Med* 36:185-193, 2006.

Cross-Reference

Nuclear Medicine: THE REQUISITES, 3rd ed, pp 88-94.

Comment

^{123}I is the preferred thyroid imaging agent because it is both trapped and organified. ^{99m}Tc is advantageous for imaging in children because of its lower radiation dose and high count rate. The adult administered dose of ^{99m}Tc is 3 to 5 mCi versus 200 to 400 µCi orally for ^{123}I. ^{123}I has the additional advantage that the percentage of iodine uptake can be calculated. ^{123}I images are obtained at approximately 4 hours after administration. Because ^{99m}Tc is not organified, it clears from the thyroid rapidly; thus, images are acquired 15 to 20 minutes after intravenous injection.

Photopenic or focal cold regions on thyroid scintigraphy scan result from various conditions other than thyroid cancer (e.g., cysts, colloid nodules, follicular nodules, new or old thyroiditis, Hashimoto's disease, hematoma, and other benign and malignant tumors). The incidence of thyroid cancer is less than 5% in a multinodular goiter and less than 1% for a hot nodule. However, a single cold nodule has a 15% to 20% incidence of malignancy.

A pinhole collimator is used with thyroid imaging for magnification. The collimator is in the shape of a cone with the lead pinhole inserted at the tip of the cone. Although parallel-hole collimation has a resolution of approximately 2 cm, pinhole collimation resolution depends on the size of the lead pinhole insert, between 2 and 6 mm. Size is difficult to judge with a pinhole collimator because of the magnification factor. The degree of magnification depends on the distance of the pinhole from the neck (i.e., the closer the distance, the greater the magnification). Size markers are sometimes used but are unreliable because of the changing magnification with depth. Physical examination is the commonly used method to estimate size, although it is subjective and open to interobserver differences. MRI would potentially be accurate but is not commonly used.

Notes

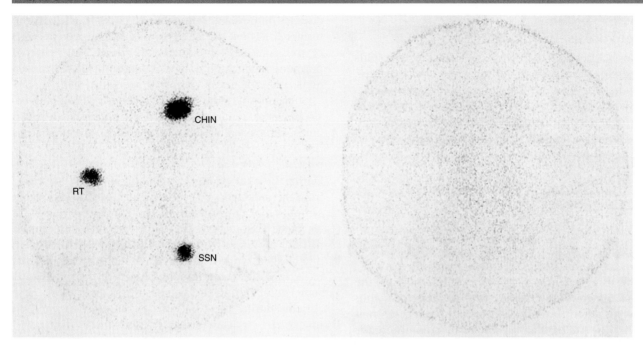

A 48-year-old woman has a recent onset of neck tenderness and thyrotoxicosis (TSH < 0.05 IU/mL); ^{123}I RAIU < 1%. Right (RT); suprasternal notch (SSN).

1. What is the differential diagnosis for thyrotoxicosis?

2. What is the clinical purpose of the thyroid scan and RAIU tests in the workup of patients with thyrotoxicosis?

3. How is the RAIU calculated?

4. What is the likely diagnosis in this patient?

Endocrine System:
Thyrotoxicosis/Thyroiditis

1. Graves' disease, toxic nodule(s), subacute thyroiditis (granulomatous, lymphocytic, silent, postpartum), iatrogenic thyroid hormone ingestion, iodine-induced hyperthyroidism (Jod-Basedow), trophoblastic tumors (hydatidiform mole and choriocarcinoma), Hashitoxicosis, ectopic hyperfunctioning thyroid tissue (struma ovarii).

2. Aid in the differential diagnosis of hyperthyroidism. To determine whether the disease is autonomous (Graves' disease, toxic nodules) (e.g., it has normal pituitary feedback [subacute thyroiditis]).

3. The RAIU is a relatively simple calculation that allows conversion of counts obtained from the patient's neck using a nonimaging probe to microcuries, the form in which the capsule was administered, thus making determination of an uptake percentage possible. The radioiodine capsule to be administered is placed in the dose calibrator (microcuries) and then counted with a nonimaging probe (counts). At 4 and 24 hours, the patient returns and has measurements of his/her neck using the probe. After correction for background (thigh) and decay, the percentage of uptake is calculated.

4. Subacute thyroiditis, based on the history of neck tenderness, suppressed TSH, and RAIU.

References

Freitas JE, Freitas AE: Thyroid and parathyroid imaging, *Semin Nucl Med* 24:234–245, 1994.

Sarkar SD: Thyroid pathophysiology. In: Sandler MP, Coleman RE, Wackers FJTh, et al (eds): *Diagnostic Nuclear Medicine,* 3rd ed. Baltimore: Williams & Wilkins, 1996, pp 899–908.

Cross-Reference

Nuclear Medicine: THE REQUISITES, 3rd ed, pp 82–87.

Comment

Thyroiditis and Graves' disease are the most common causes of thyrotoxicosis and can sometimes be difficult to distinguish clinically. A suppressed TSH (usually <0.1) is diagnostic of thyrotoxicosis. Thyroxine and triiodothyronine may or may not (subclinical) be elevated. The scan and RAIU aid in the differential diagnosis. The scan can distinguish focal nodular disease from the diffusely increased uptake of Graves' disease. The RAIU differentiates diseases with increased uptake (e.g., Graves', toxic nodule) from those with low uptakes (most other diseases listed in answer 1, e.g., thyroiditis). These latter diseases do not have autonomous function, whereas the former do. The RAIU value may also be reduced because of the presence of exogeneous iodine from thyroid hormone medication, iodine in foods, medications, vitamins, and radiographic contrast agents.

Subacute thyroiditis initially manifests as thyrotoxicosis and neck tenderness. Silent thyroiditis has no pain but a clinical course similar to that of granulomatous thyroiditis, which does have neck tenderness. The patient history may suggest postpartum thyroiditis. During the acute phase of thyroiditis, hormone is released from the inflamed cells, suppressing TSH and producing symptoms of thyrotoxicosis. Antithyroid antibodies are elevated. Hashimoto's thyroiditis is quite different. It usually presents with goiter and hypothyroidism in middle-aged women; however, a subgroup of patients have an acute hyperthyroid phase (Hashitoxicosis) at some point during the course of the disease. In these patients during the toxic phase, the thyroid scan and uptake are indistinguishable from those of Graves' disease.

Notes

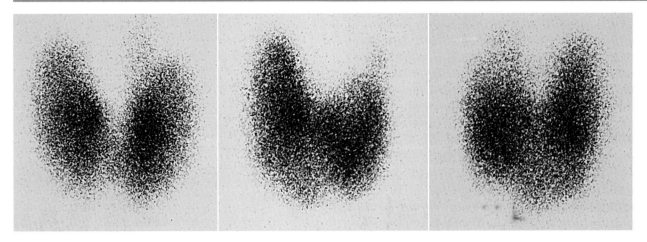

A 35-year-old woman has thyrotoxicosis. RAIU is 94% (4 hours) and 81% (24 hours).

1. Describe the difference between Graves' disease and a euthyroid scan appearance.

2. What is appropriate therapy for Graves' disease?

3. What are the usual administered doses of radiotracer for ^{131}I uptakes, ^{123}I scans, and therapy for Graves' disease and toxic nodules?

4. What are the short-term and long-term side effects of ^{131}I therapy for hyperthyroidism?

C A S E 5 6

Endocrine System: Graves' Disease

1. The scans at first glance may appear similar; however, the background is much reduced with Graves' disease, the gland tends to have a plumper appearance with convex borders, and often a pyramidal lobe is seen, as in this case. However, the uptake calculation is needed to confirm this. The amount of apparent thyroid uptake and background can be altered with different workstation intensity settings and background subtraction.

2. Surgery is seldom performed today because of good alternative therapies and its higher risk of complications/morbidity. Propylthiouracil and methimazole (Tapazole) sometimes are used initially, particularly in patients with severe disease who require "cooling down" and in young children. Today, many patients are treated initially with ^{131}I. Patients not treated initially with radioactive iodine are usually treated after 6 to 12 months of antithyroid medication.

3. ^{131}I uptake (10-20 µCi), ^{123}I scan and uptake (200-400 µCi), Graves' disease therapy (5-15 mCi ^{131}I), toxic nodules (20-30 mCi ^{131}I).

4. Short-term: occasional transient exacerbation of thyrotoxicosis, cardiac symptoms (e.g., tachycardia, angina; in the elderly, rarely thyroid storm). Long-term: hypothyroidism. There is no increased incidence of secondary cancers, reduction in fertility, or congenital defects in offspring.

References

Iagaru A, McDougall IR: Treatment of thyrotoxicosis, *J Nucl Med* 48:379-389, 2007.

Kaplan MM, Meier DA, Dworkin HJ: Treatment of hyperthyroidism with radioactive iodine, *Endocrinol Metab Clin North Am* 27:205-223, 1998.

Cross-Reference

Nuclear Medicine: THE REQUISITES, 3rd ed, pp 80, 82-87.

Comment

The normal percentage of radioiodine uptake increases progressively over 24 hours. Normal uptake is approximately 10% to 30%. With Graves' disease, the uptake typically increases more rapidly and to higher levels; it may plateau between 4 and 24 hours. However, in some cases, the 24-hour uptake is lower than that at 4 hours because of rapid iodine turnover. This has therapeutic implications and is the reason both 4- and 24-hour RAIU values are often obtained.

For Graves' disease therapy, an arbitrary dose (e.g., 10-15 mCi) is used by some clinicians. Others adjust for the two variables that determine the radiation dose to the gland: gland size and the percentage of RAIU. Many others use an equation to calculate the therapy dose that includes these factors: gland size (grams) × 120 to 150 µCi/g divided by the percentage of RAIU. With lower µCi/g doses, the radiation dose is minimized, but the recurrence rate is higher. With higher µCi/g doses, the need for retreatment is lower, but onset of hypothyroidism is earlier and more likely. Many endocrinologists today prefer the higher dose range because of the lack of serious side effects and the inevitability of hypothyroidism.

Notes

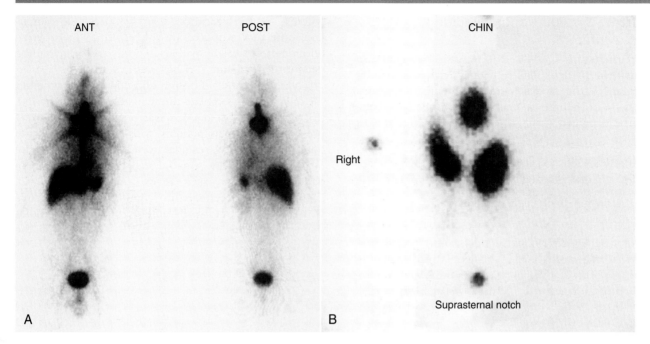

ANT POST CHIN

Right

Suprasternal notch

A

B

A 39-year-old woman underwent total thyroidectomy 6 weeks before ^{131}I therapy for thyroid cancer. The scan was performed 7 days after ablation therapy with 75 mCi of ^{131}I.

1. Describe the scintigraphic images.

2. What is the name of the characteristic scintigraphic pattern in the neck seen in scan A? What is the cause?

3. What collimators were used for image A and for image B?

4. Why is the liver seen in image A?

Endocrine System: ^{131}I Radioiodine "Star" Artifact

1. A, Post-therapy ^{131}I whole-body scan shows intense uptake in the neck, diffuse liver activity, and bladder clearance. The mediastinum is difficult to visualize because of the intense neck uptake. B, Pinhole collimator magnified image of the neck with three foci of uptake.

2. Star artifact due to septal penetration of high-energy ^{131}I gamma rays through the collimator septa.

3. A, Parallel-hole high-energy collimator. B, Pinhole collimator centered on the thyroid.

4. Radiolabeled thyroid hormone is produced in the thyroid and metabolized in the liver. This is seen only on the post-therapy scans because of the high administered dose relative to pretherapy scans.

References

Cooper DS, Doherty GM, Haugen BR, et al: Revised American Thyroid Association management guidelines for patients with thyroid nodules and differentiated thyroid cancer, *Thyroid* 19:1167–1214, 2009.

Elisei R, Schlumberger M, Driedger A, et al: Follow-up of low risk differentiated thyroid cancer patients who underwent radioiodine ablation of postsurgical thyroid remnants after either recombinant human thyrotropin or thyroid hormone withdrawal, *J Clin Endocrinol Metab* 94:4171–4179, 2009.

Cross-Reference

Nuclear Medicine: THE REQUISITES, 3rd ed, pp 79–80, 85, 101.

Comment

The star artifact makes interpretation of the neck and upper chest difficult. The pinhole collimator only has a single hole; therefore, septal penetration is not possible; there are no septa. The pinhole collimator in this case made interpretation of the neck possible, but the upper chest region can still be problematic. The pinhole collimator cannot correct for the considerable scatter into the mediastinum, and is not effective for whole-body imaging because the collimator would have to be a considerable distance away (and resolution falls off precipitously).

The reason for near-total thyroidectomies for thyroid cancer is to remove tumor and as much other thyroid tissue as possible, but preserve the parathyroids, which usually requires leaving some adjacent tissue. Removal of normal thyroid in thyroid cancer permits follow-up with reliable measurements of serum thyroglobulin and ^{131}I scans postoperatively. Preparation of the patient for whole-body thyroid cancer scans requires TSH stimulation to maximize uptake, by either withholding thyroid hormone to make the patient hypothyroid or giving the patient recombinant TSH before the scan.

The therapeutic ^{131}I dose is chosen based on whether the indication is to ablate the remaining normal thyroid, to treat thyroid cancer that was not removed or likely present, or both. In patients with thyroid cancer, the dose for ablation of residual normal tissue ranges from 30 to 100 mCi. The thyroid cancer therapy dose in patients with metastases ranges from 100 to 200 mCi. Higher doses sometimes are administered in patients with metastases but usually only after dosimetric studies that ensure no excess radiation to the bone marrow, the critical organ.

Notes

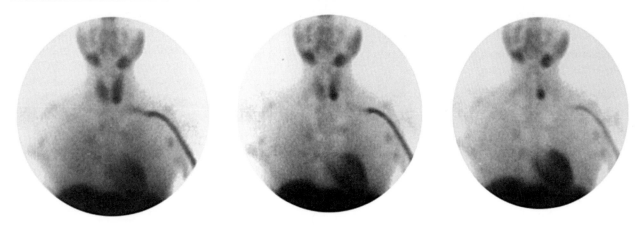

A 55-year-old man with hypercalcemia has an elevated serum parathormore (PTH). In this case, planar anterior mages were acquired at 5 minutes and 1 and 2 hours after injection of the radiopharmaceutical.

1. Which radiopharmaceutical is most commonly used for this study?

2. What is the diagnostic advantage and mechanism of this radiopharmaceutical?

3. What is your interpretation?

4. What is the most common cause of a false-positive study result?

Endocrine System: Parathyroid Adenoma—Planar Early and Delayed Imaging Method

1. ^{99m}Tc-sestamibi, the same radiopharmaceutical that is often used for cardiac imaging.

2. Sestamibi distributes according to blood flow and localizes intracellularly in the region of mitochrondria. It is taken up initially by both the thyroid and parathyroid tissue, but usually washes out more rapidly from the thyroid.

3. Parathyroid adenoma in the region of the left lower lobe of the thyroid.

4. Thyroid adenoma. The radiopharmaceutical is taken up by many benign and malignant tumors and may have a clearance pattern similar to that of parathyroid adenomas. Furthermore, not all parathyroid adenomas have slower washout than the thyroid. In those cases, increased early focal uptake is diagnostic.

References

Eslamy HK, Ziessman HA: Parathyroid scintigraphy in patients with primary hyperparathyroidism: 99mTc sestambi SPECT and SPECT/CT, *Radiographics* 28:1461–1476, 2008.

Taillefer R, Boucher Y, Potvin C, et al: Detection and localization of parathyroid adenomas in patients with hyperparathyroidism using a single radionuclide imaging procedure with ^{99m}Tc sestamibi (double-phase study), *J Nucl Med* 33:1801–1805, 1992.

Cross-Reference

Nuclear Medicine: THE REQUISITES, 3rd ed, pp 101–108.

Comment

In the past, parathyroid surgery consisted of four gland bilateral neck exploration. Preoperative localization was not always requested because good surgeons claimed to have greater than 90% accuracy in localizing the offending parathyroid adenoma. However, today with minimally invasive surgery in which a small incision is made, preoperative localization is more important and has become routine. An intraoperative serum PTH level is obtained before and after removal of the adenoma. If PTH has decreased significantly after the adenoma removal, the successful surgery is finished. If the intraoperative PTH level is still elevated after adenoma removal, there is further search for another hyperfunctioning parathyroid. Approximately 10% of patients have hyperplasia of all four glands.

^{99m}Tc-sestamibi has a higher accuracy for the detection of parathyroid tumors than other imaging modalities (e.g., ultrasonography, MRI). However, anatomic imaging methods are sometimes used in combination with the radionuclide study. Various different scintigraphic methodologies are currently used, including computer subtraction of ^{123}I thyroid images and SPECT. SPECT/CT has shown improved accuracy over planar images or SPECT alone.

Notes

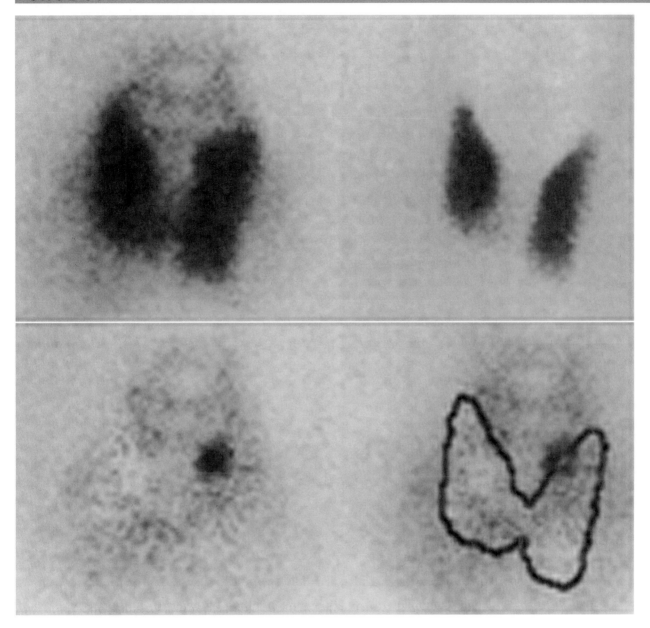

Patient with elevated serum calcium and PTH levels. ^{99m}Tc-sestamibi (*upper left*); ^{123}I (*upper right*); subtraction image (*lower left*); subtraction image with ^{99m}Tc-sestamibi outline superimposed (*lower right*).

1. What is the principle behind this methodology?

2. Describe the likely protocol.

3. Describe findings in the upper and lower panel.

4. What is the sensitivity compared with the delayed imaging method?

Endocrine System: Parathyroid Adenoma—Subtraction Method

1. ^{99m}Tc-sestamibi is taken up by the thyroid and parathyroid. ^{123}I is taken up only by the thyroid. Subtracting the ^{123}I thyroid image from the sestamibi image should show only the hyperfunctioning parathyroid.

2. ^{123}I is ingested. After a delay of 2 to 3 hours, an anterior ^{123}I thyroid scan is performed. Without moving the patient, an image is obtained after intravenous injection of ^{99m}Tc-sestamibi. The ^{123}I image is computer subtracted from the ^{99m}Tc-sestamibi image.

3. The ^{99m}Tc-sestamibi and ^{123}I thyroid scans in the upper images appear normal at first glance, except that the sestamibi image shows a slight bulge superomedially. The subtraction image confirms this abnormality and demonstrates a likely parathyroid adenoma.

4. The sensitivity for parathyroid adenoma detection (approximately 90%) is similar to that of the delayed imaging method (i.e., images at 5–10 minutes and 2 hours after sestamibi).

References

Hindie E, Melliere D, Perlemuter L, et al: Primary hyperparathyroidism: higher success rate of first surgery after preoperative Tc-99m sestamibi-I-123 subtraction imaging, *Radiology* 204:221–228, 1997.

Lavely WC, Goetze S, Friedman KP, et al: Comparison of SPECT/CT, SPECT, and planar imaging with single- and dual-phase (99m)Tc-sestamibi parathyroid scintigraphy, *J Nucl Med* 48:1084–1089, 2007.

Cross-Reference

Nuclear Medicine: THE REQUISITES, 3rd ed, pp 101–105.

Comment

Parathyroid scintigraphy may be performed successfully using a variety of different protocols. ^{99m}Tc-sestamibi has replaced ^{201}Tl for parathyroid imaging because of its better image resolution. Either ^{99m}Tc-pertechnetate or ^{123}I can be used for the thyroid imaging portion of the subtraction technique. ^{123}I has the advantage of a different photopeak (159 keV) compared with ^{99m}Tc-sestamibi.

Some variability in washout occurs with the two-phase sestamibi technique. The addition of the thyroid scan and subtraction images offers some advantages. It can confirm thyroid rather than parathyroid origin of the uptake (e.g., follicular adenomas) and can be helpful in patients with anatomic variants, those having undergone previous thyroid surgery, or those receiving thyroid hormone causing thyroid suppression. However, subtraction techniques sometimes produce artifacts because of patient motion or misregistration of images. Computer subtraction images should always be interpreted as an adjunct to image analysis, not in isolation.

SPECT and SPECT/CT are increasingly being used to localize parathyroid adenomas. These methods are somewhat more sensitive than planar imaging. Various different methods have been used (e.g., early SPECT imaging, delayed SPECT imaging, and a combination of early and delayed). SPECT/CT performed early and late appears to be somewhat more accurate.

Notes

Fair Game

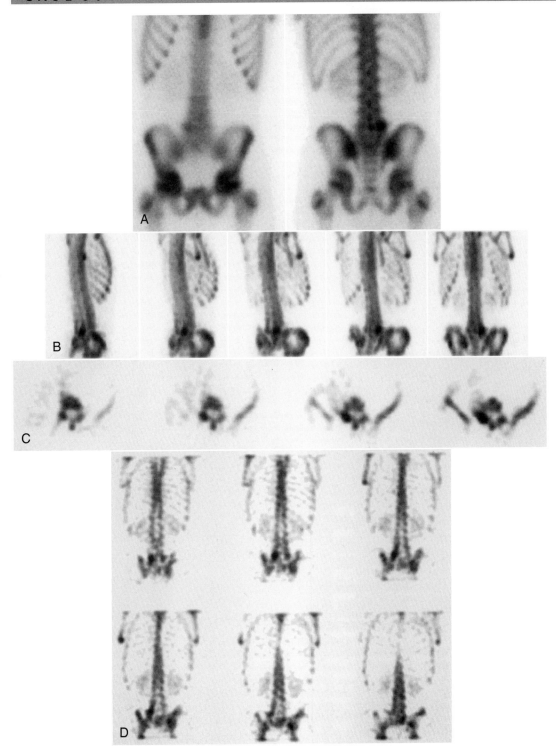

A 12-year-old boy has a recent onset of back pain. Findings of radiographs obtained at another institution were reported as negative.

1. Describe the bone scan findings on the planar (A) and maximum intensity projection (MIP) SPECT (B) images shown at different projections.

2. Describe the findings on the transverse and coronal SPECT slices (C and D).

3. Provide a differential diagnosis and the most likely diagnosis.

4. This entity may be associated with an abnormality of alignment. Describe it.

Skeletal System: L5 Pars Interarticularis Defect

1. There is focal increased uptake in the region of the lateral aspect of the L5 vertebra.

2. The finding is best demonstrated and localized on the cross-sectional SPECT images where abnormal uptake is seen in the region of the right pars interarticularis/facet joint.

3. L5 unilateral pars interarticularis defect, degenerative, or post-traumatic facet disease. Pars defect is the most likely diagnosis in this age group.

4. Spondylolisthesis or slippage of the vertebrae out of normal alignment can occur if the defect is bilateral.

References

Collier BD, Krasnaw AZ, Hellman RS: Bone scanning. In: Collier BD, Fogelman I, Rosenthall L (eds): *Skeletal Nuclear Medicine*. St. Louis: Mosby, 1996, pp 51–56.

Ruiz-Cotorro A, Balius-Matas R, Estrch-Massana AE, Vilaro Angulo J: Spondylolysis in young tennis players, *Br J Sports Med* 40:441–446, 2006.

Cross-Reference

Nuclear Medicine: THE REQUISITES, 3rd ed, pp 117–118.

Comment

Spondylolysis is a fracture of the neural arch of the vertebra involving the pars interarticularis. It is believed to represent a stress fracture caused by repetitive injury between infancy and early adult life, rather than a single trauma, although the latter may occur. Spondylolysis occurs most frequently in the lumbar spine; the majority of cases involve the fifth vertebra, as in this case. It may be unilateral or bilateral and may be associated with slippage or spondylolisthesis of the vertebra with respect to adjacent vertebrae.

Spondylolysis may cause symptoms, prompting an imaging diagnosis, but it may be asymptomatic and discovered incidentally on radiographic studies. Localization of increased uptake on planar images is often difficult. SPECT allows determination of whether abnormal uptake is in the body, pedicle, or posterior elements. SPECT has significantly higher sensitivity than planar imaging (85% vs. 62%) for detection of a pars defect. SPECT should be performed even after negative planar study findings when the diagnosis is suspected, particularly in young patients with low back pain. An abnormality seen on bone scintigraphy has significant patient management implications. Inappropriate early manipulation or too early a return to sports could convert the stress-related parts defect into a frank fracture, possibly leading to unstable spondylolisthesis. Spondylolysis without bone scan uptake suggests that the bone defect is not the cause of the patient's pain.

Notes

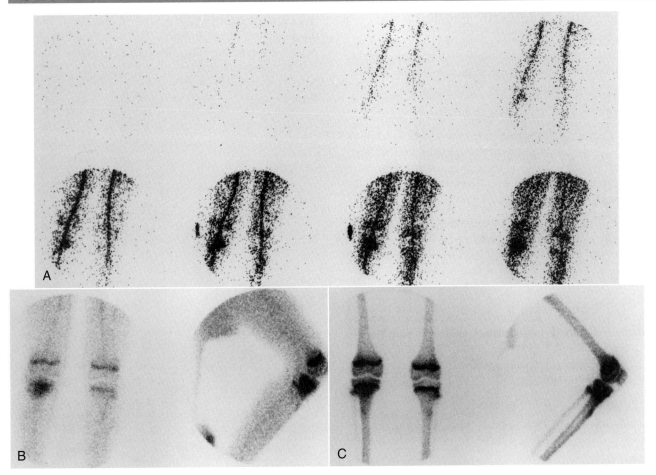

A 5-year-old boy presented with low-grade fever and pain in the right knee.

1. Describe the three-phase scintigraphic findings.

2. Provide a differential diagnosis.

3. What bone scan scintigraphic findings would be typical of septic arthritis?

4. What other radionuclide study could confirm or exclude infection?

CASE 61

Skeletal System: Tibial Osteomyelitis— Three-Phase Bone Scan

1. Increased blood flow (A), blood pool (B), and uptake on delayed images (C) in the proximal metaphyseal region of the right tibia.

2. Osteomyelitis, fracture, osteotomy, bone tumor.

3. Septic arthritis shows increased flow and blood pool to the joint and increased uptake at the end of long bones symmetrically on both sides of the joint. An asymmetrical appearance may be seen if osteomyelitis and septic arthritis coexist.

4. Radiolabeled white blood cell study. ^{99m}Tc-HMPAO leukocytes might be preferable over ^{111}In-oxine leukocytes in a child because of the lower radiation dose to the spleen.

References

Palestro CJ, Love C: Radionuclide imaging of musculo-skeletal infection: conventional agent, *Semin Musculoskelet Radiol* 11:335–352, 2007.

Stumpe KD, Strobel K: Osteomyelitis and arthritis, *Semin Nucl Med* 39:27–35, 2009.

Cross-Reference

Nuclear Medicine: THE REQUISITES, 3rd ed, pp 147–152.

Comment

Bone infection is usually bacterial in origin, often staphylococcal, and reaches the bone by direct extension from a contiguous skin site of infection, hematogenous spread, or direct introduction by surgery or trauma. Direct extension from contiguous sites of infection is a very common cause of osteomyelitis, usually as a result of soft-tissue infection after trauma, radiation therapy, burns, or pressure sores. Direct introduction of bacteria may occur during open fractures, open surgical reduction, or penetrating trauma by foreign bodies. In acute hematogenous osteomyelitis, infection involves the red marrow of long bones as a result of the relatively slow blood flow in metaphyseal sinusoidal veins and the relative lack of phagocytes. In adults, the long bones rarely are affected because adipose tissue has replaced red marrow. Infection occurs in the spine most frequently secondary to septicemia.

The bone scan is very sensitive for diagnosing osteomyelitis. However, a positive three-phase bone scan is not specific for osteomyelitis. Fracture, tumor, and Charcot joints may be three-phase positive. The specificity of the bone scan is particularly poor in patients with underlying conditions such as previous bone infection, fractures, and orthopedic implants or devices. The patient's history, radiographs, radiolabeled leukocytes, and biopsy frequently are necessary to make a definitive diagnosis in non-virgin bone. The bone scan has a high negative predictive value, and thus a negative study can rule out osteomyelitis.

Notes

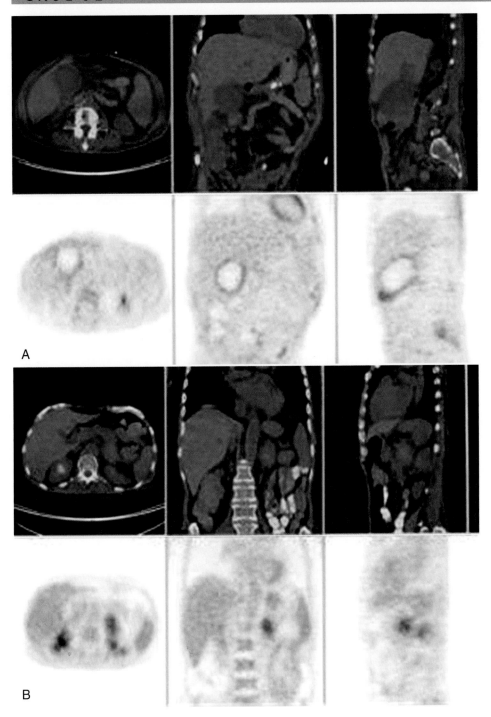

A

B

Patients A and B both have multiple myeloma. They were referred for FDG-PET/CT restaging evaluations without specific or localizing symptoms.

1. Describe the abnormal uptake in patient A.

2. What are possible causes of this uptake?

3. Describe the abnormal uptake in patient B.

4. What are possible causes of this uptake?

FDG-PET/CT: Gallbladder Visualization

1. Ring-shaped increased FDG uptake in the right upper quadrant.

2. Acute or chronic cholecystitis, liver abscess, centrally necrotic liver tumor, gallbladder cancer, inflammatory cyst of the liver (e.g., hydatid cyst, hematoma). Histopathology after cholecystectomy showed chronic cholecystitis.

3. FDG uptake anterior to the left kidney.

4. Metastatic lymphadenopathy, adrenal metastasis or primary tumor, focal pancreatitis, primary pancreatic tumor or metastasis to the pancreas. This was proven to be pancreatic adenocarcinoma.

References

Bang S, Chung HW, Park SW, et al: The clinical usefulness of [18]FDG PET in the differential diagnosis, staging, and response evaluation after concurrent chemoradiotherapy for pancreatic cancer, *J Clin Gastroenterol* 40:923–929, 2006.

Corvera CU, Blumgart LH, Akhurst T, et al: 18F-fluorodeoxyglucose positron emission tomography influences management decisions in patients with biliary cancer, *J Am Coll Surg* 206:57–65, 2008.

Cross-Reference

Nuclear Medicine: THE REQUISITES, 3rd ed. pp 331–332, 335.

Comment

Gallbladder wall uptake is occasionally an incidental finding on PET/CT scans in patients referred for oncologic reasons. Correlative imaging with CT and ultrasonography can often clarify the cause. Asymptomatic acute cholecystitis would be unlikely. Chronic cholecystitis, as seen in this case, is not rare. However, other etiologies of gallbladder uptake must be considered. Gallbladder cancer is the most common neoplasm of the biliary tract. It occurs most often in patients older than 60 years of age. As many as 50% of patients have nodal metastases at the time of diagnosis, and 70% involve the liver. The most common tumors to metastasize to the gallbladder are melanoma and lung cancer. Most biliary tract tumors are FDG avid. PET can alter management, primarily through upstaging, in 24% of cholangiocarcinomas and 23% of gallbladder carcinomas compared with the combination of CT, MRI/magnetic resonance cholangiopancreatography, and ultrasonography.

The normal pancreas typically has minimal if any uptake on FDG-PET. Pancreatitis shows diffuse homogeneous FDG uptake, although focal pancreatitis (e.g., autoimmune pancreatitis) may demonstrate intense uptake that may mimic pancreatic cancer. It is reported that FDG-PET can detect adenocarcinoma superimposed on chronic inflammation with good accuracy, superior to that of CT alone. PET is more sensitive than other imaging modalities for the detection of hepatic metastases. FDG-PET is less sensitive for detection of well-differentiated tumors of the endocrine pancreas (e.g., carcinoid, gastrinoma, insulinoma, glucagonoma) due to their indolent, slow-growing nature.

Notes

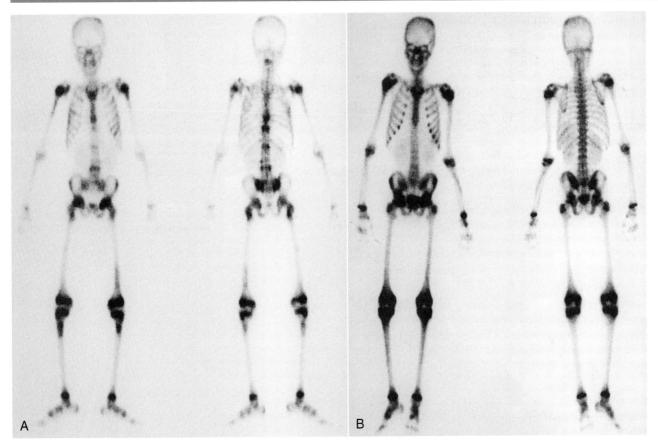

A 13-year-old girl with sickle cell disease was referred with low-grade fever and arm, leg, and back pain (A). The scan was repeated 1 year later with arm and back pain (B).

1. Describe the scintigraphic soft-tissue findings.

2. Describe the scintigraphic bone findings.

3. What is the likely diagnosis?

4. How can osteomyelitis be differentiated from bone infarct?

C A S E   6 3

Skeletal System: Sickle Cell Disease

1. Mild soft-tissue uptake is present in the region of the spleen.

2. A, Abnormal increased uptake in the proximal right humerus, left distal femur, multiple sites in the thoracic and lumbar spine. B, Uptake in the right ulna and left posterior ninth rib. The previous abnormalities have resolved.

3. Sickle cell crises with infarcts.

4. Radiolabeled leukocyte study combined with a bone marrow scan, ^{99m}Tc sulfur colloid (^{99m}Tc-SC).

References

Rifai A, Nyman R: Scintigraphy and ultrasonography I differentiating osteomyelitis from bone infarction in sickle cell disease, *Acta Radiol* 38:139–143, 1997.

Skaggs DL, Kim SK, Greene NW, et al: Differentiation between bone infarction and acute osteomyelitis with sickle cell disease with use of sequential radionuclide bone marrow and bone scans, *J Bone Joint Surg Am* 83A:1810–1813, 2001.

Cross-Reference

Nuclear Medicine: THE REQUISITES, 3rd ed, pp 142–143, 146–151.

Comment

Bone and joint complaints are common in patients with sickle cell hemoglobinopathies. Symptoms may be transient, but they are often related to marrow infarctions that occur as part of a sickle crisis. Many resolve without radiographic changes. Radionuclide scans are the most sensitive imaging technique for early detection and evaluation of the extent of damage. During the first few days after a vaso-occlusive crisis with infarction, decreased uptake may be seen on the bone scan. Soon increased uptake becomes evident, starting as a rim of increased activity around the infarct. Often, only increased uptake will be seen because the bone scan is usually not obtained during the acute phase. A ^{99m}Tc-SC bone marrow scan is reported to be able to detect bone marrow infarctions early; the lesion appears as a cold defect. In infection, a radiolabeled leukocyte study would show increased uptake but no or low uptake with infarction. Splenic uptake is often seen on a bone scan due to microcalcifications before autoinfarction.

Notes

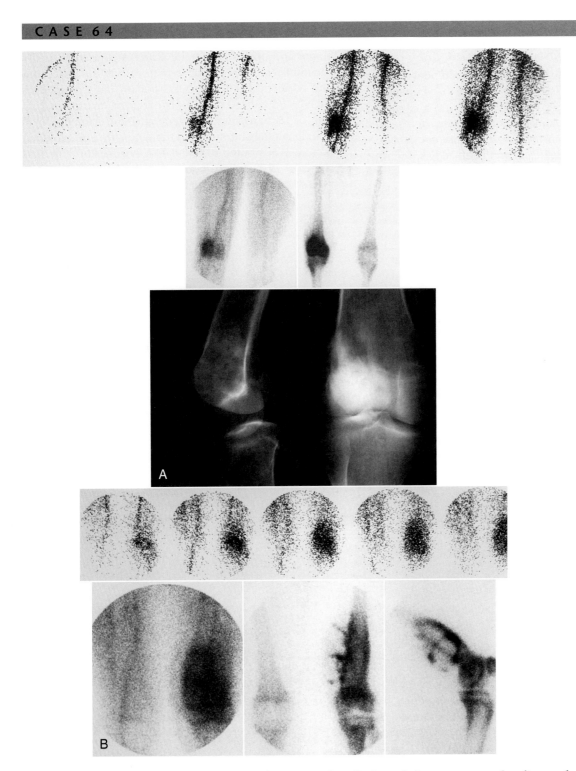

A

B

Two patients have knee pain, with no fever or calor. Patient A, bone scan and radiograph; patient B, bone scan.

1. Describe the abnormal three-phase bone scan findings for patients A and B.

2. What other general information about the patients is evident from the bone scans?

3. Provide a differential diagnosis and the most likely diagnoses for each patient.

4. What term is commonly used to describe the pattern seen on delayed images in patient B?

CASE 64

Skeletal System: Osteosarcoma

1. A, Increased blood flow (*top*) and blood pool (*bottom left*) to the right distal femur and increased uptake on delayed images in the distal femoral metaphysis extending to the joint surface (*bottom right*). Mild increased uptake in the proximal tibia, probably the result of hyperemia. Radiograph: mixed lytic-sclerotic lesion of the distal femur with cortical destruction and indistinct margins. No periosteal reaction. B, Abnormal increased flow and blood pool to the left distal femur with delayed increased uptake in a spiculated pattern extending beyond the femoral contour.

2. The patients are skeletally immature but near the mature stage. Physes are seen faintly on delayed images, indicating that fusion is imminent. These are teenagers.

3. A, Monostotic primary neoplasm (e.g., osteosarcoma, secondary neoplasm, osteomyelitis). B, Osteosarcoma.

4. Sunburst pattern.

References

Costellowe CM, Macapinlac HA, Madewell JE, et al: 18F-FDG PET/CT as an indicator of progression-free and overall survival in osteosarcoma, *J Nucl Med* 50:340–347, 2009.

Meyer JS, Nadel HR, Marina N, et al: Imaging guidelines for children with Ewing sarcoma and osteosarcoma: a report from Children's Oncology Group Bone Tumor Committee, *Pediatr Blood Cancer* 51:163–170, 2008.

Cross-Reference

Nuclear Medicine: THE REQUISITES, 3rd ed, pp 127–128, 134.

Comment

Osteosarcoma (osteogenic sarcoma) is the most common malignant primary tumor in children and adolescents. The intraosseous tumor usually arises in the metaphyses of long bones, the distal femur (44%), proximal tibia (22%), and proximal humerus (9%). It can extend into the diaphysis, epiphysis, or both. Two thirds of patients initially are seen with a large metaphyseal tumor as the primary focus. Radiographically the lesion may be predominantly osteosclerotic (25%), osteolytic (25%), or mixed (50%). A coexisting soft-tissue mass characterized by the production of osteoid or bone usually is present. A periosteal reaction of interrupted or spiculated type frequently occurs.

Bone scintigraphy is indicated before initiation of therapy to detect skip lesions, multicentric osteosarcoma, or a primary lesion with multiple metastases. In the presence of multiple lesions, limb amputation is no longer appropriate. On bone scan, osteosarcoma avidly accumulates the radiotracer with or without extension into adjacent soft tissue. Occasionally, an extended or augmented pattern may imply extensive marrow extension or transarticular involvement. Bone scintigraphy is poor in defining intraosseous tumor length. The extended pattern is attributed to circulatory changes in bone that simulate regional osteoblastic activity. Preoperative assessment is now based on MRI.

Notes

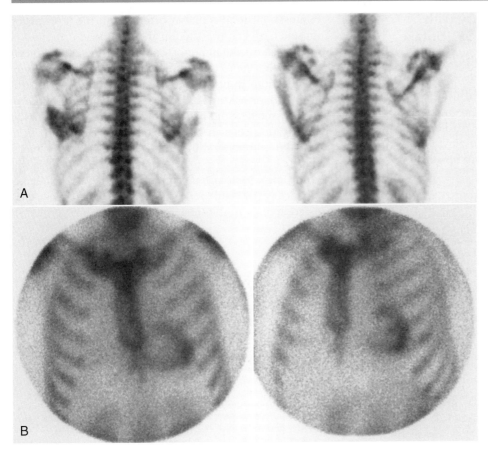

Two patients were referred for a bone scan. Both had thoracic pain.

1. Describe the soft-tissue scintigraphic findings in both patients.

2. What is the diagnosis and cause of this soft-tissue pattern of uptake?

3. What is the mechanism of radiopharmaceutical uptake?

4. What are other causes of soft-tissue uptake on bone scan?

Skeletal System: Muscle Injury with ^{99m}Tc–Methylene Diphosphate (MDP) Uptake

1. A, Uptake in teres major muscles bilaterally. B, Myocardial uptake.

2. Soft-tissue muscle injury caused by repetitive stress (A) and myocardial uptake of the entire left ventricle (B), which could be caused by cardiomyopathy, cardiotoxic drugs, myocarditis, or amyloidosis. A myocardial infarction would not have uptake in the entire ventricle.

3. Soft-tissue deposition of ^{99m}Tc-labeled diphosphonates is caused by binding to microcalcifications at sites of injury and possibly binding to injured immature collagen.

4. In muscle: rhabdomyolysis, iron dextran injection, polymyositis, myositis ossificans, ischemia, electrical injuries, direct trauma, myocardial infarction. Uptake of bone scan agents is sometimes seen in tumors (e.g., neuroblastoma, liver metastases from mucinous carcinoma of the colon, and others).

References

Brill DR: Radionuclide imaging of nonneoplastic soft tissue disorders, *Semin Nucl Med* 11:277–288, 1981.

Loutfi I, Collier BD, Mohammed AM: Nonosseous abnormalities on bones scans, *J Nucl Med Technol* 31:154–156, 2003.

Cross-Reference

Nuclear Medicine: THE REQUISITES, 3rd ed, pp 124–125.

Comment

A good general rule when reviewing bone scans is to first scrutinize the scan for renal and soft-tissue abnormalities before focusing on the bones. Although kidney abnormalities are more commonly noted, soft-tissue abnormalities are not uncommon. Patients usually are referred to confirm or exclude bone abnormalities (e.g., stress fractures and shin splints); however, the bone scan occasionally provides specific soft-tissue diagnosis. Overexertion injuries to the musculoskeletal system are common.

The proposed mechanism of uptake is absorption to denatured proteins or binding to mitochondrial calcium, which is increased in ischemic tissues. The cause of muscle localization is believed to be rhabdomyolysis. Muscle localization of bone tracers has been reported after a variety of exercises. In downhill runners, uptake occurs in the buttocks, hamstrings, and quadriceps, whereas uphill runners have increased uptake in the thigh adductors. Uptake in the thighs can be seen in bicycle riders and in the abdominal muscles after push-up

contests. Bilateral activity posteriorly in the teres major muscle has been reported in weight lifters.

Normal uptake in nonosseous structures often is seen on bone imaging, including uptake in thyroid cartilage, calcifications in blood vessels, and calcified costal cartilages. Abnormal uptake occurs in patients with heterotopic calcification, rhabdomyolysis, and soft-tissue calcification seen in scleroderma and dermatomyositis, in addition to more diffuse lung uptake caused by metastatic calcification (e.g., hyperparathyroidism, milk-alkali syndrome). Some primary and metastatic tumors characteristically take up bone radiotracers (e.g., metastatic osteosarcoma to the lung and neuroblastoma).

Notes

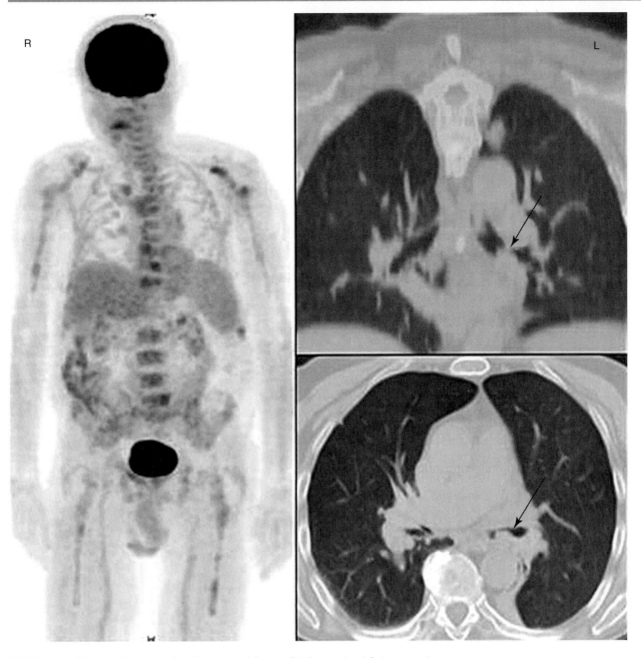

A 70-year-old man has newly diagnosed bronchial carcinoid (*arrows*).

1. Describe the abnormal findings on this FDG-PET/CT study.

2. Name at least other 3 tumor types that may have very low FDG uptake.

3. Why is FDG uptake low in some types of tumors?

4. How might tumor lesion size affect quantified FDG uptake in various tumors?

Oncology: FDG-PET/CT—Bronchial Carcinoid

1. No FDG uptake above background (mediastinum) is seen in the endobronchial lesion (*arrows*). The maximal intensity projections (MIPs) image shows a very heterogeneous pattern of uptake as well as focal areas of intense uptake throughout the bony skeleton suggestive of bone metastases.

2. Renal cell, prostate carcinoma, bronchoalveolar carcinoma, low-grade glioma, neuroendocrine tumors.

3. FDG uptake is generally low in low-grade tumors in contrast to high-grade tumors. This may be due to their lower mitotic rate and low cellularity. FDG uptake is closely related to GLUT transporter expression in malignant tumors and their increased utilization of glucose. FDG accumulation also depends on its rate of transport across cell membranes, phosphorylation by hexokinase, and intracellular entrapment.

4. If a lesion is below PET camera resolution (6–8 mm full-width half-maximum), the uptake and quantitative uptake values (SUV) will be artificially lower due to partial volume effect.

References

Park CM, Goo JM, Lee HJ, et al: Tumors in the tracheobronchial tree: CT and FDG PET features, *Radiographics* 29:55–71, 2009.

Soret M, Bacharach SL, Buvat I: Partial-volume effect in PET tumor imaging, *J Nucl Med* 48:932–945, 2007.

Cross-Reference

Nuclear Medicine: THE REQUISITES, 3rd ed, pp 66, 279–283.

Comment

Bronchial carcinoids often have low uptake similar to mediastinal background activity. Low-grade neuroeuroendocrine tumors in general are better imaged with ^{111}In-pentetreotide (OctreoScan), which targets serotonin receptors. PET radiopharmaceuticals that are ^{18}F-labeled serotonin receptor agents are under active investigation (^{18}F-DOPA as well as generator produced ^{68}Ga-tetraazacyclododecanetetraacetic acid. Poorly differentiated high-grade neuroendocrine tumors may be better detected with FDG-PET.

Due to the partial volume effect, small lesions will appear to have less FDG uptake (lower SUV) than larger lesions, which have the same FDG per gram of tissue. This effect is seen in lesions up to at least twice the size of the resolution of the camera system (~5–7 mm for modern PET cameras). Counts are spread over a volume that is determined by the intrinsic resolution of the imaging system. If the volume is larger than 1 pixel, the apparent activity of a small source will be distributed over several pixels, effectively decreasing the activity within each pixel and falsely lowering the calculated SUV.

Notes

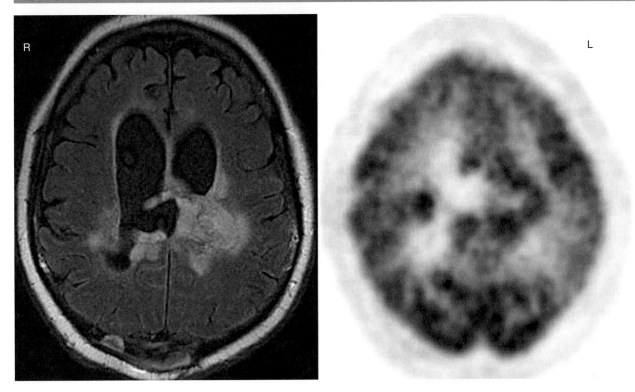

A 55-year-old patient has glioblastoma multiforme and presents for follow-up imaging after radiation and chemotherapy.

1. Describe the abnormality seen on the FDG-PET image of the brain.

2. Correlate the FDG-PET findings with those of the MRI shown. The head is tilted differently on the two studies.

3. What additional important diagnostic information does the FDG-PET add?

4. What are some potential causes of false-positive FDG-PET brain imaging?

CASE 67

FDG-PET: Glioblastoma Multiforme

1. Increased FDG uptake in the mid-left cerebral hemisphere in a semicircular pattern. There is also focal increased uptake in the right mid-hemisphere.

2. The FDG uptake correlates with hyperintense signal on the flair-weighted MRI along the periatrial white matter and splenium of the corpus callosum.

3. MRI with enhancement could not differentiate radiation-induced necrosis or viable tumor. The increased FDG uptake indicates that this is active malignancy. Radiation necrosis has reduced uptake on PET.

4. Infection, inflammation, seizure focus, surgically resected area causing asymmetry on the contralateral side, infiltration of the necrotic area by macrophages, which take up FDG.

References

Dresel S: *PET in Oncology*. Berlin: Springer, 2007, pp 33–37.

Floeth FW, Pauleit D, Sabel M, et al: 18F-FDG PET differentiation of ring-enhancing brain lesions, *J Nucl Med* 47:776–782, 2006.

Glantz MJ, Hoffman JM, Coleman RE, et al: Identification of early recurrence of primary central nervous system tumors by (18F) fluorodeoxyglucose positron emission tomography, *Ann Neurol* 29:347–355, 1991.

Cross-Reference

Nuclear Medicine: THE REQUISITES, 3rd ed, pp 438–440.

Comment

FDG-PET brain imaging is less sensitive than CT or MRI for initial detection of primary or metastatic tumors of the brain because of the high normal brain FDG uptake. However, it is very useful for differentiating postradiation necrosis from recurrent malignancy. Uptake outside normal cortex is always abnormal. Increased uptake within cortex is abnormal. FDG-PET is a better predictor of outcome than surgical brain biopsy and superior to intravenous contrast-enhanced CT in these cases.

There is a strong correlation between the tumor grade and the degree of FDG uptake in gliomas. High-grade tumors have very high FDG uptake, whereas low-grade gliomas tend to have low or no uptake. Thus, low-grade gliomas may not be detected on PET.

FDG-PET scans should not be performed within 3 months of major surgery or radiation therapy. Inflammatory uptake may mask focal tumor uptake. Potential causes of false-negative findings on FDG-PET brain imaging include small size, non–FDG-avid tumor type, and steroid administration, which can cause globally decreased cerebral glucose metabolism.

Notes

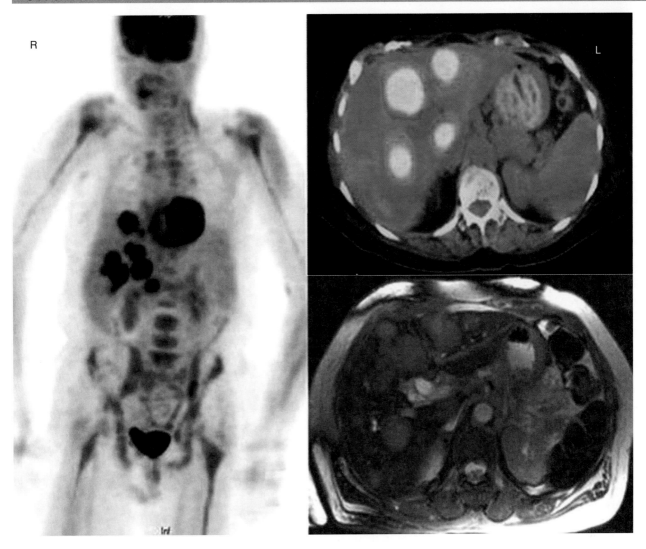

A 50-year-old man with right upper quadrant pain. *Left,* MIP; *upper right,* PET/CT; *lower right,* MRI.

1. Describe the abnormal findings on the FDG-PET/CT and the correlative abdominal MRI slice.

2. What is the differential diagnosis for the abnormal uptake in the liver?

3. How useful is FDG-PET in detecting primary hepatocellular carcinoma (HCC)?

4. What are the most common primary tumors metastatic to the liver?

FDG-PET/CT: Liver Metastases

1. Multiple lesions are seen in the liver on MRI that demonstrate abnormally increased FDG uptake on PET.

2. Both primary and metastatic liver carcinoma can present as multifocal disease. This patient has multifocal HCC.

3. FDG uptake in HCC is variable and often low, probably related to the level of hexokinase and glucose-6-phosphatase in hepatocytes (phosphorylation/dephosphorylation ratio). FDG-PET uptake is seen in 50% to 70% of HCCs.

4. Colon/rectum, pancreas, stomach, breast, and lung.

References

Cantwell CP, Setty BN, Holalkere N, et al: Liver lesion detection and characterization in patients with colorectal cancer: a comparison of low radiation dose non-enhanced PET/CT, contrast-enhanced PET/CT, and liver MRI, *J Comput Assist Tomogr* 32:738–744, 2008.

D'Souza MM, Sharma R, Mondal A, et al: Prospective evaluation of CECT and 18F-FDG-PET/CT in detection of hepatic metastases, *Nucl Med Commun* 30:117–125, 2009.

Cross-Reference

Nuclear Medicine: THE REQUISITES, 3rd ed, pp 331–332.

Comment

The most common cause of malignant liver lesions in the Western world is metastasis, 20-fold more common than a primary hepatic malignancy. Metastatic disease to the liver most commonly originates from colorectal cancer. Both liver lobes are involved in 77%; solitary metastases occur in 10%. HCC is the most common primary liver cancer worldwide and is often associated with chronic hepatitis B or C infection.

Data are mixed regarding the relative accuracy for detection of liver metastases by FDG-PET compared with contrast-enhanced CT or MRI. All have high accuracy. FDG-PET has the added advantage of whole-body imaging. Nearly all metastatic malignant tumors to the liver, cholangiocarcinomas, and gallbladder cancers are FDG avid. Approximately one third to one half of hepatocellular carcinomas do not accumulate FDG. Although FDG-PET may be useful in the diagnosis and management of small cholangiocarcinomas in patients with primary sclerosing cholangitis, FDG-PET has a high false-negative rate for infiltrating cholangiocarcinoma and for the detection of low-volume peritoneal carcinomatosis. Inflammation along biliary stents can reduce specificity for FDG-PET for residual or recurrent carcinoma.

FDG-PET/CT imaging is superior to contrast-enhanced CT in both sensitivity and specificity for detecting metastatic disease in the liver regardless of the primary tumor type, despite the fact that lesions less than 1 cm in the liver are sometimes difficult to detect on PET. The combination of contrast-enhanced CT and FDG-PET provides the highest diagnostic accuracy. In contrast, other studies have compared MRI with contrast- and non–contrast-enhanced PET/CT and found that MRI was superior for detecting and characterizing liver lesions in patients with metastatic colorectal cancer.

Notes

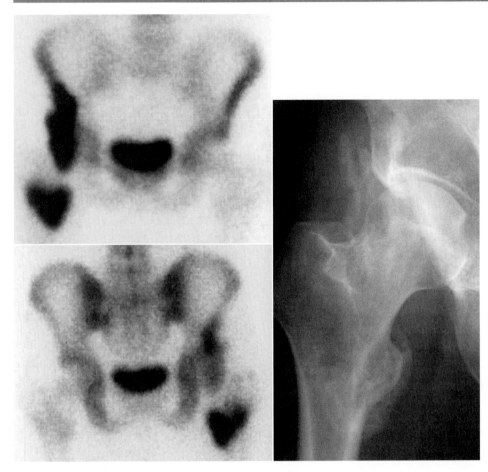

The bone scan image and radiograph of a paraplegic patient are shown.

1. Describe the bone scan findings.

2. Provide a bone scan differential diagnosis.

3. What interventions could be performed if artifact is suspected?

4. Radiograph of the right hip obtained after the bone scan. What is the most likely diagnosis?

Skeletal System: Heterotopic Ossification

1. Intense uptake is seen overlying the right acetabulum with a separate area of uptake overlying the proximal right femur. Radiotracer is seen in the urinary bladder.

2. Urinary contamination, fracture with exuberant callus, heterotopic ossification or myositis ossificans, soft-tissue injury (contusion).

3. If urinary contamination is suspected, remove clothing and overlying bedsheets; wash the patient's skin in the area of suspected contamination.

4. Heterotopic ossification.

Reference

Shehab D, Elgazzar AH, Collier BD: Heterotopic ossification, *J Nucl Med* 43:346–353, 2002.

Cross-Reference

Nuclear Medicine: THE REQUISITES, 3rd ed, pp 142, 149.

Comment

The terms *heterotopic ossification of myositis ossificans* and *heterotopic bone formation* frequently are used interchangeably. Some restrict the term *myositis ossificans* to cases in which new bone arises as a result of inflammation of muscle and reserve *heterotopic ossification* or *heterotopic new bone formation in soft tissue* in the absence of well-defined cause. The proposed mechanism is that primitive mesenchymal cells differentiate into osteoblasts that deposit matrix that ossifies. The radiographic appearance in this patient is typical. The lesion frequently is seen adjacent to the cortex of a long bone or flat bone. It shows dense, well-organized bone at the periphery with less organized bone at the center. A well-defined separation of the lesion from the cortex of the adjacent bone is present. Alternatively, the condition looks like a veil-like lesion that is less well delineated. Biopsy of myositis ossificans/heterotopic ossification early after onset can lead to histologic confusion with sarcoma. Appropriate correlation with the radiographic appearance is critical to avoid unnecessary biopsy or further intervention if biopsy is inadvertently performed.

Notes

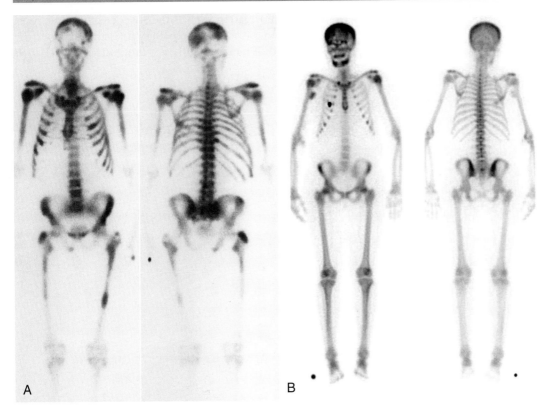

A   B

Two patients referred for a whole-body bone scan.

1. Describe the bone findings.

2. Name two other nonosseous systems that should be evaluated on the bone scan.

3. Describe any other findings.

4. What descriptive term could be applied to this case?

Skeletal System: Superscans

1. A, Increased radiotracer uptake is seen in the large majority of the visualized bones, with nonuniform involvement particularly evident in both femurs, both humeri, and skull. B, Homogeneous, normal-appearing uptake throughout the skeleton, except for increased uptake in the skull and mandible.

2. Soft tissues and genitourinary tract.

3. The kidneys are not visualized in either patient. Faint activity is seen in the urinary bladder in patient A, none in patient B. Little soft-tissue activity is seen for either patient.

4. Superscan.

Reference

Buckley O, O'Keeffe S, Geoghegan T, et al: 99mTc bone scintigraphy superscans: a review, *Nucl Med Commun* 28:521–527, 2007.

Cross-Reference

Nuclear Medicine: THE REQUISITES, 3rd ed, pp 123, 126.

Comment

The term *superscan* refers to a bone scan pattern with increased radiopharmaceutical uptake relative to soft-tissue background. Soft tissue, kidneys, and bladder usually have no or minimal visualization. The superscan can occur in any diffuse skeletal disorder in which tracer uptake is markedly increased in the skeleton. Thus, less radiotracer is available for renal excretion, resulting in faint or no visualization of the kidneys. Optimization of imaging parameters for the skeletal activity level contributes to the apparent nonvisualization of renal activity.

Widespread metastatic disease is the most frequent cause of a superscan. The primary tumors responsible include carcinomas of the breast, lung, and prostate, although it may occur with lymphoma and bladder cancer. Superscan occurs in late-stage metastatic disease of bone with diffuse involvement. Patient A had prostate cancer. Usually some inhomogeneity or hot spots in the pattern suggest tumor as the cause. A single radiograph of an involved bone such as the pelvis or femur usually provides easy confirmation of metastatic involvement. The other major causes of a superscan are metabolic bone diseases (e.g., renal osteodystrophy, osteomalacia, and severe hyperparathyroidism). Patient B had tertiary hyperparathyroidism with renal failure. Myelofibrosis and systemic mastocytosis can result in a similar pattern. These causes usually have more uniform uptake throughout the bones. In this case, additional clinical information such as the absence of chronic renal failure and primary hyperparathyroidism increases the likelihood of metastatic disease as the diagnosis.

Notes

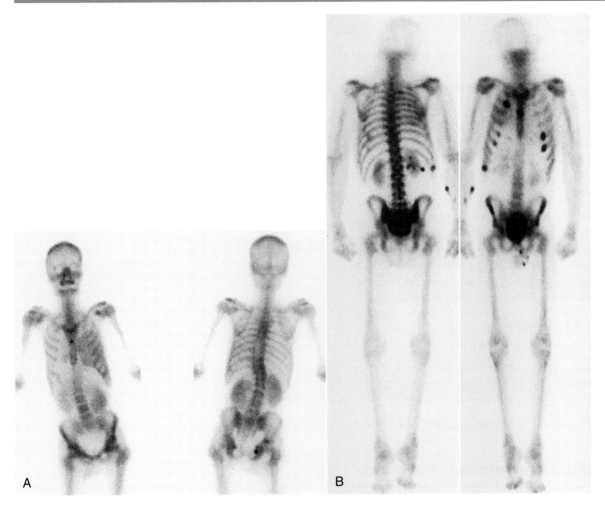

A, A 43-year-old patient with a history of left-sided empyema. B, A 56-year-old man had a recent seizure and fall.

1. Describe the skeletal abnormalities in both studies.

2. Describe soft-tissue abnormalities.

3. What is the differential diagnosis the soft-tissue and bone uptake?

4. Name primary and metastatic tumors that have increased bone tracer uptake.

Skeletal System: Pleural and Lung Mass with ^{99m}Tc-MDP Uptake

1. A, Scoliosis, apparent increased uptake in ribs of left chest. Mild arthritic changes in both hips. B, Focal abnormal uptake in the right and left anterior ribs, right upper posterior rib, and sternum.

2. A, Abnormal soft-tissue uptake in the anterior left hemithorax; B, Abnormal diffuse radiotracer uptake in the right upper chest on the anterior and posterior views, which does not conform to normal bone configuration.

3. Starting on the inside working outward: in lung parenchyma, in a primary or secondary lung tumor, in the pleura or pleural effusion, in the soft tissue of the chest wall. Differential diagnosis includes lung cancer, pleural calcification, fibrothorax, post-radiation inflammation/calcification. Bone scan abnormalities (B) are likely traumatic because of the distribution and history of a fall. The diagnoses in these cases were fibrothorax (A) and lung cancer (B).

4. Osteosarcoma, lung, breast, prostate, and colon cancer. Renal cell, thyroid, and myeloma often do not have bone uptake because of their primary lytic properties.

References

Gray HW, Krasnow AZ: Soft tissue uptake of bone agents. In: Collier DB Jr, Fogelman I, Rosenthall L (eds): *Skeletal Nuclear Medicine.* St. Louis: Mosby, 1996, p 383.

Peller PJ, Ho VB, Kransdorf MJ: Extraosseous Tc-99m MDP uptake: a pathophysiologic approach, *Radiographics* 13:715–734, 1993.

Cross-Reference

Nuclear Medicine: THE REQUISITES, 3rd ed, pp 119–126.

Comment

Bone scintigraphy may demonstrate abnormal soft-tissue uptake in a wide variety of nonosseous disorders, including neoplastic, hormonal, inflammatory, ischemic, traumatic, excretory, and artifactual entities. Thoracic uptake on bone scans often is seen in patients with lung cancer. However, in contrast to study B, which was lung cancer, it is more commonly the result of pleural involvement and malignant pleural effusion. The distribution characteristically extends to the diaphragmatic costal margin, particularly if the patient is standing or sitting up. On the other hand, benign effusions typically cause attenuation and thus decreased uptake is seen on that side.

The curvilinear inferior margin in study A follows the contour of the diaphragm, suggesting that the uptake relates to pleura. The finding is evident on the anterior view only, indicating that it is located anteriorly; therefore, pleural effusion is unlikely unless it is loculated anteriorly. Previous radiation is unlikely to involve the anterior and spare posterior structures or have a rounded superior margin, as in this case. Similarly, uptake in a soft-tissue mass within the thorax or arising from the chest wall is unlikely to have an inferior margin that parallels the diaphragm. This patient had a history of left-sided empyema and subsequently a fibrothorax developed.

In general, the most common reason for unilateral uptake in soft tissues within the thorax is malignant pleural effusion. If the effusion is free flowing, the scintigraphic pattern can change with changes in patient position, as it does when radiographs are taken with the patient erect and supine or in the decubitus position.

Notes

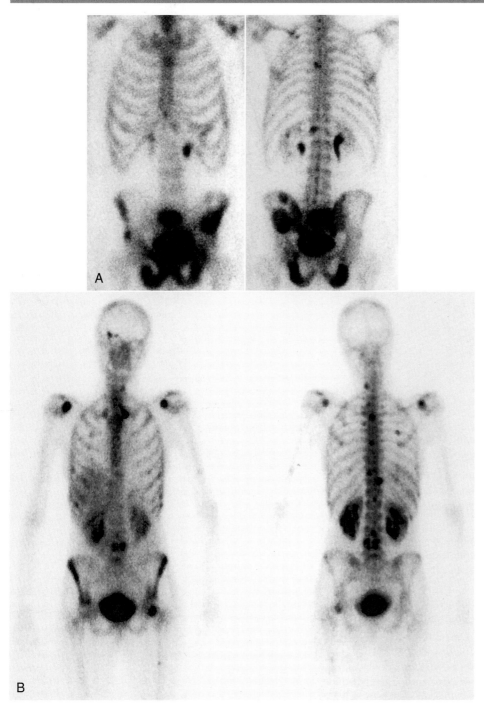

Two elderly nonsmoking male patients (A and B) have low back pain.

1. Provide a distribution for the bone abnormalities in both patients.

2. Describe the findings.

3. List three factors that help limit the differential diagnosis.

4. List the three most common etiologies. What is the most likely diagnosis?

Skeletal System: Prostate Cancer Bone Metastases, Axial Distribution

1. Spine and pelvis.

2. A, Abnormal focal and regional uptake in multiple sites in the sacrum, both ilia, both inferior pubic rami, right superior pubic ramus, mid-thoracic and lower thoracic spine. B, Abnormal focal uptake in the skull, scapulae, ribs, spine, pelvis, and left femur. Diffuse uptake in the liver.

3. Multiple lesions, axial predominance, older adult man, nonsmoker.

4. Breast, colon, lung cancers. Most likely are skeletal metastases from prostate cancer.

Reference

Hricak H, Choyke PL, Eberhardt SC, et al: Imaging prostate cancer: a multidisciplinary perspective, *Radiology* 243:28-53, 2007.

Cross-Reference

Nuclear Medicine: THE REQUISITES, 3rd ed, pp 120–125.

Comment

The bone radiotracer must be delivered to the bone surface for uptake to occur. The amount of uptake depends somewhat on the amount of blood flow. The greater the flow is, the higher the uptake. ^{99m}Tc-phosphonates become adsorbed to the hydroxyapatite matrix. The radiopharmaceutical localizes in the mineral phase of bone at active sites of bone formation (remodeling), particularly at the osteoid mineral interfaces, and is incorporated into the crystalline structure. The binding sites for the bone agent can be saturated by diphosphonates.

The polyostotic distribution of multiple focal abnormalities strongly suggests skeletal metastases. To ascribe all the findings to one disease entity, the liver abnormality should be considered as an additional site of involvement. In addition, the long list of tumors that metastasize to bone and liver can be shortened by considering only those whose soft-tissue metastases are likely to show uptake of bone radiotracer. Many of these are adenocarcinomas. Therefore, the shortened differential diagnosis list includes common malignancies such as breast, colon, and lung and the less common malignancies such as ovarian and adenocarcinomas arising from other gastrointestinal organs (e.g., pancreas, gastric).

General agreement exists that the vertebral venous plexus is an important factor in the predilection of bone metastases to the axial skeleton. Tumor cells originating below the diaphragm can move through the vertebral venous plexus to the pelvis, abdomen, and chest while bypassing the inferior vena cava. Interconnections between the Batson plexus and the intercostal veins provide a route of spread to ribs. Retrograde flow through the valveless plexus can occur from increased pressure resulting from coughing or straining. In this case, radiographs of the pelvis revealed multiple sclerotic lesions, and prostate biopsy confirmed the diagnosis.

Notes

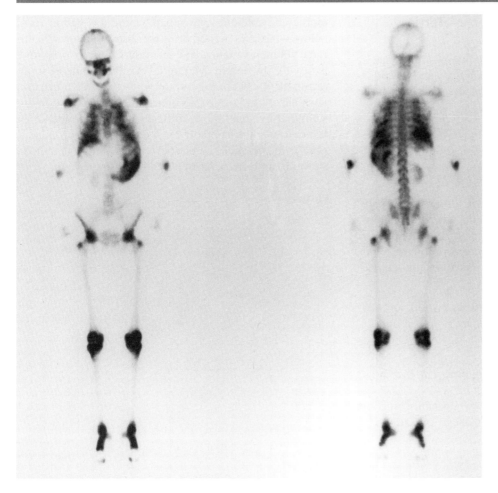

A 53-year-old woman with hypercalcemia was referred for possible metastatic bone disease.

1. Describe the bone scan findings.

2. Provide a differential diagnosis.

3. What is the most likely diagnosis?

4. Could this pattern be caused by free ^{99m}Tc-pertechnetate? Why or why not?

Skeletal System: Hypercalcemia—Tertiary Hyperparathyroidism

1. Abnormal diffuse uptake in the lungs and stomach. Poor visualization of small kidneys and bladder, increased uptake in the shoulders, elbows, hips, knees, and ankles.

2. Metastatic calcification caused by hypercalcemia, renal failure, metabolic bone disease, severe hyperparathyroidism.

3. This particular pattern of metastatic calcification is characteristic of long-standing or tertiary hyperparathyroidism, usually seen in patients with renal failure. Although other causes of metabolic bone disease (e.g., osteomalacia, renal osteodystrophy) result in abnormal bone scans, they do not have this characteristic soft-tissue pattern.

4. Free ^{99m}Tc-pertechnetate has gastric, thyroid, and salivary gland uptake. The last two are not seen here.

References

Ryan PJ, Fogelman I: Bone scintigraphy in metabolic bone disease, *Semin Nucl Med* 27:291–305, 1997.

Siegel BA (ed): *Nuclear Radiology* (syllabus, second series). Reston, VA: American College of Radiology, 1978, pp 410–424.

Cross-Reference

Nuclear Medicine: THE REQUISITES, 3rd ed, pp 131–132, 143.

Comment

The mechanism of altered bone radiotracer uptake in hyperparathyroidism is related to the increase in bone resorption and secondary increased bone turnover, causing increased osteoblastic activity in the skeleton with less radiotracer available for renal excretion. The bone scan in primary hyperparathyroidism usually appears normal or may have subtle abnormalities of diffusely increased bone uptake detectable only by quantitative techniques. When present, bone scan abnormalities usually correspond to areas with radiographic demineralization or erosion (e.g., in the calvaria, mandible, acromioclavicular areas, sternum, lateral humeral epicondyles, and hands). If brown tumors are present, they are seen as focal hot spots.

As the disease advances, extraskeletal mineralization of soft tissues can occur in the cornea, cartilage, joint capsules, tendons, and periarticular regions. Bone scans in patients with severe, long-standing or severe hyperparathyroidism may have soft-tissue uptake, characteristically in the lungs, stomach, and often kidneys as a result of metastatic calcification. These patients often have increased calcium phosphate products and renal failure—tertiary hyperparathyroidism. Patients with renal failure invariably have secondary hyperparathyroidism with low serum calcium levels. When one or more of the glands becomes autonomous, the serum calcium normalizes and then becomes elevated. In addition, scintigraphy may show diffusely increased uptake in bone, low soft-tissue and renal activity, and prominent uptake in the skull, acromioclavicular joints, mandible, sternum, and the periarticular areas of large joints.

Notes

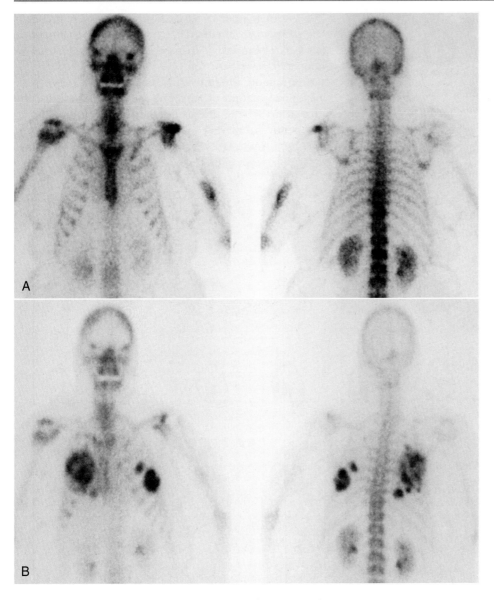

An initial bone scan (A) and repeat study 2 years later (B).

1. Describe the bone scan abnormalities on the initial study (A).

2. Describe the skeletal abnormalities on the follow-up study (B).

3. List the differential diagnoses.

4. Provide the most likely diagnosis.

CASE 74

Skeletal System: Osteosarcoma Metastatic to the Lung

1. A, Abnormal decreased and increased uptake in the left humerus (proximal and mid, respectively).

2. B, Irregular uptake in a similar pattern in the chest anterior and posterior views indicates a location likely midway between in the lung parenchyma. Uptake is nodular and masslike. Rib abnormalities cannot be excluded, but the pathological condition extends across the rib spaces. Left shoulder arthroplasty is shown by photopenia.

3. The differential diagnosis for abnormal lung activity in a focal pattern includes primary lung tumors and metastases, especially for tumors with calcific or ossific components. For abnormal lung activity in a regional pattern, not evident in this case, the differential diagnosis includes malignant pleural effusion, fibrothorax, and radiation therapy–induced pneumonitis.

4. Osteosarcoma of the left proximal humerus, status post-arthroplasty, with lung metastases.

References

Divisi D, Gizzonio D, Crisci R: Multimodal treatment of osteosarcoma of lung metastases, *Thorac Cardiovasc Surg* 54:328–331, 2006.

Manaster BJ, May DA, Disler DG: *Musculoskeletal Imaging*, 3rd ed. St. Louis: Mosby, 2007, pp 429–441.

Cross-Reference

Nuclear Medicine: THE REQUISITES, 3rd ed, pp 127–128.

Comment

Distant metastases are found at initial staging of osteosarcoma in only 2% of patients. Osseous metastases occur at a rate of 1% per month between 5 and 29 months after diagnosis with a decrease in the rate thereafter. Before the advent of adjuvant chemotherapy, bone metastases usually were detected before pulmonary metastases. However, the natural course of the disease has been altered; bone metastases now appear before pulmonary metastases in only 15% of cases. Metastases to other sites, including the liver, kidney, and lymph nodes, occasionally are demonstrated by skeletal scintigraphy.

The primary tumor and metastases avidly produce osteoid that results in bone tracer uptake. Although bone scintigraphy often can demonstrate lung metastases, both planar imaging and SPECT are less sensitive than CT for the detection of lung metastases in osteosarcoma.

The increasing use of surgical resections of lung metastases, especially in children, has contributed to improved survival. The most widely used excisional procedures for lung metastases are for osteosarcoma. The surgery is rather unique: the individual metastasis is excised with a minimal margin of surrounding lung tissue with the goal of preserving the maximum amount of lung tissue. One study comparing sensitivity/specificity for diagnosing lung metastases found 86%/66% with CT and 80%/100% with SPECT.

Notes

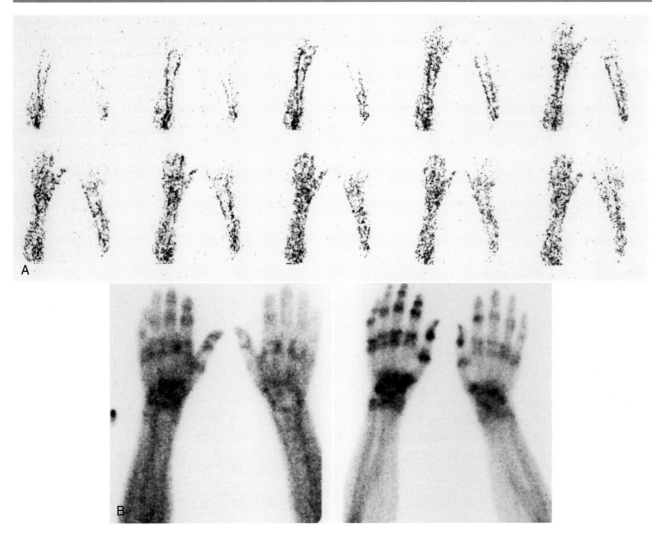

A

B

Right hand pain began 3 months after thoracotomy. Hand radiographs are normal.

1. Describe the scintigraphic bone scan findings in this case (A, flow; B *left,* blood pool; B *right,* 3-hour delayed images; palms are down on the camera).

2. Provide the differential diagnosis.

3. What is the most likely diagnosis in this case?

4. What is the pathogenesis of this pathophysiologic process?

C A S E 7 5

Skeletal System: Complex Regional Pain Syndrome

1. Three-phase study demonstrates abnormal increased blood flow and blood pool to most of the right upper extremity. Delayed image shows increased uptake in the bones with a striking increase in periarticular activity causing the joints to stand out.

2. Complex regional pain syndrome (formerly referred to as reflex sympathetic dystrophy), shoulder-hand syndrome, or multiple-joint synovitis.

3. Shoulder-hand syndrome, a frequently encountered form of complex regional pain syndrome.

4. Neurogenic origin with loss of sympathetic autonomic tone is the generally accepted explanation, although not firmly established. This often occurs after recent loss of use of a limb, for example, stroke or immobilization by orthopedic cast or splint. Sometimes there is a history of trauma.

References
Intenzo CM, Kim SM, Capuzzi DM: The role of nuclear medicine in the evaluation of complex regional pain syndrome type I, *Clin Nucl Med* 30:400–407, 2005.

Manaster BJ, May DA, Disler DG: *Musculoskeletal Imaging: THE REQUISITES*. St. Louis: Mosby, 2007, pp 394–396.

Cross-Reference
Nuclear Medicine: THE REQUISITES, 3rd ed, pp 137–138.

Comment
Other causes of increased periarticular uptake include inflammatory osteoarthritis (e.g., rheumatoid, early post-arthroplasty changes, prosthesis complicated by infection or loosening). However, these entities generally do not involve the entire limb, so they would be inappropriate considerations in this case. Also referred to as Sudeck's atrophy or causalgia, reflex sympathetic dystrophy syndrome is an entity that includes pain, swelling, osteoporosis, and late atrophy of the limb. The cause is thought to be neurogenic, and often it is associated with trauma, surgery, or illness.

Radiographs may demonstrate soft-tissue swelling and osteoporosis. Bone scintigraphy often demonstrates abnormalities before clinical or radiographic findings. Classically, the entire distal extremity demonstrates scintigraphic abnormalities. The typical pattern of complex regional pain syndrome is increased perfusion, blood pool, and uptake on delayed images in the affected extremity. Typically, prominent and characteristic diffuse periarticular uptake is present. All were seen in this case. The perfusion and blood pool phases are not always as reliable as the delayed images. Increased flow and blood pool is seen in approximately 50% of patients with reflex sympathetic dystrophy syndrome, whereas more than 95% are abnormal on delayed images.

Notes

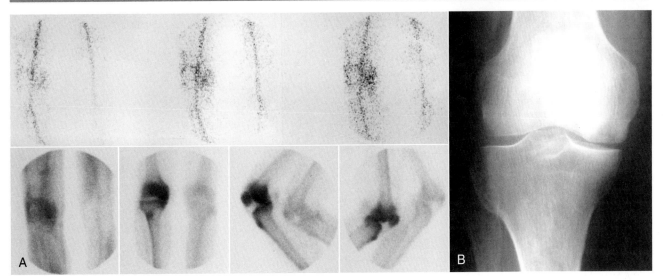

An elderly patient has had right knee pain for 3 months.

1. Describe the bone scan findings. A *top,* flow; A *bottom,* blood pool and delayed images.

2. Based on the scan findings, provide a differential diagnosis.

3. A radiograph then was obtained (B). Given all available information, what is the most likely diagnosis?

4. What are common causes of this condition in the femoral head?

Skeletal System: Spontaneous Osteonecrosis of the Femur

1. Increased flow, blood pool, and uptake in the right medial femoral condyle.

2. Osteonecrosis, fracture, osteoarthritis, primary bone neoplasm (unlikely with previous normal radiograph).

3. Spontaneous osteonecrosis of the medial femoral condyle.

4. Trauma, steroid therapy, vasculitis, infarction (sickle cell, Gaucher's disease), alcoholism, Caisson disease.

Reference

Manaster BJ, May DA, Disler DG: *Musculoskeletal Imaging: THE REQUISITES*. St. Louis: Mosby, 1996, pp 347–354.

Cross-Reference

Nuclear Medicine: THE REQUISITES, 3rd ed, pp 143–150.

Comment

Juxta-articular lesions that are three-phase positive on scintigraphy and result in subchondral sclerosis and deformity of the articular contour on radiographs include osteonecrosis and osteochondritis desiccans. Most bones have a dual blood supply that includes a network of periosteal vessels and one or more nutrient arteries that supply the marrow, the trabecular bone, and an endosteal portion of the cortex. Bones that lack the periosteal supply because they are covered with articular cartilage or enclosed within the joint capsule are more vulnerable to ischemic insults and osteonecrosis (also called avascular necrosis). Osteonecrosis can be idiopathic or result from an underlying cause. This patient demonstrates idiopathic osteonecrosis, a spontaneous disorder of the knee that occurs with sudden onset in older patients. It usually involves the medial femoral condyle. Bone scan abnormalities may precede the development of radiographic abnormalities. Osteonecrosis resulting from an underlying cause such as steroid use can create a similar pattern, but it usually involves multiple sites, including the medial and lateral femoral condyles, humeral and femoral heads, and talus. Osteochondritis dessicans is a condition that occurs in children and adults; it usually involves the lateral surface of medial femoral condyle, although it may involve other bones, including the talus and capitellum.

Notes

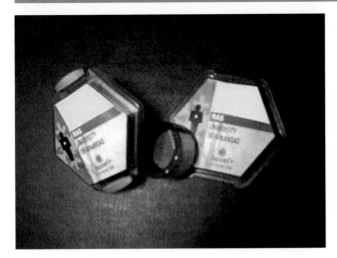

1. Describe how film badge and thermoluminescent ring detect radiation exposure.

2. What are the Nuclear Regulatory Commission (NRC) occupational annual dose limits for adults and minors?

3. What is the radiation dose limit to pregnant women?

4. What does ALARA mean?

Radiation Safety: Radiation Personal Protection Detectors—Film Badge, Ring, Dosimeter

1. The film badge detects radiation with a radiosensitive film inside a plastic holder. The amount of x-ray film blackening is used to determine the radiation dose. The thermoluminescent ring consists of a small crystal that absorbs energy from gamma or high-energy beta emitters and gives off light when heated that can be measured to estimate radiation exposure.

2. Adult occupational workers are limited to a total effective dose equivalent of 5 rem (50 mSv) per year. For minors, the annual occupational dose limit is 10% of the adult limit (NRC 10 CFR Part 20).

3. Once pregnancy is established, the radiation dose limit for the entire gestation period must be limited to 0.5 rem (5 mSv). The embryo/fetus is most sensitive to ionizing radiation during the first trimester of pregnancy (days 11–56).

4. ALARA stands for "as low as is reasonably achievable."

References

Cherry SR, Sorenson JA, Phelps ME: *Physics in Nuclear Medicine*, 3rd ed. Philadelphia: WB Saunders, 2003, pp 431, 433, 435–436, 439–440.

Siegel JA: *Guide for Diagnostic Nuclear Medicine and Radiopharmaceutical Therapy*. Reston, VA: Society of Nuclear Medicine, 2004.

Cross-Reference

Nuclear Medicine: THE REQUISITES, 3rd ed, pp 16–17.

Comment

The film badge consists of x-ray film placed inside a plastic holder with filters that can differentiate gamma rays, x-rays, high-energy beta particles, but not low-energy beta emitters. If the film inadvertently becomes exposed to light, the results become invalid. When the crystals (lithium fluoride or manganese-activated calcium fluoride) of a thermoluminescent ring are heated, the stored or absorbed energy is released in the form of visible light that can be measured and radiation exposure determined.

To minimize radiation exposure to personnel, it is important to maximize the worker's distance from a radiation source whenever possible. Where r is your distance from a radiation point source, the exposure rate decreases as $1/r^2$. This is known as the "inverse square law" (i.e., radiation intensity is inversely proportional to the square of the distance from the radiation source). For example, at 10 cm, a 5-mCi ^{125}I source has an exposure rate of 75 mR/hr. By moving it to 20 cm, the exposure rate is reduced: $(75 \text{ mR/hr})(10/20)^2 = 18.75$ mR/hr.

The NRC dose limits are legal requirements not to be exceeded. However, there is potential radiation hazard below those limits. ALARA is an NRC requirement for licensees to not simply keep radiation doses within legal limits but to keep them as low as reasonably achievable, taking into account the state of the technology and economics of improvement in relation to benefits to the public health and safety. This is achieved through a good radiation protection plan, education, laboratory practices, and administrative controls.

Notes

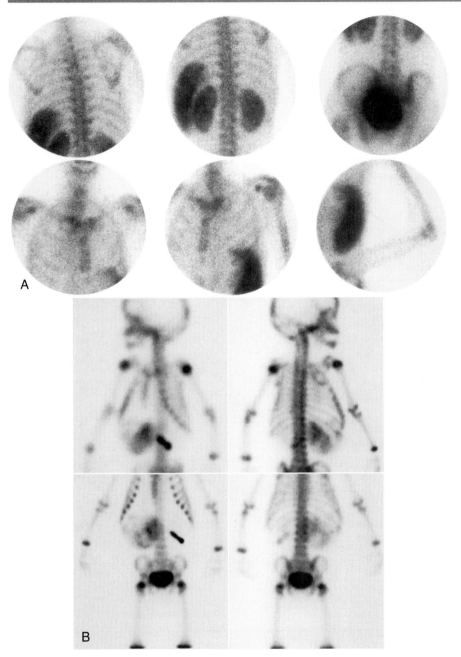

A

B

A, A 20-year-old patient referred for a bone scan. B, A hepatic mass is found on ultrasonography in an 11-month-old child.

1. Describe the scintigraphic findings.

2. What would be the likely cause of abnormal uptake in the two patients?

3. Besides a neoplastic process, what conditions could be associated with the findings in patient B?

4. What is the most likely diagnosis for patient B?

Skeletal System: Bone Scans with Spleen and Hepatoblastoma Uptake

1. A, Uniform intense uptake in a structure that appears to be an enlarged spleen by its location and configuration and increased diffuse uptake in both kidneys; B, Nonuniform abnormal soft-tissue right upper quadrant uptake.

2. A, Blood dyscrasias, including sickle cell disease, sickle thalassemia, thalassemia major; hemosiderosis; extensive subcapsular splenic hematoma. B, Hepatoblastoma, neuroblastoma.

3. Trauma to soft tissue or organs, in this case, the liver, resulting in contusion or hematoma, ischemic injury (although the pattern appears round rather than suggestive of a vascular distribution), chronic abscess.

4. Hepatoblastoma is most likely based on the patient's age and uptake of bone radiotracer in a hepatic mass.

References

Blickman H: *Pediatric Radiology: THE REQUISITES*, 2nd ed. St. Louis: Mosby, 1998, pp 137-138.

Silberstein EB, McAfee JG, Spasoff AP: *Diagnostic Patterns in Nuclear Medicine*. Reston, VA: Society of Nuclear Medicine, 1998, p 228.

Cross-Reference

Nuclear Medicine: THE REQUISITES, 3rd ed, pp 124-125, 142-143.

Comment

A common cause of splenic uptake of bone tracer is sickle cell disease. The spleen is usually shrunken from autoinfarction in a patient who is skeletally mature. In a child, it may not be small. Kidneys may have increased uptake. Bone findings suggesting bone infarcts would support the diagnosis. If multiple fractures or uptake in soft-tissue contusions were noted, splenic trauma would be a possibility. Sickle thalassemia, thalassemia major, and hemosiderosis are the likely diagnoses. This patient (A) had sickle thalassemia.

After the kidney and adrenals, the liver is the third most common site of abdominal malignancies in infants and children. In children younger than 5 years of age, the most likely tumors are hepatoblastoma, mesenchymal hamartoma, and hemangioma. Hepatoblastoma is the most common primary hepatic tumor of childhood; two thirds of cases occur in children younger than 2 years of age. Abdominal radiographs of patients with hepatoblastoma show calcification in up to 50% of cases,

similar to patients with neuroblastoma. This accounts for the deposition of bone radiopharmaceutical. The bone scan is used to diagnose metastases.

Notes

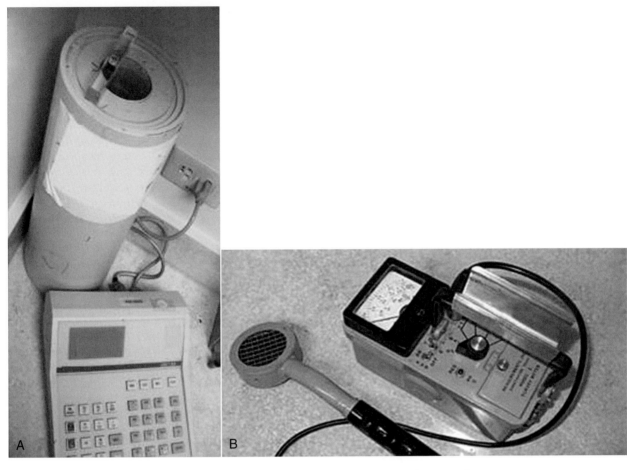

1. What are the instruments pictured and for what purposes are they used?

2. Are the procedures for measuring ^{99m}Tc activity the same as those for measuring ^{111}In for both instruments (A and B)? If not, how are they different?

3. How often should they be recalibrated and undergo routine quality control?

4. What is the function of the switch indicated by the *arrow* in figure B?

Radiation Safety: Radiation Detection Instrumentation—Dose Calibrator, Geiger-Müller (G-M) Counter

1. A, Dose calibrator, a gas-filled ionization chamber used to measure the activity of patient doses before injection. B, G-M counter with "pancake" probe used for detection of contamination and area surveys.

2. Dose calibrator: no. It requires the user to select the radionuclide being counted because different energies and types of radiation produce different amounts of ionization. The same activity from different isotopes produces different amounts of current. G-M counter: yes. The procedure is the same. The G-M counter cannot differentiate between different energies and isotopes.

3. Dose calibrator: constancy check daily, accuracy and linearity checks quarterly and after service, geometry-dependent response at installation and after service. G-M counter: battery check daily, check of background counting rate, constancy check daily, calibration at installation, annually, and after service.

4. This switch changes the multiplier (e.g., ×0.1, ×10, ×100) and, thereby, allows a wide range of counts.

References

Range NT: The AAPM/RSNA physics tutorial for residents: radiation detectors in nuclear medicine, *Radiographics* 19:481–502, 1999.

Zanzonico P: Routine quality control of clinical nuclear medicine instrumentation: a brief review, *J Nucl Med* 49:1114–1131, 2008.

Cross-Reference

Nuclear Medicine: THE REQUISITES, 3rd ed, pp 17–18, 35.

Comment

The National Institute of Standards and Technology provides certified, long-lived isotopes to use for accuracy checks of nuclear medicine equipment. Dose calibrator accuracy should be measured using more than one (at least two) different long-lived isotopes, such as cobalt-57 ($t_{1/2}$ = 271 days) and cesium-137 ($t_{1/2}$ = 30 years), and should not vary from the certified value by more than 10%. ^{137}Cs is used for the calibration of G-M counters.

G-M counters operate in the Geiger region in which the higher voltages result in the production of an avalanche of interactions such that the measured current is identical regardless of the number of ion pairs produced by the incident radiation. Ionization chambers (dose calibrator) operate in the saturation region in which the measured current depends on the primary ion pairs generated by the incident ionizing radiation and individual events are not being detected; α, β, and γ radiation produces different ionizations and therefore different amounts of current. G-M counters are more sensitive than dose calibrators. The gain switch on the G-M counter allows adjusting the current multiplying factor. The actual number of counts detected by the G-M counter will be the dial value times the multiplier, for example, if the dial needle is resting on 2.5 K with the multiplier set to ×10, the actual counts will be 2500 cpm × 10, which equals 25,000 cpm. Conversely, if the needle rests on 2.5 K with the multiplier set to ×0.1, the actual number of detected counts is 2500 cpm × 0.1, which equals 250 cpm.

Notes

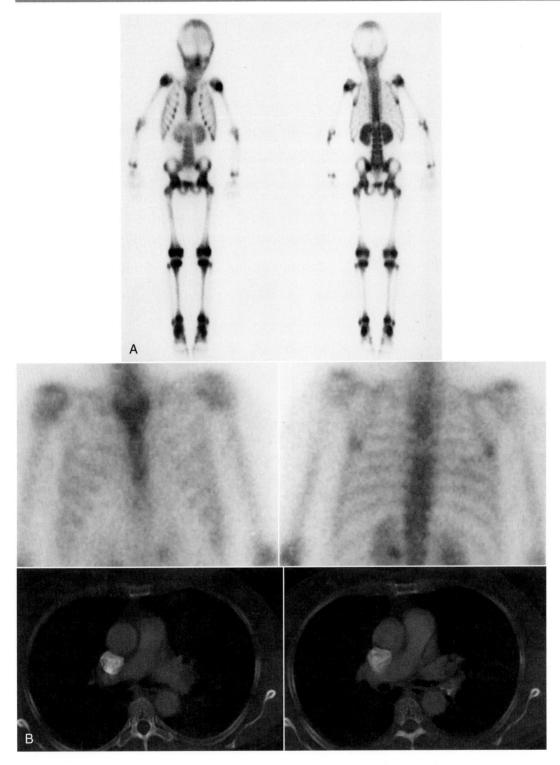

Two patients are shown. A, A 10-year-old boy referred for back pain. B, A 60-year-old man with recently diagnosed lung cancer. Bone scans and CT scan are provided.

1. Describe the bone scan findings in both patients.

2. Give a differential diagnosis for these abnormalities.

3. Describe the extraosseous soft-tissue abnormality in patient B.

4. What are the two most likely causes of the soft-tissue abnormality?

Skeletal System: Bone Scan Cold Spine Defects

1. A, Cold defect at T11. B, Decreased activity at approximately T6.

2. Benign or malignant tumor, osteomyelitis, avascular necrosis, congenital or surgical defect, artifact, radiation therapy.

3. Intense renal cortical uptake (cortical staining).

4. Nephrotoxic antibiotics or chemotherapeutic agents associated with interstitial nephritis.

Reference

Sopov V, Liberson A, Gorenberg M, et al: Cold vertebrae on bone scintigraphy, *Semin Nucl Med* 31:82-83, 2001.

Cross-Reference

Nuclear Medicine: THE REQUISITES, 3rd ed, p 124.

Comment

Patient A had leukemia, the cause of the cold defect in this case. Patient B had a hemangioma. Common causes of a cold defect on a bone scan are avascular necrosis (e.g., post-traumatic, sickle cell disease), but also radiation therapy–induced fibrosis, malignant tumors, particularly osteoclastic or lytic lesions (e.g., multiple myeloma, renal cell and thyroid cancer). Osteomyelitis may appear as a cold defect, particularly in children. Chordoma, plasmocytoma, and previous orthopedic surgery are other causes of cold defects. Attenuation cold artifacts may be caused by jewelry, belt buckles, clothing snaps, coins, or barium in the gastrointestinal tract.

Renal cortical uptake is not an uncommon finding on bone scans, particularly in patients receiving nephrotoxic chemotherapy or metastatic calcification. High-grade bilateral renal obstruction may show this renal pattern. In that case, no activity would be seen in the bladder and background would be high. Patients with sickle cell anemia may have increased cortical uptake as a result of microcalcifications due to sluggish flow.

The CT shows an intact vertebral body with prominent trabeculae, widely spaced and sclerotic without a soft-tissue component. Hemangiomas often cause no symptoms and usually represent an incidental finding. On bone scans, they display the full spectrum of uptake, are most commonly isointense, and are unrecognized; however, they may be photopenic (as in patient B) or even have increased uptake. Intraosseous hemangiomas are most commonly found in the spine (75%) but also occur in skull and facial bones.

Notes

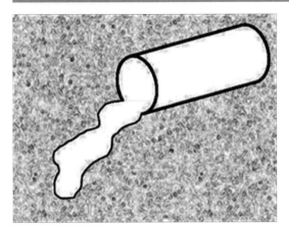

1. What are the three important steps to follow after a radioactive spill?

2. With what substance should a floor surface or countertop be cleaned when contaminated with a radio-active material?

3. What is a minor spill? What is a major spill?

4. What should be done if clothing is contaminated?

Radiation Safety: Radioactive Spills

1. Inform personnel in the area of the spill and the radiation safety officer. Contain the spill, usually with absorbent paper towels. Decontaminate.

2. Soap and water. Wear gloves, disposable lab coat, and booties.

3. Most diagnostic dose spills in nuclear medicine are minor. Minor means that it involves a small restricted area with activity and exposure limited. Major spills involve either a large area or escape from a restricted area, pose an external or internal hazard, and are airborne (>5 mrad/hr at 1 m).

4. Remove the article of clothing and place it in a plastic bag. Rinse contaminated body area with lukewarm water and wash with soap.

References

Cherry SR, Sorenson JA, Phelps ME: *Physics in Nuclear Medicine*, 3rd ed. Philadelphia: WB Saunders, 2003, pp 431, 433, 435–436, 439–440.

Lombardi MH: *Radiation Safety in Nuclear Medicine*. Boca Raton, FL: CRC Press, 2006, p 58.

Siegel JA: *Guide for Diagnostic Nuclear Medicine and Radiopharmaceutical Therapy*. Reston, VA: Society of Nuclear Medicine, 2004, pp 40–41.

Cross-Reference

Nuclear Medicine: THE REQUISITES, 3rd ed, pp 16–17.

Comment

When there is a radioactive spill, first inform those in the immediate work area, then inform those outside this area and the radiation safety officer. To contain the spilled radioactivity, use absorbent pads; wear gloves, a lab coat, eye protection, and booties; close doors; segregate contaminated individuals; and use a low-range radiation detector survey meter to monitor the contamination of the area and individuals. Decontaminate personnel first, then the work area. Place the contaminated materials in a plastic bag and into a radioactive waste container.

Major and minor radioactive spills are essentially handled in the same manner with exceptions for a major spill. Clear the area of persons not involved in the spill, vacate the area, close the room and secure the area, and try to shield the source if possible. Spills should be reviewed by the department and institution to determine whether corrective actions are necessary (e.g., modification of operating procedures, additional radiation safety instruction).

Notes

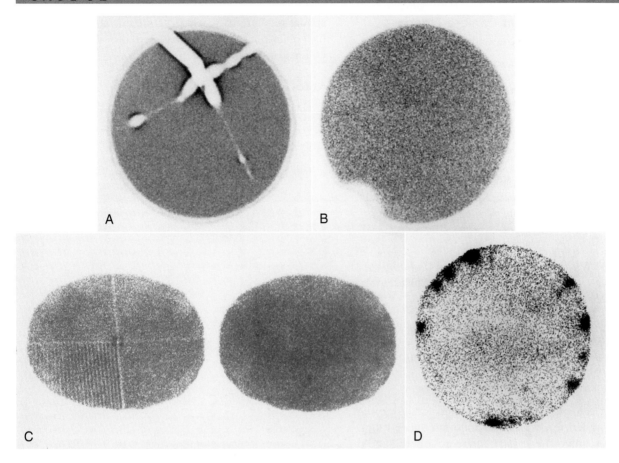

Provide the probable cause and give your recommendations for the abnormal gamma camera quality-control floods.

1. A.

2. B.

3. C. What is the difference in methodology between the left and right images?

4. D.

C A S E 8 2

Quality Control: Gamma Camera Floods

1. A, Cracked crystal (buy a new crystal).

2. B, Nonfunctioning photomultiplier tube (call service).

3. C, Distorted (not circular) and nonuniform images. *Left,* Lead bars for linearity and resolution placed on top of flood. *Right,* Flood only. Electronic tuning required. The power went off overnight. Call the service representative.

4. D, Contamination of crystal with radiopharmaceutical. (Clean camera or allow radiotracer to decay 10 half-lives.)

Reference

Christian PE, Waterstram-Rich K: *Nuclear Medicine and PET/CT Technology and Techniques*. Philadelphia: Elsevier/Mosby, 2007, pp 88–98.

Cross-Reference

Nuclear Medicine: THE REQUISITES, 3rd ed, pp 44–51.

Comment

The gamma camera consists of a sodium iodide crystal optically coupled to an array of photomultiplier tubes. Gamma rays enter the crystal, undergo photoelectric and Compton interactions, and are absorbed. The gamma camera's response should be uniform across the field. However, the response is inherently nonuniform because of spatial distortions, systematic errors in location determination, variation in light transit efficiency, and so on. Digital microprocessors correct for this inherent nonuniformity. The output of the photomultiplier tubes is thereby adjusted to yield maximum uniformity.

Gamma camera quality-control floods are performed on a daily basis each morning before patient studies. The method used varies. Daily floods are obtained either by placing a ^{99m}Tc source at a standard distance (3–5 feet) from the camera (usually hanging from above) with the collimator off (intrinsic flood). Alternatively, with the collimator on (extrinsic flood), the flood source is placed directly on the camera. ^{57}Co (122 keV; half-life, 270 days) fixed in Plexiglas is often used or, alternatively, ^{99m}Tc is mixed in water and placed in a fillable Plexiglas disk.

The flood image from a well-tuned gamma camera with working photomultiplier tubes and uniformity correction circuitry should have a uniform appearance. The flood image evaluates the crystal, photomultiplier tubes, preamplifiers, pulse height analyzer, position electronics, and display system. The four-quadrant lead bar phantom (image C) is used to evaluate linearity and spatial resolution; weekly assessment is adequate. The bar phantom is placed between the source and the collimator.

Notes

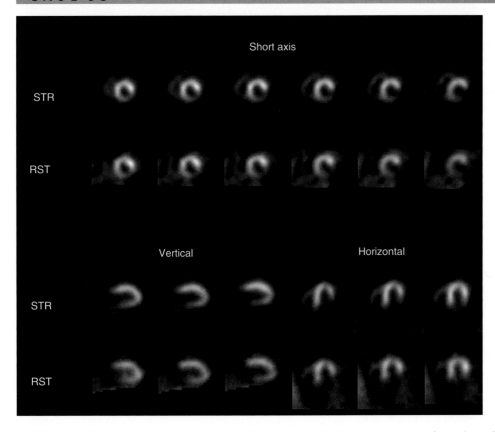

A 50-year-old patient with a history of myocardial infarction was referred with recent onset of chest pain. He achieved 4.0 METS (metabolic equivalents) and 60% of maximum age-predicted heart rate on an exercise treadmill stress test before stopping due to weakness.

1. What are the indications to discontinue the exercise treadmill stress test?

2. Describe the myocardial stress and rest perfusion SPECT image findings.

3. Provide the differential diagnosis and any likely involved vessel(s).

4. Discuss any other factor important to the interpretation of the scan.

Cardiovascular System: Inferior Lateral Wall Myocardial Infarction

1. Severe anginal chest pain, a decrease in blood pressure, frequent premature ventricular contractions (PVCs), or ST-T wave elevation suggestive of acute infarction. The patient can walk no further because of general fatigue, leg pain, or dyspnea.

2. Severe fixed stress and rest fixed defect in the basal lateral, inferior, and inferolateral walls, sparing the apex.

3. Myocardial infarction. Circumflex coronary artery.

4. The exercise stress level was inadequate.

Reference

Wackers FJTh: Coronary artery disease: exercise stress. In: Zaret BL, Beller GA (eds): *Clinical Nuclear Cardiology*, 3rd ed. Philadelphia: Elsevier, 2005, pp 215–232.

Cross-Reference

Nuclear Medicine: THE REQUISITES, 3rd ed, pp 461–467.

Comment

The principle underlying stress perfusion imaging is that the degree of cardiac work must be sufficient to unmask ischemia abnormalities. The adequacy of exercise and the amount of cardiac work are indicated by the blood pressure and heart rate response. The most common indicator of adequate exercise is achieving greater than 85% of the age-adjusted maximum age-predicted heart rate (220 − patient's age). Indirect measures of oxygen consumption frequently are used because oxygen uptake parallels cardiac work. At rest, a healthy subject consumes approximately 3.5 mL/kg/min or 1 METS. A good correlation exists among oxygen uptake, METS, and exercise duration on the standard Bruce exercise protocol. Because exercise provides valuable clinical cardiopulmonary information, treadmill stress testing generally is preferred to pharmacologic stress, whenever possible. The Bruce protocol is the most common exercise protocol. However, other exercise protocols are sometimes used that have different workload increments. Ideally, exercise testing should be maximal for the patient and only discontinued because of physical symptoms. When patient safety is of concern (e.g., after myocardial infarction), a submaximal exercise stress test is used. This patient had suboptimal stress. Thus, ischemia has not been ruled. Pharmacologic stress would have been a better choice for this patient. A patient can be converted to pharmacologic stress if exercise is suboptimal.

Notes

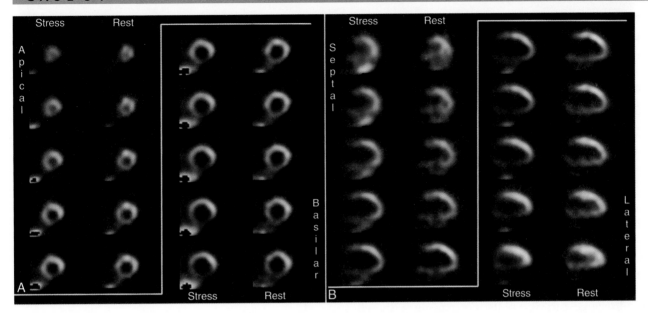

A 53-year-old man with a recent myocardial infarction had a dipyridamole stress myocardial SPECT study before hospital discharge. SPECT short-axis (A) and vertical long-axis (B) images are shown.

1. Describe the SPECT findings.

2. Name the likely coronary artery or arteries involved.

3. Interpret the study.

4. What prognostic information does the scan provide?

Cardiovascular System: Dipyridamole-Induced Inferior Wall Ischemia

1. A perfusion defect involving the entire inferior wall extending to the apex shows partial reversibility in the more distal apical inferior region.

2. Right coronary artery.

3. Inferior wall ischemia with incomplete reversibility. The latter may represent infarction or possibly hibernating myocardium with evidence of mild ischemia.

4. The patient is at risk of a further cardiac event, either myocardial infarct or death.

Reference

Brown KA, Heller GV, Landin RS, et al: Early dipyridamole Tc-99m sestamibi SPECT imaging 2 to 4 days after acute myocardial infarction predicts in-hospital and postdischarge cardiac events: comparison with submaximal exercise imaging, *Circulation* 100:2060–2066, 1999.

Cross-Reference

Nuclear Medicine: THE REQUISITES, 3rd ed, pp 461–465.

Comment

Myocardial perfusion scintigraphy can be performed safely early after myocardial infarction using submaximal exercise treadmill stress or vasodilators. Dipyridamole can risk stratify patients better than submaximal exercise treadmill. The SPECT images show reversibility, but a portion of the abnormality does not normalize. This raises the possibility that ischemic regions may coexist with areas of fibrosis or even hibernating myocardium (i.e., viable but dysfunctional myocardium with reduced blood flow). The amount of viable myocardium could be further evaluated with a gated SPECT study to evaluate wall motion, metabolic imaging using FDG, or a 2D1 thallium rest study.

The normal male pattern of myocardial perfusion shows decreased inferior wall uptake, which is attributed to diaphragmatic attenuation, which refers to attenuation by soft tissue and organs below the diaphragm. Usually attenuation appears as a fixed defect and cannot always be differentiated from an inferior wall infarct. Normalization with attenuation correction or a gated SPECT study showing normal wall motion and myocardial thickening could confirm that it is caused by attenuation and not infarct.

SPECT provides prognostic information for this patient. Multiple studies have shown that any rest perfusion abnormality and any stress-induced perfusion abnormality are independent adverse prognostic indicators.

This patient is at risk of an adverse event (e.g., myocardial infarct or death). Consideration of revascularization is warranted.

Notes

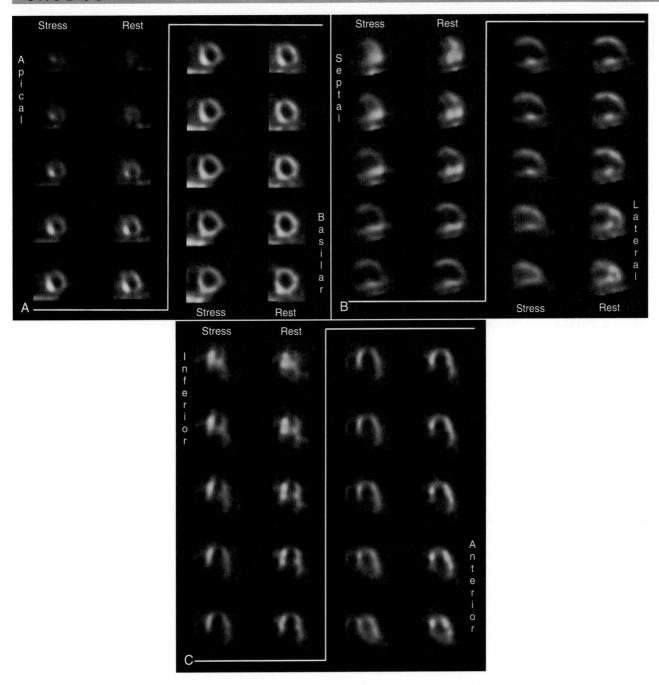

SPECT adenosine stress/rest myocardial perfusion images (short-axis [A], vertical long-axis [B], and horizontal long-axis [C] images).

1. What are clinical indications for adenosine stress?

2. List contraindications to the use of intravenous adenosine.

3. Describe the procedure for adenosine stress (A), adenosine's duration of action (B), and the procedure to deal with side effects of adenosine (C).

4. Describe the SPECT findings and the diagnosis.

Cardiovascular System: Adenosine Stress—Apical Infarction, Anterolateral Wall Ischemia

1. Whenever adequate exercise stress is not possible.

2. Second- or third-degree atrioventricular block, bronchospastic lung disease, adenosine allergy.

3. A, Adenosine is infused intravenously for 6 minutes (140 μg/kg/min). After 3 minutes, the radiotracer is injected and adenosine is continued for 3 more minutes. B, Adenosine is cleared rapidly from the circulation ($t_{1/2}$ of 10 seconds). Return to baseline blood flow levels occur within 2 to 3 minutes after stopping the infusion. C, Stop the infusion.

4. Small, moderately severe fixed defect at the apex on both stress and rest images consistent with infarct. Some improvement in perfusion of the anterior and lateral walls at rest compared with stress, consistent with mild/moderate anterolateral ischemia.

Reference

Botvinick EH: Current methods of pharmacologic stress testing and the potential advantages of new agents, *J Nucl Med Technol* 37:14–25, 2009.

Cross-Reference

Nuclear Medicine: THE REQUISITES, 3rd ed, pp 461–466.

Comment

Adenosine, a potent coronary artery vasodilator, demonstrates regional disparity of coronary blood flow reserve in patients with CAD. Partially occluded vessels cannot dilate to the same degree as normal vessels, thus producing nonuniform tracer distribution. The resulting images are similar to those obtained with exercise; however, the physiology is quite different. Exercise stress maximizes cardiac work to bring out ischemic regions of the heart. The accuracy of the two techniques is similar. Pharmacologic stress is used in patients unable to exercise (e.g., those with claudication, severe arthritis, general fatigue, physical deconditioning).

Theophylline-type drugs and caffeine block the effect of adenosine and dipyridamole and are thus prohibited before the study. Side effects of adenosine and dipyridamole are similar because both agents act through the stimulation of the adenosine receptors. Common side effects are chest pain, headache, and dizziness. The frequency of side effects is greater with adenosine, but their duration is short-lived and thus more easily controlled compared with dipyridamole. Conduction abnormalities may occur with adenosine: first-degree atrioventricular block in 10% of patients, transient second-degree block in 4%, and third-degree block in less than 1%. Because of adenosine's short duration of action, side effects are transient and generally not serious.

Notes

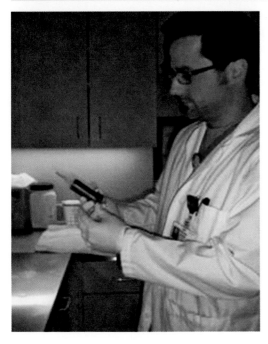

Scenario 1: A 35-year-old patient was prescribed a dose of 7 mCi of ^{131}I but was administered 27 mCi instead.

Scenario 2: A 55-year-old patient was prescribed 5 mCi ^{111}In-leukocytes but was administered 5 mCi of ^{99m}Tc-HMPAO leukocytes instead.

Scenario 3: An 18-year-old patient was prescribed 10 mCi of ^{99m}Tc-SC, but this was administered to a different patient than the one for whom it was prescribed.

Scenario 4: A 56-year-old patient was prescribed a dose of 40 mCi ^{99m}Tc-DTPA for inhalation, but the radiopharmaceutical was administered intravenously instead.

Scenario 5: A 45-year-old patient was prescribed a dose of 20 mCi ^{99m}Tc-MDP but was given 40 mCi instead.

1. Which of the scenarios is considered a reportable *medical event* by the NRC?

2. What is a reportable medical event regarding radioactive material?

3. What was the previous terminology used for a reportable medical event?

4. What action should be taken if there is a nuclear medicine medical event?

Radiation Safety: Medical Event

1. All the scenarios except scenario 5 represent a reportable medical event.

2. The NRC defines a reportable medical event in 10 CFR Part 35 as having to meet both of two criteria: (a) The difference between the dose administered and prescribed exceeds annual occupation dose limits (5 rem in adults, 0.5 rem in embryo, fetus, or nursing child) *and* (b) one of the following occurs regarding the administered radiopharmaceutical: wrong drug, wrong route of administration, wrong patient, differs from prescribed dose by 20% (more than or less than).

3. Misadministration. This term is no longer used.

4. Minimize adverse effects immediately (e.g., enema, laxative, emesis, gastric lavage, diuresis, hydration, administer blocking agent for thyroid glands, salivary gland, stomach). Inform the responsible nuclear medicine physician, patient, and Radiation Safety Officer immediately. Report to the NRC/Agreement state.

References
Siegel JA: *Guide for Diagnostic Nuclear Medicine and Radiopharmaceutical Therapy*. Reston, VA: Society of Nuclear Medicine, 2004, pp 10-11.
U.S. Nuclear Regulatory Agency: Medical Use of Bypass Material, 10 CFR Part 35.3045. Revised 2002.

Cross-Reference
Nuclear Medicine; THE REQUISITES, 3rd ed, pp 16-17.

Comment
The NRC requires licensees to report a medical event because it indicates technical or quality assurance problems in administering the physician's prescription. Dose errors (e.g., 20%) may indicate treatment delivery problems in the medical facility's operations that need correcting. However, this does not mean that the error necessarily results in harm to the patient. Harm to the patient, whether injury from overexposure or inadequate treatment due to underexposure, must be determined through separate evaluation done by a physician.

The following are methods to minimize the incidence of reportable medical events: Ensure proper labeling, patient identification, and check system; handle paperwork carefully, including request forms; educate and train all workers in emergency procedures; clearly define responsibilities; minimize distractions in a busy environment; establish efficient quality assurance; properly measure radioactivity; establish clear lines of communication for reporting.

Notes

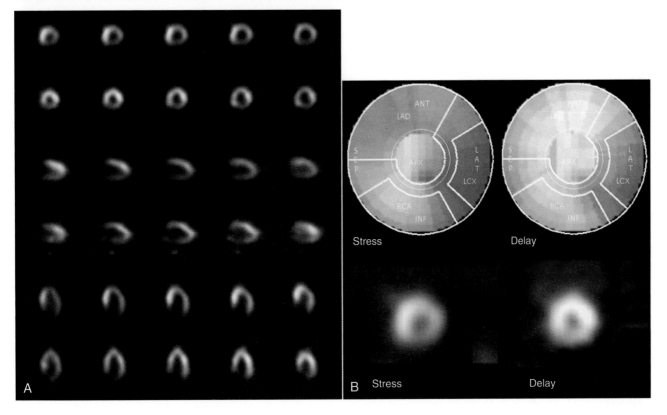

1. Describe the image findings on the stress (A, *top*) and rest (A, *bottom*) perfusion images.

2. Describe how the bull's-eye format (B, *top*) is obtained. Does it confirm your image description?

3. List possible errors that may occur when applying a bull's-eye quantitative analysis technique to myocardial perfusion SPECT.

4. Describe the likely culprit coronary artery or arteries. List the characteristics of perfusion scan abnormalities that should be included in any report.

Cardiovascular System: Polar Plot, Results Reporting

1. Stress: Hypoperfusion of the anterior, lateral, and inferior walls. Rest: Normalized perfusion of the anterior and lateral walls and incomplete normalization of the inferior wall. Most consistent with ischemia of the left circumflex and possible infarction of the right coronary artery.

2. A polar plot is constructed by layering short-axis slices one on top of the other, with the apex forming the center and the base of the heart being the outermost portion. Yes.

3. Misregistration/misalignment, use of inappropriate reference database.

4. Include location and extent, severity, and reversibility for each perfusion abnormality. If gated SPECT is performed, include left ventricular ejection fraction (LVEF), wall motion with or without wall thickening fractions. Note ancillary signs of significant CAD (e.g., stress-induced dilation of the left ventricle).

References

Cooke CD, Faber TL, Areeda JS, et al: Advanced computer methods in cardiac SPECT. In: DePuey G, Garcia EV, Berman DS (eds): *Cardiac SPECT Imaging*, 2nd ed. Philadelphia: Lippincott Williams & Wilkins, 2001, pp 65–80.

Watson DD: Quantitative SPECT techniques, *Semin Nucl Med* 29:298–318, 1999.

Cross-Reference

Nuclear Medicine: THE REQUISITES, 3rd ed, pp 480–481.

Comment

Polar maps or "bull's-eye" displays were developed to illustrate in one image the normalized stress and rest data of the entire left ventricle. The display is produced by layering short-axis slices one on top of the other with the apex forming the center and the base of the heart the periphery. Circumferential count profiles from all slices are combined into a color-coded image, allowing a quick and comprehensive overview. The points of each circumferential profile are assigned a color based on normalized count values. Abnormal areas can be identified at a glance. The polar plot is most useful if it includes quantification of the degree of perfusion defects and the percentage of change from rest to stress (not shown here). However, this requires a normal database for comparison, which is supplementary software available for purchase from commercial vendors but not available at many hospitals. Even without quantitation, the display still serves an important purpose (i.e., showing the difference between stress and rest images that can be used to confirm image interpretation). As in other areas of nuclear medicine, quantitative data should be used only as an adjunct to image analysis and not interpreted in isolation. Now, three-dimensional quantitative displays also are available.

Notes

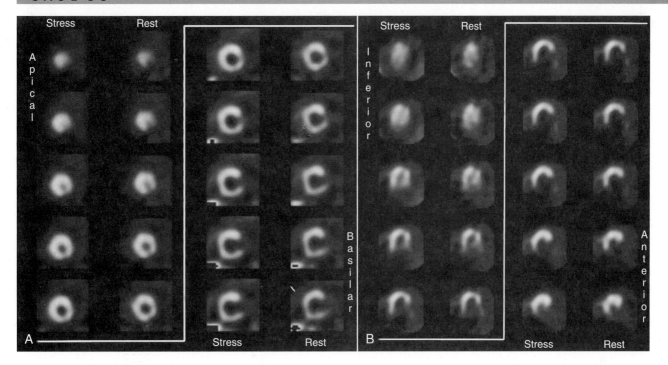

This patient had atrial fibrillation and a high baseline resting heart rate. The patient exercised for only 3.5 minutes, achieved 3.0 METS, and reached 60% of age-predicted maximum heart rate. SPECT short-axis (A) and horizontal long-axis (B) perfusion images.

1. Describe any perfusion abnormalities.

2. Describe any other findings.

3. What is the most likely culprit coronary artery?

4. Discuss the significance of failure to achieve adequate exercise.

Cardiovascular System: Inadequate Stress

1. Severe fixed defect involving the entire lateral wall.

2. Suggestive of dilated left ventricular cavity at both stress and rest.

3. Left circumflex coronary artery.

4. False-negative findings on studies for ischemia may result.

Reference

Wackers FJTh: Coronary artery disease: exercise stress. In: Zaret BL, Beller GA (eds): *Clinical Nuclear Cardiology*, 3rd ed. Philadelphia: Elsevier, 2005, pp 215–232.

Cross-Reference

Nuclear Medicine: THE REQUISITES, 3rd ed, pp 458–466.

Comment

Significant coronary stenoses involving less than 90% of vessel diameter may appear as normal regional perfusion under resting conditions. Because flow reserve across a fixed stenosis is limited, augmentation of blood flow by exercise or pharmacologic intervention is necessary to unmask blood flow heterogeneity caused by coronary artery stenosis. Failure to achieve adequate exercise stress can result in false-negative findings on studies for ischemia. Even if ischemia is demonstrated, it may be underestimated in extent or severity without adequate stress. Therefore, the dictated report should include a statement indicating that the patient reached only a low exercise level, which could decrease the sensitivity of the examination for demonstration of ischemia. Low METS is consistent with low workload and short exercise duration.

Medications can result in a false-negative scan. For example, β-blockers can prevent the achievement of maximum heart rate during exercise. Nitrates or calcium channel blockers may mask or prevent cardiac ischemia. In some cases, it may not be feasible for the patient to stop the medications. At other times, medications are deliberately continued to assess the adequacy of drug therapy in blocking ischemia. In those circumstances, detection of CAD is not the goal, as these patients are already being treated medically for CAD.

Notes

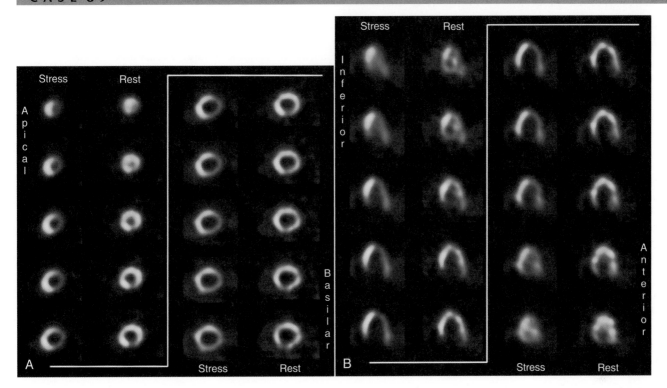

A 60-year-old diabetic patient with severe chronic obstructive pulmonary disease (COPD) was referred because of an abnormal ECG, denies chest pain. He uses a walker. Short-axis (A) and horizontal long-axis (B) SPECT myocardial perfusion images are shown.

1. What form of stress is indicated for this patient and why?

2. Describe the perfusion abnormalities.

3. What is the likely culprit coronary artery?

4. Explain the discrepancy between the findings and patient's lack of symptoms.

Cardiovascular System: Silent Lateral Wall Ischemia

1. Dobutamine. The need for a walker precludes adequate exercise stress, and severe bronchospastic disease is a contraindication to adenosine or dipyridamole use.

2. Moderately severe perfusion defect involving the entire lateral wall extending to the anterolateral and inferolateral regions and apex on the stress images that nearly normalizes on the rest images. There is incomplete reversibility of a small portion of the inferior wall.

3. Left circumflex coronary artery.

4. Silent myocardial ischemia, which is not rare in diabetic patients.

Reference

Wackers FJ, Young LH, Inzucchi SE, et al: Detection of silent myocardial ischemia in asymptomatic diabetic subjects: the DIAD study, *Diabetes Care* 27:1954-1961, 2004.

Cross-Reference

Nuclear Medicine: THE REQUISITES, 3rd ed, pp 501-503.

Comment

Silent myocardial ischemia is defined as the presence of significant CAD without anginal symptoms. Thus, CAD may go undetected until severe consequences have occurred, such as massive myocardial infarction, ischemic cardiomyopathy, and death. Patients with diabetes are at increased risk of silent ischemia as a result of autonomic neuropathy. Studies have shown that any perfusion abnormality or any stress-induced perfusion abnormality is an independent adverse prognostic indicator. Based on the scan findings, this patient is at risk of an adverse event (e.g., acute myocardial infarction, death) despite the lack of anginal symptoms. Consideration of further revascularization is warranted.

In this case, coronary vasodilator stress with dipyridamole or adenosine is contraindicated because of the severe COPD, because the drugs may induce bronchospasm. Dobutamine is a synthetic catecholamine that increases cardiac workload by increasing the heart rate and blood pressure. This patient is a typical candidate for dobutamine (i.e., one who cannot exercise and has bronchospastic pulmonary disease). Before stress, a patient should be checked for relative contraindications to dobutamine such as recent myocardial infarction or unstable angina, hemodynamically significant left ventricular outflow tract obstruction, atrial tachyarrhythmias, ventricular tachycardia, uncontrolled hypertension, aortic dissections, or large aneurysms.

Notes

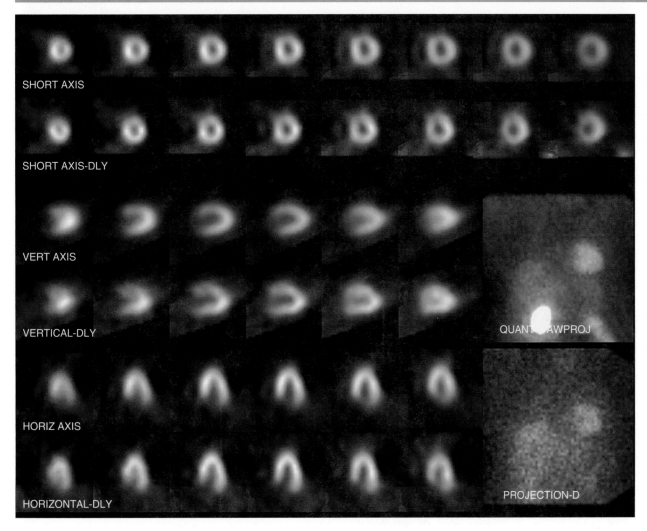

SHORT AXIS

SHORT AXIS-DLY

VERT AXIS

VERTICAL-DLY

QUANT AWPROJ

HORIZ AXIS

HORIZONTAL-DLY

PROJECTION-D

A 55-year-old woman with abnormal baseline ECG and left bundle branch block (LBBB) is referred for a SPECT study. LVEF and wall thickening by gated SPECT are normal.

1. Name the appropriate stress technique that should be performed in this patient.

2. List stress methods that would be disadvantageous for this patient. Why?

3. What is the explanation for this problem referred to in question 2?

4. Describe the scintigraphic findings in this case.

CASE 90

Cardiovascular System: LBBB

1. Cardiac vasodilator drugs (e.g., dipyridamole, adenosine, regadenoson).

2. Exercise or dobutamine may produce false-positive findings of septal reversibility suggestive of ischemia in patients with LBBB without CAD.

3. An explanation is that the stress-induced decrease in septal blood flow is secondary to asynchronous relaxation of the septum, which is out of phase with diastolic filling of the ventricle when coronary perfusion is maximal.

4. The mild decreased activity in the anterior wall appears fixed and likely is caused by breast attenuation in light of the reported normal wall motion.

Reference

DePuey EG: Artifacts in SPECT myocardial perfusion imaging. In: Gordon EG, Garcia EV, Berman DS (eds): *Cardiac SPECT Imaging*, 2nd ed. Philadelphia: Lippincott Williams & Wilkins, 2001, pp 232–262.

Cross-Reference

Nuclear Medicine: THE REQUISITES, 3rd ed, p 474.

Comment

Exercise-induced reversible perfusion defects involving the septum mimicking septal ischemia are seen in 30% to 90% of patients with LBBB. Coronary blood flow occurs primarily during diastole; therefore, flow to the septum is compromised by its asynchrony and by the shortening of diastole at high heart rates. At rest when the heart rate is not increased, no regional disparity in radiotracer activity is apparent, so the defect appears reversible. However, fixed perfusion abnormalities have also been described. Stress-induced perfusion defects caused by LBBB without CAD do not usually involve the apex and anterior wall, a pattern uncommon with true left anterior descending artery ischemia.

Both exercise and dobutamine increase cardiac work by increasing myocardial oxygen demand as a result of increasing the heart rate and systolic blood pressure and contractility. Therefore, these stress methods should not be used in patients with LBBB because the scan may be falsely positive for septal ischemia. However, regardless of the stress method, stress-induced perfusion abnormalities outside the septum have the same significance as that in patients without LBBB and indicate CAD. Abnormal septal wall motion on gated images is seen consistently after coronary artery bypass graft surgery as a result of disruption of the pericardium in the absence of LBBB.

Notes

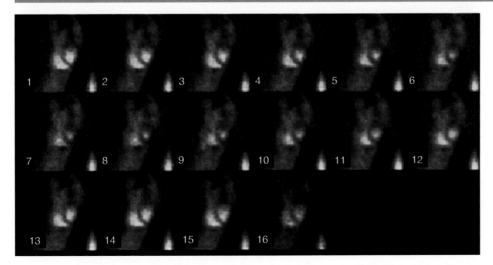

A gated resting radionuclide ventriculogram (RVG) or multiple gated acquisition (MUGA) study is shown.

1. Name the radiopharmaceutical used.

2. What is the advantage of this cardiac technique over perfusion imaging gated SPECT?

3. Describe the three major methodologies of radiolabeling RBCs.

4. List the advantages and disadvantages of the different labeling methods.

Cardiovascular System: RBC Labeling for RVG

1. ^{99m}Tc-RBCs.

2. High count blood pool images allow for accurate quantification of LVEF.

3. In vivo: tin (SN^{++}) in the form of stannous pyrophosphate is administered intravenously, followed in 20 minutes by intravenous injection of ^{99m}Tc-pertechnetate. Modified in vivo: stannous pyrophosphate is administered intravenously and 15 to 30 minutes later, 3 to 5 mL of blood is withdrawn into an attached shielded syringe containing ^{99m}Tc-pertechnetate. After a few minutes of mild agitation, it is infused. The syringe is left attached to the indwelling intravenous line during the procedure so that the entire system is closed. In vitro: blood is withdrawn and placed in a vial containing stannous chloride and sodium hypochlorite to oxidize excess extracellular stannous ion and thus prevent extracellular reduction of ^{99m}Tc-pertechnetate. Labeling occurs when ^{99m}Tc-pertechnetate is added, followed by a 20-minute incubation before reinjection of labeled cells.

4. The in vivo method is simplest and least costly, but has the lowest labeling efficiency of approximately 75%. The modified method has a labeling efficiency of 85%. The in vitro commercial kit method (Ultra-Tag) has the highest labeling efficiency (>97%).

Reference

Chilton HM, Callahan RJ, Thrall JH: Radiopharmaceuticals for cardiac imaging: myocardial infarction, perfusion, metabolism, and ventricular function (blood pool). In: Chilton HM, Callahan RJ, Thrall JH: *Pharmaceuticals in Medical Imaging*. New York: Macmillan, 1990, pp 442–450.

Cross-Reference

Nuclear Medicine: THE REQUISITES, 3rd ed, pp 490–495.

Comment

The poorer the labeling efficiency, the more free ^{99m}Tc-pertechnetate, the higher the background activity and poorer accuracy for calculation of the LVEF are. Various causes exist for poor RBC labeling. The most common are drug-drug interactions (e.g., with heparin, doxorubicin, iodinated contrast media, and quinidine). Other causes include circulating antibodies from previous transfusions, transplantation, or antibiotics. Insufficient or too much stannous ion, too short a "tinning" interval, and too short an incubation period for technetium (VII) reduction. These are less of a problem for the in vitro method.

Wall motion studies are acquired in the left anterior oblique (LAO), anterior, and left lateral views. The LAO view is used for quantification. Quantification is possible because of ECG gating and the acquisition of counts into 16 separate sequential bins during each QRS interval so that temporal data are available. The final images are a summation of many cardiac cycles over 5 to 10 minutes. Wall motion studies can be performed with gated myocardial perfusion studies (e.g., ^{99m}Tc-sestamibi or tetrofosmin). Advantages of the labeled RBC method are the high count rate, better certainty of the region of the ventricular cavity, and the greater number of bins (16 vs. 8) during each R-R interval, made possible by the higher count rate. This patient's LVEF is clearly normal. Note the good contraction of the peak end-systolic frame 8 compared with the end-diastolic frame 16.

Notes

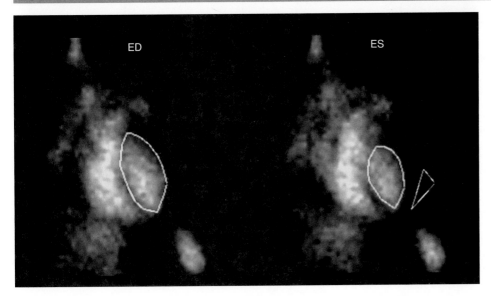

1. Describe and explain the processing performed on this equilibrium gated blood pool (RVG) or MUGA study.

2. How are the regions of interest (ROIs) selected?

3. List the nuclear medicine techniques by which left ventricular function can be assessed.

4. Provide the equation for determination of LVEF.

Cardiovascular System: Calculation of LVEF for RVG

1. Left anterior oblique end-diastolic and end-systolic images show left ventricular and background ROIs drawn on a computer and used for calculation of the LVEF.

2. The LAO view with best separation of the left and right ventricles is chosen. ROIs are drawn for the left ventricle at end-systole, at end-diastole, and for adjacent background.

3. RVG or MUGA; first-pass RVG; gated perfusion SPECT or PET.

4. Percentage of LVEF = end-diastolic counts − end-systolic counts ÷ end-diastolic counts, all corrected for background counts × 100%.

Reference

Borges-Neto S, Coleman RE: Radionuclide ventricular function analysis, *Radiol Clin North Am* 31:817–830, 1993.

Cross-Reference

Nuclear Medicine: THE REQUISITES, 3rd ed, pp 490–495.

Comment

The RVG or MUGA is a time-tested accurate method for calculating an LVEF. To obtain cardiac images that show wall motion, the patient's heart rhythm must be regular and electrically gated. Each cardiac cycle is divided into 16 frames to maximize temporal resolution so that end-diastolic and end-systolic frames can be identified for LVEF quantification. To obtain sufficient counts for high-quality images, approximately 300 cardiac cycles are acquired. The first-pass radionuclide angiocardiogram method quantifies ventricular function during radiotracer bolus transit through the heart, during approximately six cardiac cycles. These volume-based methods (radioactive counts are proportional to ventricular volume) are more accurate than geometric methods (e.g., echocardiography or contrast ventriculography).

The normal LVEF ranges from approximately 50% to 75%. Calculation of right ventricular ejection fraction using the gated blood pool technique is subject to some potential error caused by overlap of the atria and ventricles; first-pass radionuclide angiocardiogram is superior because only cycles in which the bolus resides within the right ventricle are used. SPECT is potentially more accurate than the conventional planar MUGA because selected ROIs can minimize overlap of the atria and ventricles. Commercial software for this method is becoming available.

Notes

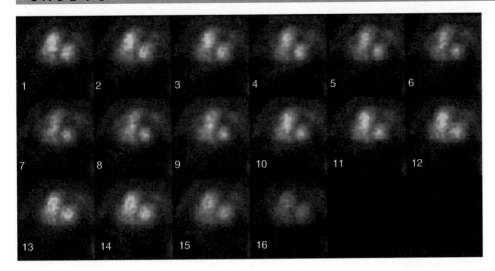

Radionuclide planar gated equilibrium blood pool study. Sequential frames are shown.

1. Estimate the LVEF based on the submitted images and explain the decreased intensity (counts) in frame 16.

2. Discuss the importance of patient positioning in the calculation of the LVEF.

3. List factors that may result in reduced accuracy of the LVEF calculation.

4. Describe the effect on the LVEF if (a) no background is subtracted, and (b) a background region is used that includes some of the spleen.

C A S E   9 3

Cardiovascular System: RVG—MUGA Technique

1. LVEF appears normal (~50%). End-diastole is seen in frame 15 or 16 and end-systole is seen at frame 7. Frame 16 shows decreased intensity compared with other frames, resulting from variability in the patient's heart rate, in this case, frequent PVCs.

2. The LAO position selected is that which provides the best separation of the left and right ventricles, approximately a 45-degree LAO view, but varies depending on the patient's anatomy (best septal view).

3. Patient-related factors: arrhythmia, inability to walk well, suboptimal RBC labeling. Technique-related: poor LAO positioning, suboptimal RBC labeling; incorrect ROI for left ventricle or background.

4. a, Falsely low; b, falsely high.

Reference

Wagner RH, Sobotka PA: Functional cardiac imaging. In: Henkin RE (ed): *Nuclear Medicine*, 2nd ed. Philadelphia: Mosby, 2006, pp 631–654.

Cross-Reference

Nuclear Medicine: THE REQUISITES, 3rd ed, pp 490–500.

Comment

The images represent the frames into which the R-R interval was divided using simultaneous cardiac gating. By visual estimation, the LVEF appears normal (calculated to be 65%). The radionuclide equilibrium gated blood pool and first-pass techniques are accurate methods for measuring the LVEF because calculation is based on volume changes and not geometric assumptions of cardiac shape as are contrast ventriculography and echocardiography. A limitation of the gated blood pool technique is cardiac arrhythmia. The LVEF becomes less reliable when the R-R interval is irregular. When ventricular premature beats occur in more than one of every six beats, quantification must be suspect. Overestimation of background activity falsely elevates the LVEF, and underestimation of background activity depresses the LVEF. The error in LVEF that results from mild arrhythmia (e.g., slow atrial fibrillation) is not large, but can be considerably greater with severe arrhythmia (e.g., rapid atrial fibrillation, frequent PVCs). When the R-R interval varies, fewer counts are shown in the terminal frames. The drop off in the intensity may appear as a flicker when viewing the gated images in cinematic display.

Notes

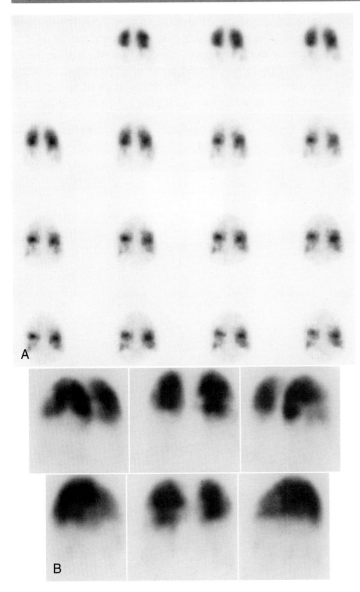

A

B

A 35-year-old man has increasing symptoms of dyspnea. A, ^{133}Xe ventilation. B, Perfusion. The chest x-ray was clear of infiltrate, effusion, mass, and pleural disease.

1. Name the three phases of a ^{133}Xe ventilation scan.

2. Describe the three phases.

3. Describe the findings of the ventilation and perfusion scans.

4. Provide an interpretation and offer a likely diagnosis for the underlying disease.

Pulmonary System: Emphysema Caused by α_1-Antitrypsin Deficiency

1. Wash-in or first single breath, equilibrium, and washout phases.

2. Single breath: patient initially breathes in and holds a single maximum deep inspiration while a 100,000-count image is acquired. Equilibrium: patient breathes a mixture of air and xenon while serial images are obtained every 60 to 90 seconds for 3 minutes. Washout: patient breathes room air and exhales xenon while serial images are obtained.

3. Ventilation: nonuniform bilaterally in the upper lung zones. Initially nearly absent at the bases. As upper lobes wash out, xenon fills and is retained in both bases, indicating delayed ventilation and severe air trapping. Perfusion: heterogeneous to both upper lung zones, which match the early ventilation images. The extensive perfusion abnormalities in both lower lung zones are matched with areas of delayed wash-in and washout.

4. Low probability of pulmonary embolism, α_1-antitrypsin deficiency.

Reference

Sostman HD, Gottschalk A: Evaluation of patients with suspected venous thromboembolism. In: Sandler MP (ed): *Diagnostic Nuclear Medicine*, 4th ed. Philadelphia: Lippincott Williams & Wilkins, 2003, pp 345–366.

Cross-Reference

Nuclear Medicine: THE REQUISITES, 3rd ed, pp 512–534.

Comment

^{133}Xe, an inert gas, demonstrates the abnormal physiology of obstructive airway disease. Initially, decreased and delayed xenon wash-in is followed by slow washout or "trapping" of the gas. The wash-in phase distribution is very similar to that on ^{99m}Tc aerosol particle images. A major advantage of ^{133}Xe is the washout phase, which is very sensitive for obstructive airway disease (e.g., COPD and asthma). A disadvantage is that images can be obtained in only one view (two if a two-headed camera is used) because of the rapid dynamic air flow. The study is best performed before the perfusion study because of the low ^{133}Xe energy photopeak (80 keV).

Emphysema is a lung disease characterized pathologically by abnormal permanent enlargement of air spaces distal to the terminal bronchial accompanied by destruction of the walls without obvious fibrosis. Panlobular emphysema is associated with α_1-antitrypsin deficiency, although it may occur in smokers and elderly patients.

α_1-Antitrypsin is a serum protein that inhibits lysosomal proteases released during inflammatory reactions and prevents their damaging effects. Patients with reduced levels of α_1-antitrypsin are at risk of emphysema. Smoking further increases the risk. Lower lobe air trapping is suggestive of α_1-antitrypsin deficiency. Upper lobe air trapping is seen more commonly in COPD.

Notes

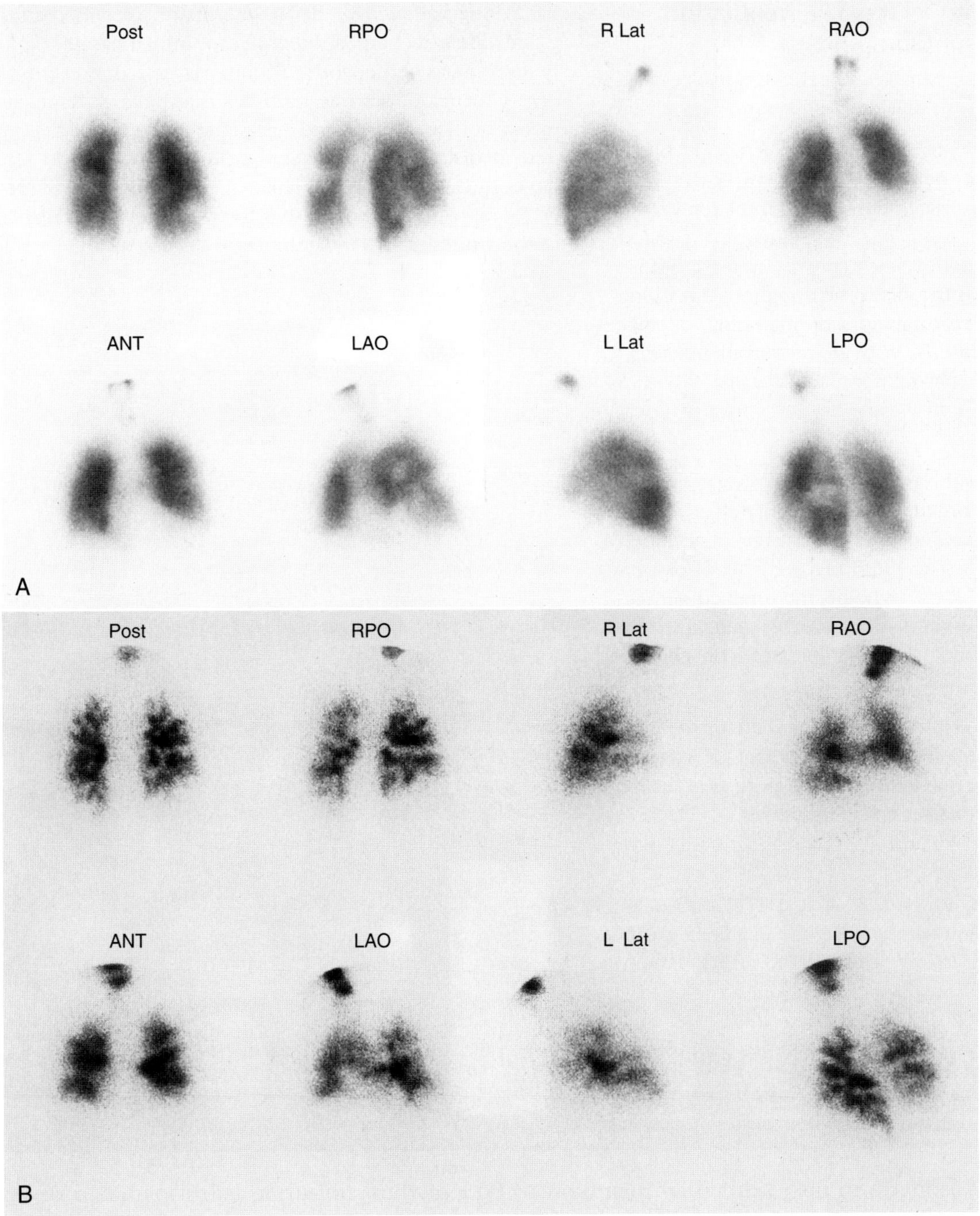

A

B

A 64-year-old man has recent onset of shortness of breath. The chest x-ray was clear.

1. What is the ventilation study radiopharmaceutical and its mechanism of distribution?

2. Describe the image findings (A, perfusion; B, ventilation). What is the likely reason for the scintigraphic appearance on this study?

3. Is the ventilation or perfusion study usually performed first, and why?

4. Provide your interpretation of the study.

C A S E   9 5

Pulmonary System: ^{99m}Tc-DTPA Ventilation Study with Aerosol Clumping

1. ^{99m}Tc-DTPA aerosol particles (0.1-0.5 μm in size) normally distribute on first impact within the distal alveoli.

2. Multiple perfusion defects in upper and lower lung fields. Many appear segmental (e.g., the lateral basal of the right lower lobe, superior segment of the left lower lobe). Ventilation study shows extensive diffuse "clumping" within the airways throughout both lung fields, making determination of matching or mismatching quite difficult. With airway turbulence (e.g., asthma or COPD), particles impact proximally within bronchi, not reaching the alveoli, and appear as focal hot spots.

3. ^{99m}Tc-DTPA aerosol ventilation study is performed first. The patient breathes in approximately 1 mCi at tidal volume until an adequate count rate is obtained (3000 counts/sec). The sixfold larger ^{99m}Tc-MAA perfusion dose (5 mCi) overwhelms the retained ventilation dose and the ventilation dose is seen, if at all, only as background, allowing for two consecutive ^{99m}Tc studies.

4. The study was interpreted as intermediate probability because the ventilation study could not be reliably interpreted; however, the segmental perfusion defect pattern is suspicious for embolus.

Reference
Trujillo NP, Pratt JP, Tahisani S, et al: DTPA aerosol in ventilation/perfusion scintigraphy for diagnosing pulmonary embolism, *J Nucl Med* 38:1781-1783, 1997.

Cross-Reference
Nuclear Medicine: THE REQUISITES, 3rd ed, pp 513-521.

Comment
Because of air turbulence in this case, the Tc-99m aerosol particles did not reach the peripheral alveoli and clumped on first impact of bronchi, making interpretation difficult. This is a case in which ^{133}Xe would have been advantageous. However, most centers exclusively use either ^{133}Xe- or ^{99m}Tc-DTPA. Patients with a history of bronchitis, asthma, or obstructive airway disease will more likely have this pattern. Advantages of ^{99m}Tc aerosol are the higher count rate, better image quality, and images obtained in the same views as the perfusion study. The ^{99m}Tc aerosols do not have the radiation safety problems of ^{133}Xe gas. Xenon is heavy and layers out on the floor if there is not enough airflow. The NRC requires negative pressure airflow for rooms using xenon. Xenon has a long half-life (5.3 days) and must be retained after exhalation in a charcoal "xenon trap" until it has decayed. In many parts of the world, Technegas is used. An aerosol generator produces fine particles that have characteristics of both an aerosol and a gas. The particles are deposited in distal alveoli. Images are excellent and do not have the troublesome proximal deposition of ^{99m}Tc-DTPA aerosol. It is hoped that this will become available in the United States in the not too distant future.

Notes

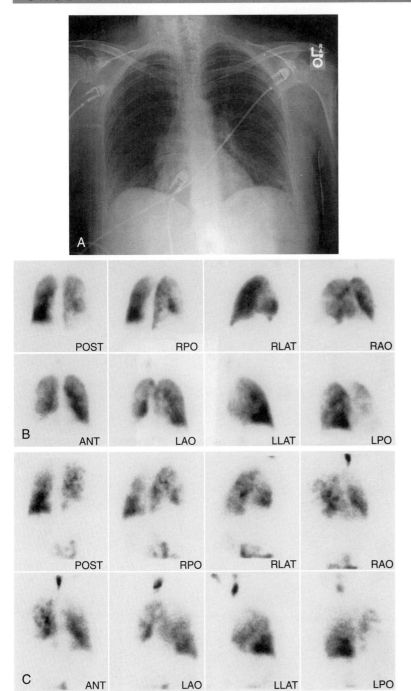

A 54-year-old man with known cardiopulmonary disease has symptoms of increasing dyspnea. A, Chest radiograph; B, perfusion; C, ventilation.

1. What are the scintigraphic findings and interpretation?

2. What is the likelihood of pulmonary embolus in this patient?

3. What is the likelihood of pulmonary embolus in a patient with a normal perfusion scan but abnormal ventilation?

4. How are perfusion defects classified as to size according to Prospective Investigation of Pulmonary Embolism Diagnosis (PIOPED) study criteria?

Pulmonary System: Low-Probability Ventilation-Perfusion Scan

1. Bilateral heterogeneous distribution. Matched perfusion and ventilation abnormalities throughout the upper and lower lobes, especially in the right lower lobe basal segments. Ventilation is worse than perfusion. Chest x-ray: minimal lower lobe atelectasis. Interpretation: low probability of pulmonary embolus.

2. Less than 20% probability of pulmonary embolus.

3. Less than 1%. If the perfusion scan is normal, pulmonary emboli have been virtually ruled out, regardless of the ventilation study.

4. Large (segmental): greater than 75% of a segment; moderate (subsegmental): 25% to 75% of a segment; small (small subsegmental): less than 25% of a segment. Two moderates equal a large.

References

Freeman LM, Stein EG, Sprayregen S, et al: The current and continuing important role of ventilation-perfusion scintigraphy in evaluating patients with suspected pulmonary embolism, *Semin Nucl Med* 38:432–440, 2008.

Gottshalk A, Stein PD, Sostman HD, et al: Very low probability interpretation of V/Q lung scans in combination with a low probability objective clinical assessment reliably excludes pulmonary embolism: data from PIOPED II, *J Nucl Med* 48:1411–1415, 2007.

Cross-Reference

Nuclear Medicine: THE REQUISITES, 3rd ed, pp 515–534.

Comment

One of the findings of the PIOPED study was that a ventilation/perfusion (V/Q) study showing extensively decreased perfusion in a lung field with matching ventilation should be interpreted as low probability as long as some perfusion exists to that lung field. Before the PIOPED study, this extensive pattern was called indeterminate. Another finding was that if the referring clinician has a high clinical suspicion for pulmonary embolus, but the scan is low probability, the clinical likelihood of pulmonary embolus increases to 40%. Conditions commonly associated with V/Q-matched abnormalities include COPD, bronchiectasis, alveolar pulmonary edema, pleural effusion, asthma, mucus plugs, and tumor.

Criteria have been proposed to define a very low probability category (i.e., <10%). They include nonsegmental perfusion defects, matched defects in two or three zones in a single lung only, and the stripe sign. The stripe sign refers to activity seen along the pleural surface of a segment that otherwise appears hypoperfused. The stripe sign lessens the likelihood of pulmonary embolus for that lung region because perfusion defects caused by vascular occlusion should extend to the pleural surface.

Notes

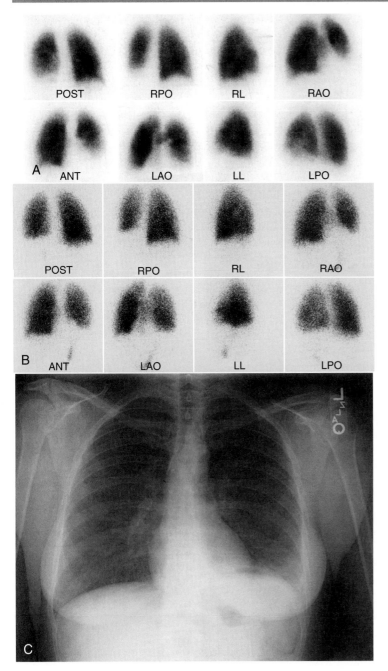

A pregnant woman in her third trimester has acute shortness of breath. She has a history of asthma.

1. Is any patient preparation indicated?

2. Would the patient's pregnancy change the V/Q protocol?

3. Describe the perfusion (A) and ventilation (B) images and radiograph findings (C).

4. Give your interpretation of the study.

Pulmonary System: Intermediate Probability—Pregnancy

1. Bronchodilator therapy before the V/Q study both as an asthmatic therapeutic trial and to minimize a bronchospastic pattern on the scan. This was done.

2. Pulmonary emboli are life threatening to the patient and fetus. The study radiation dose to patient fetus is relatively low. The benefit/risk ratio is high. However, there is reasonable concern for radiation protection of the fetus. Policies vary. Some imaging centers reduce the mCi dose. In young, nonsmoking patients without cardiopulmonary disease, some clinics perform a perfusion only study.

3. Hypoperfusion of the left lower lobe. Perhaps slightly better lower lobe ventilation than perfusion in the anterior basal and part of the lateral basal segments. The costophrenic angle loss seen on the left lateral and LPO views. Radiograph: effusion with elevation of the left diaphragm.

4. Because of the chest x-ray abnormality in the region of the perfusion abnormality, this study is intermediate probability of pulmonary embolus (35%).

References

Cronin P, Weg JG, Kazerooni EA: The role of multidetector computed tomography angiography for the diagnosis of pulmonary embolism, *Semin Nucl Med* 38:418–431, 2008.

Miniati M, Sostman HD, Gottschalk A, et al: Perfusion lung scintigraphy for the diagnosis of pulmonary embolism: a reappraisal and review of the prospective investigative study of acute pulmonary embolism diagnostic methods, *Semin Nucl Med* 38:450–461, 2008.

Cross-Reference

Nuclear Medicine: THE REQUISITES, 3rd ed, pp 515–534.

Comment

This case emphasizes the importance of comparing the perfusion study and the chest x-ray. If there is an acute abnormality of effusion, atelectasis, or infiltrate that corresponds to a perfusion defect of at least a moderate size (25–75%) segment, the interpretation must be intermediate probability of pulmonary embolus. A second bronchodilator therapy after the study was effective in relieving the patient's shortness of breath.

A normal V/Q scan excludes the diagnosis of pulmonary embolus. Patients with low-probability scans and a low clinical likelihood do not require anticoagulation or further evaluation. Patients with low-probability scans, but an intermediate or high clinical likelihood of disease should have lower extremity Doppler. If results are negative and the patient has a low clinical suspicion, anticoagulation is unnecessary; if results are positive, the patient requires treatment. Patients with an intermediate-probability V/Q scan should have a Doppler exam of the lower extremities; if results are positive, treatment is indicated, and if negative, clinical factors determine therapy.

CT angiography is often used today to diagnose pulmonary embolism. It has a high negative predictive value and can often make the diagnosis, and clinical outcome studies find that it is an accurate technique. However, CT angiography is contraindicated in patients with a definite history of allergic reaction to contrast or renal insufficiency. There is increasing concern for the high radiation dose received, particularly in children and women, the latter because of breast dose.

Notes

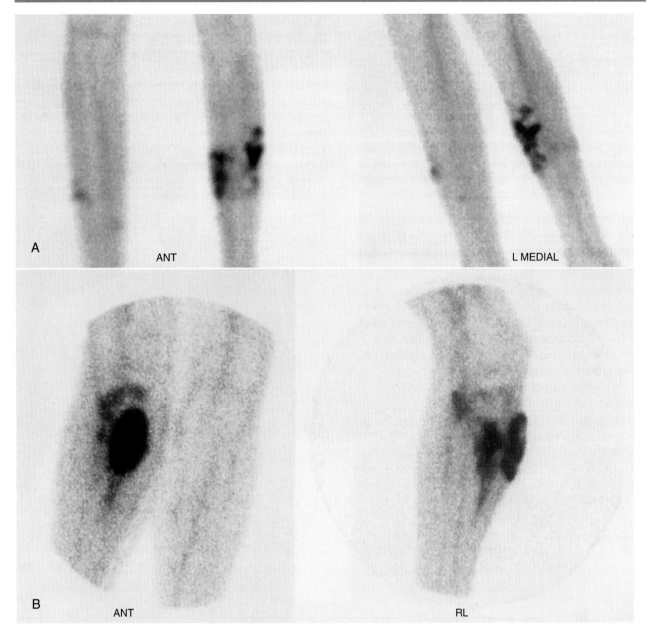

A   ANT   L MEDIAL

B   ANT   RL

Two patients (A and B) have similar histories of persistent soft-tissue infection overlying the tibia. ^{99m}Tc-HMPAO leukocyte studies were ordered to confirm or exclude underlying osteomyelitis.

1. Describe the findings. What is your interpretation of the two studies?

2. Would a bone scan be useful as the initial study in these cases?

3. Would a bone marrow study with ^{99m}Tc-SC be useful in this clinical setting?

4. Would an ^{111}In-oxine leukocyte study or ^{67}Ga-citrate study be useful?

Inflammatory Disease: ^{99m}Tc-HMPAO Leukocytes—Osteomyelitis

1. Patient A: Soft-tissue uptake. No bone uptake rules out osteomyelitis; the study is consistent with cellulitis. Patient B: Soft-tissue and bone localization consistent with osteomyelitis and overlying soft-tissue infection.

2. A negative bone scan rules out osteomyelitis with a high degree of certainty. Thus, it would be useful in a patient without previous bone disease, surgery, orthopedic hardware, or any insult to bone.

3. Not by itself. A bone marrow study can improve the specificity of a leukocyte study if there is the potential for displaced normal marrow as seen in the situations discussed in answer 2.

4. ^{111}In-leukocytes may be able to make the same diagnosis. However, the superior imaging resolution of ^{99m}Tc-HMPAO often better differentiates soft-tissue and bone infection in the distal extremities. ^{67}Ga is less specific because increased uptake occurs with bone remodeling from any cause.

References

Auler MA, Bagg S, Gordon L: The role of nuclear medicine in imaging infection, *Semin Roentgenol* 42;117–121, 2007.

Palestro CJ, Love C: Radionuclide imaging of musculoskeletal infection: conventional agents, *Semin Musculoskelet Radiol* 11:335–352, 2007.

Cross-Reference

Nuclear Medicine: THE REQUISITES, 3rd ed, pp 404–410.

Comment

The most common cause of osteomyelitis in adults is direct extension from a soft-tissue infection. Although hematogenous spread occurs in adults, it occurs most commonly in children. Long bone metaphyses commonly are affected in children because of the relatively slow blood flow in its sinusoidal veins and the paucity of phagocytes. Adult hematogenous acute osteomyelitis rarely involves the long bones. In adults, osteomyelitis is often the result of direct introduction of bacteria from soft-tissue wounds, compound fractures, and contamination of bone during surgery.

A negative three-phase bone scan rules out osteomyelitis with a high degree of accuracy in adults without previous fracture, infection, or orthopedic hardware. A ^{99m}Tc-SC bone marrow study in conjunction with leukocyte scintigraphy is useful for evaluating proximal marrow-filled bones (e.g., hip or knee prosthesis) or in patients with orthopedic hardware that results in marrow displacement. Similar distribution of leukocytes and ^{99m}Tc-SC is against infection. Leukocyte uptake where there is normal or reduced marrow is consistent with infection. ^{111}In-oxine and ^{99m}Tc-HMPAO leukocytes have similar accuracy for the diagnosis of osteomyelitis. Image quality is better with ^{99m}Tc-HMPAO and the radiation dose is lower, which is an advantage in children. However, both have a high false-negative rate for osteomyelitis of the spine; thus, ^{67}Ga or ^{18}F-FDG is preferable for the spine.

Notes

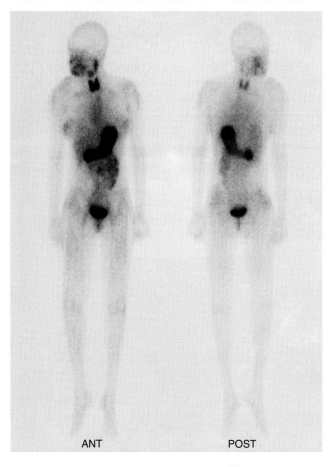

ANT   POST

A 49-year-old man is referred for a ^{99m}Tc-HMPAO leukocyte study to locate the source of *Staphylococcus aureus* sepsis.

1. What are the scintigraphic findings?

2. What is your interpretation of the study?

3. What are causes of false-positive radiolabeled leukocyte studies?

4. What are the potential advantages and disadvantages of ^{99m}Tc-HMPAO leukocytes rather than ^{111}In-oxine leukocytes for infection imaging?

Inflammatory Disease: ^{99m}Tc-HMPAO Leukocytes—Poor Radiolabeling

1. Activity in the salivary glands, thyroid, stomach, bowel, and bladder.

2. Free ^{99m}Tc-pertechnetate. Poor radiolabel. Nondiagnostic study.

3. Gastrointestinal bleeding, swallowed leukocytes from oropharyngeal, sinus, or lung inflammation/infection, uninfected postoperative surgical wounds, intestinal stomas, and catheter sites.

4. ^{99m}Tc-HMPAO is preferable in children because of its considerably low radiation dose to the spleen. It has a higher count rate and better image resolution, and imaging can be performed the same day. The major disadvantage is its genitourinary and hepatobiliary clearance. The major advantage of ^{111}In is that there is no abdominal or pelvic uptake except for the liver and spleen, making it superior for the detection of intra-abdominal infection.

References

Beeker-Rovers CP, Van der Meer JWM, Oyen WJG: Fever of unknown origin, *Semin Nucl Med* 39:81–87, 2009.

Kumar V, Yeates PG, Baker RJ: Radiopharmacy. In: Ell PJ, Gambhir SS (eds): *Nuclear Medicine in Clinical Diagnosis and Treatment*, 3rd ed. New York: Churchill Livingstone, 2004, pp 1737–1745.

Cross-Reference

Nuclear Medicine: THE REQUISITES, 3rd ed, pp 388–396.

Comment

Free ^{99m}Tc-pertechnetate is caused by poor leukocyte labeling. This is not commonly seen with white blood cell labeling. It more commonly occurs with bone scintigraphy. Poor cell labeling results in a suboptimal scan, thus limiting infection detection because of the reduced number of labeled leukocytes, poor count density where it matters, and intra-abdominal clearance of pertechnetate that complicates detection of infection. Careful attention to proper methodology is critical. Radiolabeling leukocytes with ^{99m}Tc or ^{111}In requires approximately 2 hours. If it is done at a regional radiopharmacy, an additional 1 to 2 hours is required to transport the patient's blood before and after labeling.

Quality control of radiolabeled leukocytes before injection is limited to microscopic examination of the leukocytes and determination of the labeling percentage of efficiency because the radiolabeled cells must be injected promptly to ensure cell viability. Leukocyte viability is difficult to evaluate but critical to diagnostic accuracy. Morphologic characteristics are checked microscopically. However, the ultimate test of viability is in vivo function. The presence of an increased blood pool indicates a high portion of the label is on the RBCs, platelets, or both. Prolonged lung uptake indicates cellular damage. Usually, the spleen has highest uptake. If the spleen/liver ratio is reversed, this suggests cell damage. Strict attention to ensuring that the reinfused cells are the patient's cells is mandatory.

Notes

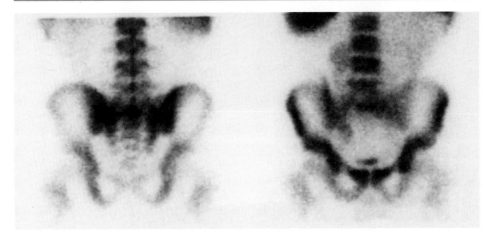

A 25-year-old man has fever and abdominal pain. ^{99m}Tc-HMPAO–labeled leukocyte images were acquired 2 hours after reinfusion of the patient's radiolabeled cells.

1. Which leukocytes are labeled with ^{99m}Tc-HMPAO compared with ^{111}In-oxine?

2. What is the explanation for the apparent skeletal uptake?

3. What is the optimal imaging time for ^{111}In-oxine–labeled leukocytes and ^{99m}Tc-HMPAO–labeled leukocytes?

4. Give an image interpretation and diagnosis in this case.

Inflammatory Disease: Intra-abdominal Abscess

1. ^{111}In-oxine binds to all leukocytes. ^{99m}Tc-HMPAO binds only to neutrophils.

2. This is normal bone marrow distribution of radiolabeled leukocytes.

3. Abdominal imaging: ^{99m}Tc-HMPAO images are acquired at 1 to 2 hours before hepatobiliary and renal clearance occurs, which could complicate interpretation. Extremity imaging can be performed later (e.g., 2-6 hours). ^{111}In-labeled leukocytes are routinely imaged at 24 hours. Four-hour imaging is possible, although leukocyte uptake is maximal and image quality is better at 24 hours. Four-hour imaging is indicated for inflammatory bowel disease because sloughing of intestinal mucosa leukocytes occurs and 24-hour location may be misleading as to the inflammatory location.

4. Infection in the right lower quadrant overlying the sacroiliac joint in the anterior view and lateral and right of the spine. The patient had a perforated appendix.

References

Annovazzi A, Bagni B, Burroni L, et al: Nuclear medicine imaging of inflammatory/infective disorders of the abdomen, *Nucl Med Commun* 26:657–664, 2005.

Bunyaviroch T, Aggarwal A, Oates ME: Optimized scintigraphic evaluation of infection and inflammation: role of SPECT/CT fusion imaging, *Semin Nucl Med* 36:295–311, 2006.

Cross-Reference

Nuclear Medicine: THE REQUISITES, 3rd ed, pp 388–396.

Comment

^{99m}Tc-HMPAO was initially approved for cerebral perfusion imaging. It is lipid soluble; this allows it to cross the blood-brain barrier and localize intracellularly. This property of HMPAO was subsequently used to transport the ^{99m}Tc into the leukocytes. ^{99m}Tc-HMPAO and ^{111}In-oxine radiolabel RBCs, platelets, and leukocytes. Cells other than leukocytes are then removed by sedimentation. Except for renal and biliary clearance, the distribution of HMPAO leukocytes is similar to that of ^{111}In-oxine-labeled leukocytes.

Greatest uptake is normally seen in the spleen, followed by liver and bone marrow. The spleen has the highest radiation dose, 15 to 20 rads with ^{111}In-oxine but only 2 rads with ^{99m}Tc-HMPAO. Thus, ^{99m}Tc-HMPAO is the preferred agent in children. An additional advantage of ^{99m}Tc-HMPAO is its better image resolution. Radiolabeled cells can be used as an alternative to repeat endoscopy or oral contrast studies. Good correlation exists between the amount and site of uptake of radiolabeled leukocytes compared with endoscopy and radiologic localization for patients with ulcerative colitis and Crohn's disease (granulomatous or regional enteritis). However, ^{99m}Tc-HMPAO is not usually used to investigate intra-abdominal disease in adults because of its intra-abdominal clearance. If imaging is performed early between 1 and 2 hours, the study can usually be diagnostic before urinary and hepatobiliary clearance occurs, but it allows less time for leukocyte accumulation.

Notes

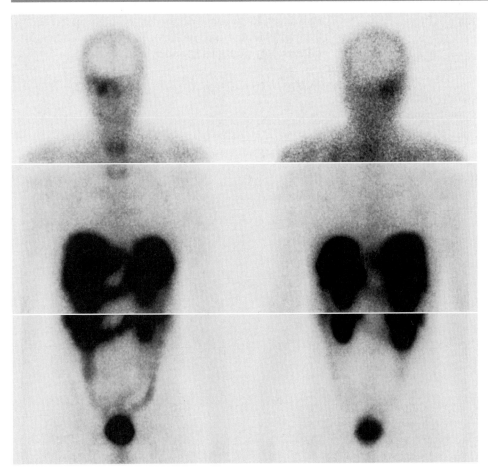

A patient with pulsatile tinnitus. CT shows mass in right temporal bone.

1. What radiopharmaceuticals are applicable?

2. Based on the biodistribution, what agent was used?

3. Describe the findings in the head and neck.

4. Provide the most likely diagnosis and a differential diagnosis.

Oncology: OctreoScan-Glomus Tympanicum

1. ^{111}In-pentetreotide (OctreoScan), ^{123}I-metaiodobenzyl-guanidine (MIBG), ^{131}I-MIBG.

2. Prominent liver, spleen, and kidney uptake is seen with ^{111}In-pentetreotide (OctreoScan).

3. Focal abnormal uptake in the right temporal bone that correlates with CT report.

4. Paraganglioma (glomus tympanicum) considering the patient's history; also meningioma or neuroendocrine tumor metastasis.

References

Krenning EP, Kwekkeboom DJ, Reubi JC, et al: 111In-octreotide scintigraphy in oncology, *Metabolism* 41:83–86, 1992.

Telischi FF, Bustillo A, Whiteman ML, et al: Octreotide scintigraphy for the detection of paragangliomas, *Otolaryngol Head Neck Surg* 122:358–362, 2000.

Cross-Reference

Nuclear Medicine: THE REQUISITES, 3rd ed, pp 279–283.

Comment

Glomus tympanicum and glomus jugulare arise from paraganglioma tissue in the middle ear. Glomus tympanicum, associated with the ninth cranial nerve, usually manifests as pulsatile tinnitus, although other entities can present similarly (e.g., high jugular bulb, aberrant carotid artery, dural arteriovenous malformation, cavernous carotid fistula, meningioma). Glomus tympanicum usually produces symptoms early in the clinical course as a small soft-tissue mass behind the tympanic membrane that markedly enhances. It is critical in preoperative assessment to distinguish among various tympanic masses to avoid a patient with a vascular abnormality being inadvertently sent to the operating room without the surgeon's foreknowledge.

[111]In-pentetreotide (OctreoScan) is a somatostatin analogue that binds to somatostatin receptors on neuroendocrine tumors and numerous other malignancies (e.g., breast cancer, small cell lung cancer, lymphoma). The radiopharmaceutical's sensitivity for detection of tumors varies by malignancy. It has a very high accuracy for carcinoid, gastrinoma, and small cell lung cancer (80–95%), but the accuracy is lower for insulinoma and medullary carcinoma of the thyroid (30–50%). The sensitivity for paragangliomas has been reported to be 86%. The ^{111}In radiolabel allows for delayed imaging at 24 to 48 hours when the target-to-background ratio is optimal.

This is an advantage because of the high uptake in the liver and kidneys (see images). Therapy with somatostatin receptor peptides is under investigation.

Notes

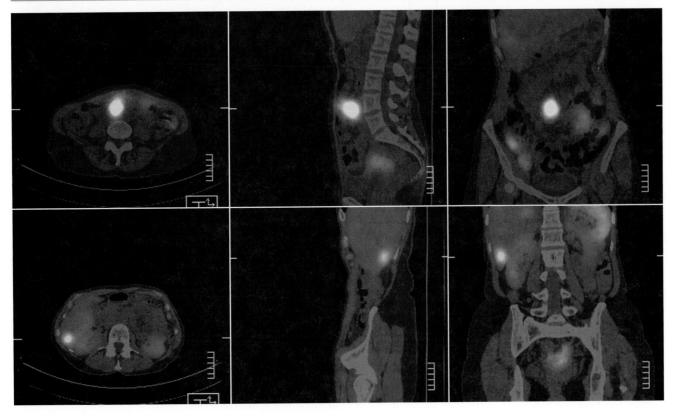

A 58-year-old woman had a carcinoid tumor diagnosed several years ago. Now she presents with recurrent symptoms of flushing and an elevated serum 5-hydroxyindoleacetic acid.

1. What is the radiopharmaceutical and what is its mechanism of uptake?

2. List the category of tumors for which this radiopharmaceutical is particularly useful.

3. Describe the image findings of this study. Provide your interpretation.

4. Name the organs that normally have greatest uptake of the radiopharmaceutical.

Oncology: SPECT-CT, OctreoScan, Carcinoid Tumor

1. ^{111}In-pentetreotide (OctreoScan). The radiopharmaceutical is a somatostatin receptor imaging radiopharmaceutical.

2. Neuroendocrine tumors.

3. SPECT/CT fused images (transverse, sagittal, and coronal slices). Intense uptake in the anterior mid-abdomen and one intense focus in the right lobe of the liver. Metastatic carcinoid tumor.

4. Kidneys and spleen.

References

Gibril F, Reynolds JC, Lubensky IA, et al: Ability of somatostatin receptor scintigraphy to identify patients with gastric carcinoids: a prospective study, *J Nucl Med* 41:1646–1656, 2000.

Krenning EP, Kwekkeboom DJ, Bakker WH, et al: Somatostatin receptor scintigraphy with [111-in-DTPA-Dphe-1] and [123 I-Tyr-3]-octreotide: the Rotterdam experience with more than 1000 patients, *Eur J Nucl Med* 20:716–731, 1993.

Cross-Reference

Nuclear Medicine: THE REQUISITES, 3rd ed, pp 279–283.

Comment

Neuroendocrine tumors are derived from neural crest cells. They can synthesize amines from precursors and produce peptides that act as hormones and neurotransmitters (APUDomas). Many neuroendocrine tumors can be difficult to detect on conventional imaging because of their small size. All have increased somatostatin receptors to varying degrees, and a great many have high tumor uptake with ^{111}In-pentetreotide (OctreoScan) scintigraphy. SPECT and SPECT/CT can help detect small tumors and improve localization compared with planar scans. Imaging is typically performed at 24 hours. Octreotide (Sandostatin), also an analogue of somatostatin, is used therapeutically to suppress tumor growth and symptoms.

Sensitivity for tumor detection with ^{111}In-pentetreotide varies depending on the neuroendocrine tumor: gastrinoma (95%), carcinoid (>80%), glucagonoma (>70%), medullary carcinoma of the thyroid (>50%), and pheochromocytoma and neuroblastoma (>90%). Other nonrelated tumors with tracer-avid somatostatin receptors include small cell lung cancer, lymphoma, and breast cancer. Seventy percent of these tumors take up the ^{111}In-pentetreotide. Uptake also occurs in astrocytomas, meningiomas, and thymomas. Therapeutic analogues labeled with beta emitters are under investigation.

Notes

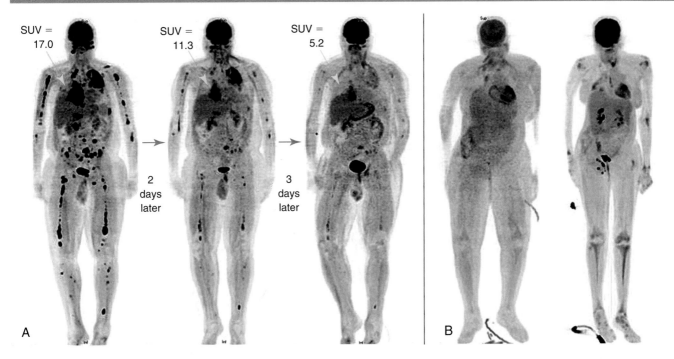

SUV =
17.0

SUV =
11.3

SUV =
5.2

2
days
later

3
days
later

A

B

A, FDG-PET MIP images of the same patient, baseline (*far left*) and subsequent postchemotherapy images.
B, A different patient, initial study (*left*) and 2 months later (*right*).

1. How can the increased abnormal FDG uptake in patient A on initial and subsequent PET imaging be evaluated for determining response to therapy, with attention to the larger chest lesion (*yellow arrows*)?

2. How can this be quantified?

3. How can the obvious weight differences between the two studies for patient B affect image interpretation, and which SUV method of calculation would have been best in this patient?

4. Name some factors that can affect SUV calculation.

FDG-PET: SUV, Body Habitus, Image Quality

1. A reduction in uptake post-therapy suggests a response to therapy (reduction in tumor metabolism). Visual interpretation is the standard accepted method. However, in addition, a semiquantitative index, the SUV, is often used. It is most useful if there is a baseline study for comparison.

2. An ROI is drawn for the focal FDG uptake (e.g., chest lesion in patient A). A ratio of tissue radioactivity concentration and injected dose (mCi) is calculated and corrected for body weight, lean body mass, or body surface area. Thus, it is a unitless value (ratio). A maximum or mean value is calculated.

3. Patient B had fluid overload initially (*left*); edema caused the hazy appearance. In the image on the right, the fluid overload has resolved. An SUV based on lean body mass would have been best for this patient. Although SUVs based on body weight are most commonly used, large changes in body weight will result in overestimation of the SUV when the patient is heavier and underestimation when lighter because of lower FDG uptake in fat.

4. The time interval between imaging and FDG injection, patient size or weight, serum glucose level and endogenous insulin at the time of injection, partial volume effect, and dense material that may be present in the patient when applying attenuation correction (e.g., contrast media).

References

Sugawara Y, Zasadny KR, Neuhoff AW, Wahl RL: Reevaluation of the standardized uptake value for FDG: variations with body weight and methods for correction, *Radiology* 213:521–525, 1999

Thie JA: Understanding the standardized uptake value, its methods, and implications for usage, *J Nucl Med* 45:8–9, 2004.

Cross-Reference

Nuclear Medicine: THE REQUISITES, 3rd ed, pp 313–314.

Comment

Controversy exists regarding the clinical utility of SUVs. There are concerns regarding standardization of the methodology within an institution and between institutions. No absolute cutoff separates benign from malignant lesions. SUVs are best used in serial measurements in the same patient and same lesions to confirm response to therapy. However, the percentage of decrease that represents a partial response is uncertain and varies between publications, institutions, and methodologies. Some centers use SUVs more extensively than others.

Serial SUVs should be calculated at the same time point after FDG injection for each scan. Uptake occurs most rapidly during the first 2 hours after injection, with slower uptake thereafter. If a patient is imaged early, the uptake seen in lesions will be lower, whereas it will be higher at later time points. Partial volume effects occur with small lesions (<1 cm), resulting in artificially low SUVs. Dense material such as barium contrast or metal can cause overcorrection when applying an attenuation-correction method and thereby may affect SUV. High endogenous serum glucose interferes with uptake. Endogenous insulin will push glucose into skeletal muscle, drawing the radiotracer away from tissues of interest and lowering their SUVs.

Notes

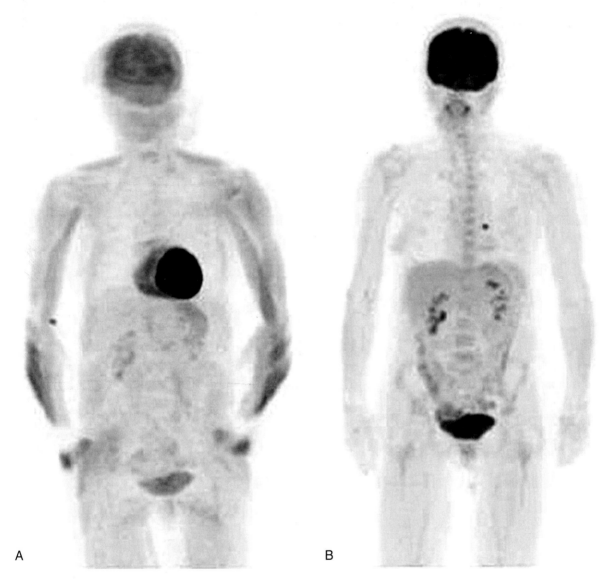

A   B

A patient with recently diagnosed breast cancer. Initial ^{18}F-FDG study (A) and repeat study 8 days later (B).

1. Describe the ^{18}F-FDG distribution and uptake in image A. Is this normal?

2. Describe the change in ^{18}F-FDG uptake from image A to B? Is image B normal?

3. What could explain this change in distribution?

4. What patient preparation is required for FDG-PET imaging?

FDG-PET: Hyperglycemia, Hyperinsulinemia

1. A, Abnormal diffuse FDG uptake in muscles, soft-tissue, and heart. Poor uptake in internal organs.

2. B, Uptake in muscles, soft tissue, and heart is considerably less than in image A. Also increased uptake in brain and internal organs (e.g., liver, kidneys). Focal uptake in the medial left chest was not seen in the previous study. Image B shows normal uptake and distribution.

3. A, Hyperglycemia, hyperinsulinemia, and, in this case, probably strenuous forearm muscular exercise. The patient ate the morning of the study. B, Fasting study.

4. Patients fast for at least 4 hours and refrain from strenuous exercise for 24 hours. Diabetic patients may take long-acting insulin the evening before the study. ^{18}F-FDG injection must be held for at least 2 hours if administration of short-acting insulin is necessary.

References

Bell GI, Kayano T, Buse JB, et al: Molecular biology of mammalian glucose transporters. *Diabetes Care* 13:198–208, 1990.

Hamblen SM, Lowe VJ: Clinical ^{18}F-FDG oncology patient preparation techniques. *J Nucl Med Technol* 31: 3–10, 2003.

Cross-Reference

Nuclear Medicine: THE REQUISITES, 3rd ed, pp 304–306.

Comment

Standardization of patient preparation is important to ensure optimal image quality. Fasting is mandatory. At least 4 hours of fasting; 8 to 12 hours is preferable. A fasting blood sugar greater than 200 mg/dL is not acceptable, and the patient should be rescheduled. At some centers, a trial of short-acting insulin is administered in an effort to decrease blood glucose levels, but not within 2 hours of FDG administration to ensure good image quality.

With hyperinsulinemia, not only is there uptake in soft tissue, there is also reduced uptake in the brain and tumors. In image B, focal uptake is seen in the left chest, the site of the known breast cancer. This was not seen in the initial study (image A). Oral hypoglycemic drugs may be taken as usual. Increased soft-tissue uptake may also be seen in patients with edema, anasarca, heart, kidney, and liver failure and in patients taking steroids.

After injection with ^{18}F-FDG, patients should be kept in a dimly lit room with minimal distractions (e.g., no magazines, music, other people). This is particularly important for brain imaging as these activities will activate regional cerebral cortex. Talking will increase uptake in the larynx. Chewing gum will increase uptake in masticator muscles. The patient should be kept warm to minimize brown fat uptake.

FDG enters muscle cells via the insulin-dependent GLUT4. This is in contrast to cancer cells, in which the primary overexpressed protein is GLUT1 (in some cases, GLUT3), which is not insulin responsive.

Notes

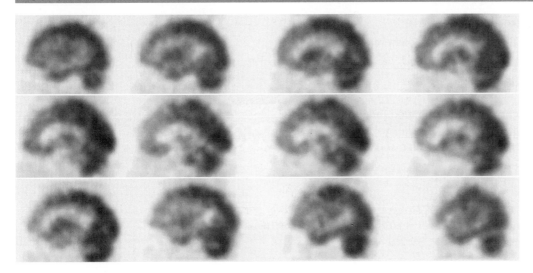

A 55-year-old man has increasing symptoms of dementia. Sagittal SPECT cross-sectional slices are shown.

1. Describe the scintigraphic findings in this patient.

2. What is the likely diagnosis?

3. Which radiopharmaceuticals are used for SPECT brain cerebral perfusion scintigraphy?

4. What is the mechanism of cortical uptake for ^{99m}Tc brain perfusion radiopharmaceuticals?

Central Nervous System: Pick's Disease

1. Reduced blood flow in the frontal cortex bilaterally.

2. Frontal lobe dementia (e.g., Pick's disease).

3. ^{99m}Tc-HMPAO, ^{99m}Tc-ECD.

4. The lipophilic agents cross the intact blood–brain barrier and have prompt intracellular uptake in proportion to cerebral blood flow. They localize and are fixed intracellularly.

Reference

Silverman DH, Mosconi L, Ersoli L, et al: Positron emission tomography scans obtained for the evaluation of cognitive dysfunction, *Semin Nucl Med* 38:251–261, 2008.

Cross-Reference

Nuclear Medicine: THE REQUISITES, 3rd ed, pp 427–432.

Comment

Pick's disease is a neurodegenerative disorder that results in altered cognition and personality changes. Symptoms may include memory loss, confusion, cognitive and speech dysfunction, apathy, and abulia. No treatment exists for Pick's disease, and progressive deterioration occurs over months or years. However, differentiation from Alzheimer's disease and other causes of dementia is important for proper therapy. Functional brain imaging using a ^{99m}Tc brain perfusion agent (HMPAO or ECD) or a metabolic agent (^{18}F-FDG) can reveal decreased function before anatomic changes have occurred. Associated anatomic atrophy may occur later in the disease. In contrast to Alzheimer's disease, which typically involves both posterior parietotemporal regions of the brain, Pick's disease affects the frontal and anterotemporal lobes and spares the posterior cortex. Multi-infarct dementia is characterized by asymmetrical defects in the cortex and deep gray matter. Lewy body disease has a pattern similar to that of Alzheimer's disease, except that there is also hypoperfusion of the occipital cortex.

Notes

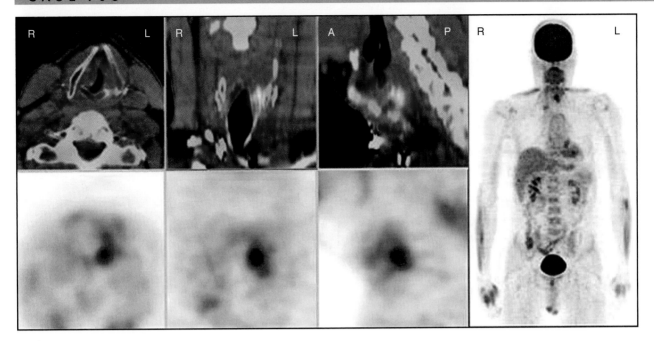

Right, MIP. *Left,* Fused FDG-PET/CT and PET (*left to right:* transverse, coronal, sagittal).

1. Describe the major abnormality on the PET/CT study.

2. What is your interpretation?

3. What are common pathologic causes of asymmetrical uptake in this area?

4. What are physiologic causes of increased vocal cord uptake with FDG?

FDG-PET/CT: Laryngeal Uptake

1. Increased focal uptake in the left arytenoid cartilage and cricoarytenoid muscles and mildly increased uptake in the left vocal cord. CT shows evidence of flaccid right vocal cord with no FDG uptake.

2. Right vocal cord paralysis and secondary compensation by the left vocal cord.

3. Laryngeal nerve damage typically produces decreased uptake on the involved side. Teflon injections, infection and inflammation, and malignancy all produce increased uptake on the involved side.

4. Coughing, humming, and any other type of phonation due to increased glucose utilization of the muscles innervated by the laryngeal nerves.

References

Lee M, Ramaswamy MR, Lilien DL, Nathan CO: Unilateral vocal cord paralysis causes contralateral false-positive positron emission tomography scans of the larynx, *Ann Otol Rhinol Laryngol* 114:202–206, 2005.

Truong MT, Erasmus JJ, Macapinlac H, et al: Teflon injection for vocal cord paralysis: false-positive finding on FDG-PET-CT in a patient with non-small cell lung cancer, *AJR Am J Roentgenol* 182:1587–1589, 2004.

Comment

In this case, a patient with head and neck cancer underwent surgery on the right side resulting in damage to his recurrent laryngeal nerve, causing right-sided vocal cord paralysis. The unaffected vocal cord appears active on FDG-PET, with intense uptake due to increased glucose consumption as a compensatory mechanism. Thus, increased FDG uptake does not always mean pathology.

Laryngeal cancers usually have prominent increased uptake. Most are of squamous cell origin. For tumor staging, the larynx is divided into three regions: the glottis (true vocal cords, anterior and posterior commissures), the supraglottis (epiglottis, arytenoids, aryepiglottic folds, and false cords), and the subglottis. Most laryngeal cancers originate in the glottis. Supraglottic cancers are less common, and the subglottic tumors least frequent. Smoking is the major risk factor. Patients with a history of head and neck cancer are at a higher risk for the development of a second head and neck cancer or lung cancer.

Most whole-body PET/CT scans are obtained from the eyes to thighs as a whole-body scan. However, for head and neck cancer, many institutions acquire separate acquisitions of the head and neck and the remainder of the body to ensure good images of the area of interest. Patients are requested to refrain from vocalization or phonation. All possible efforts should be made to ensure that the patient is comfortable and still and in a quiet room before injection so that movement and talking after FDG injection can be minimized.

Notes

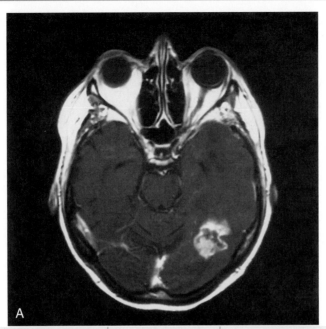

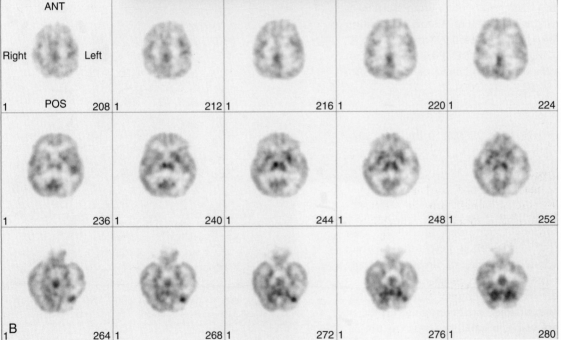

A 54-year-old patient with bronchogenic carcinoma metastatic to the brain was treated with stereotactic radiosurgery for a metastasis in the left temporoparietal region 6 months previously. A, Subsequent MRI could not differentiate post-therapy changes from viable tumor. B, FDG brain scan transaxial slices.

1. What is the relative accuracy of FDG-PET versus CT or MRI for initial diagnosis of malignant brain tumor?

2. What is the relative accuracy of FDG-PET versus CT/MRI for differentiating recurrent or persistent tumor versus postradiation necrosis?

3. Describe the image findings and interpret the transaxial images (B) of FDG-PET of the brain.

4. List clinically useful single-photon radiotracers for brain tumor imaging and describe the expected findings.

Oncology: ^{18}F-FDG-PET—Bronchogenic Cancer Metastatic to the Brain

1. CT and MRI are more sensitive for tumor detection. Normal brain uses only glucose for metabolism and has higher ^{18}F-FDG uptake than any other organ. This high background can make tumor detection difficult.

2. FDG-PET is more accurate than CT or MRI for determining whether post-therapy changes are the result of residual/recurrent tumor or radiation necrosis.

3. Focal increased uptake in the left temporoparietal region that correlates with the lesion on MRI. This is consistent with viable residual or recurrent tumor.

4. ^{201}Tl- and ^{99m}Tc-sestamibi have increased uptake in tumors. Tumors usually are cold on ^{99m}Tc-HMPAO/ECD.

References

Griffeth LK, Rich KM, Dehdasti F, et al: Brain metastases from non-central nervous system tumors: evaluation with PET, *Radiology* 186:37–44, 1993.

Hagge RJ, Wong TZ, Coleman RE: Positron emission tomography: brain tumors and lung cancer, *Radiol Clin North Am* 39:871–882, 2001.

Cross-Reference

Nuclear Medicine: THE REQUISITES, 3rd ed, pp 302–323.

Comment

The brain has the greatest FDG uptake of any organ. This results in high background, making detection of increased uptake in primary or metastatic tumors difficult. Because FDG-PET is insensitive for initial detection of brain metastases, PET whole-body imaging does not usually include the whole brain at most centers.

After surgery and radiation therapy, CT and MRI often have difficulty differentiating post-therapy necrotic or fibrotic masses from viable residual or recurrent tumor. Surgical biopsy is not always possible and has associated morbidity. Increased uptake in a previously treated region suggests recurrence. Abnormal increased uptake in white matter is always abnormal. FDG-PET can be diagnostic and thus can direct therapy. If positive on PET/CT, biopsy may follow, if possible. FDG-PET also is proving useful for radiation therapy planning. Fusion of FDG-PET and MRI or CT studies can help direct the radiation beam to the residual tumor within a heterogeneous tumor mass.

Notes

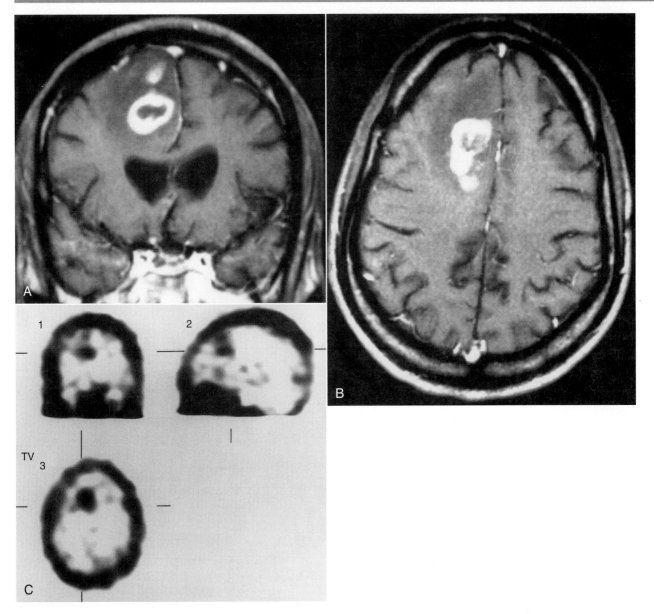

A 35-year-old-man with AIDS has a new intracranial abnormality on MRI (A and B) of uncertain etiology. SPECT study (C1, coronal; C2, sagittal; C3, transverse) was ordered to assist in the differential diagnosis.

1. What is the single-photon radiopharmaceutical?

2. What is the differential diagnosis before the SPECT study?

3. What is the likely diagnosis after the radionuclide study?

4. What is the accuracy of the radionuclide method?

Oncology: ^{201}Tl—Intracranial Lymphoma in AIDS

1. ^{201}Tl is the standard single-photon radiopharmaceutical used in these cases and was used in this instance. ^{99m}Tc-sestamibi also can be used; however, it is taken up by the choroid plexus and could pose interpretative problems in some cases.

2. Tumor, particularly malignant lymphoma, versus infection, usually toxoplasmosis, or other opportunistic infections (e.g., cytomegalic inclusion virus, herpes simplex, *Cryptococcus*).

3. Malignant lymphoma.

4. 85% to 90%.

References

Hoffman JM, Waskin HA, Shifter T, et al: FDG-PET in differentiating lymphoma from non-malignant CNS lesions in patients with AIDS, *J Nucl Med* 34:567–575, 1993.

O'Malley JP, Ziessman HA, Kumar PN, et al: Diagnosis of intracranial lymphoma in patients with AIDS: value of 201-Tl single-photon emission computed tomography, *AJR Am J Roentgenol* 163:417–421, 1994.

Skiest DJ, Erdman W, Chang WE, et al: SPECT thallium-201 combined with toxoplasma serology for the presumptive diagnosis of focal central nervous system lesions in AIDS patients, *J Infect* 40:274–281, 2000.

Cross-Reference

Nuclear Medicine: THE REQUISITES, 3rd ed, pp 314–316, 418.

Comment

Toxoplasma gondii is the most common cause of focal encephalitis in patients with AIDS. However, intracranial lymphoma is increasing in incidence and is the second most common cause; it is a very aggressive and often lethal disease. CT and MRI are not reliable for distinguishing between tumor and infectious causes. Both may appear as ring-enhancing lesions on MRI. Often, patients are treated empirically for toxoplasmosis, and biopsy is performed only if therapy yields no response. However, a clinical response may take at a minimum several days and as long as many weeks. Drug toxicity is high. Prompt therapy of these aggressive tumors would be optimal. ^{201}Tl has also been used to distinguish radiation necrosis from viable tumor in patients with treated brain tumors who have equivocal or suspicious MRIs. ^{201}Tl is taken up in many benign and malignant tumors. Although resolution is not high, the ^{201}Tl target-to-background ratio is very high, allowing straightforward interpretation. Tumors have high uptake, whereas infections usually have poor uptake. SPECT is mandatory.

Notes

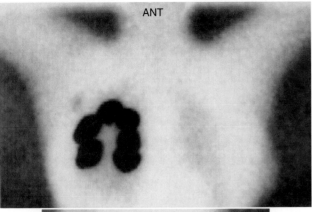

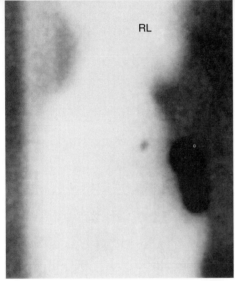

A 49-year-old woman was referred for breast sentinel node lymphoscintigraphy after recent right breast mass biopsy that was diagnostic of breast cancer.

1. What prognostic information is provided by axillary node dissection in newly diagnosed breast cancer?

2. What is a sentinel node? What is the purpose of radionuclide sentinel node scintigraphy?

3. What is the purpose of sentinel node biopsy?

4. What is the radiopharmaceutical used, and how is the study performed?

Oncology: Breast Cancer
Lymphoscintigraphy

1. Metastasis to axillary nodes is the best predictor of post-treatment recurrence and death. Adjuvant chemotherapy is indicated.

2. A sentinel node is the first node drained by the lymphatics in a nodal basin. Lymphoscintigraphy can detect the sentinel node.

3. If the sentinel node biopsy is tumor negative, no further axillary node dissection is needed. If positive, axillary dissection is performed.

4. The pharmaceutical most commonly used is filtered ^{99m}Tc-SC. It is injected around the lesion or biopsy site. Imaging is usually but not always performed. At surgery, a specialized small gamma probe is used to help locate the sentinel node.

References

Aarsvold JN, Alazraki NP: Update on detection of sentinel lymph nodes in patients with breast cancer, *Semin Nucl Med* 35:116–128, 2005.

Krag D, Weaver D, Ashikaga T, et al: The sentinel lymph node in breast cancer: a multicenter validation study, *N Engl J Med* 339:941–974, 1998.

Cross-Reference

Nuclear Medicine: THE REQUISITES, 3rd ed, pp 299–300.

Comment

In the absence of systemic adjuvant therapy, the chance for recurrence within 10 years is 24% in patients without nodal metastasis on histologic examination and 76% for patients with nodal metastasis. Clinical evaluation of the axilla for abnormal nodes is not predictive; almost 40% of patients have metastases to axillary nodes that are not detected clinically. More than 80% of women who undergo axillary node dissection have at least one postoperative complication, commonly, lymphedema, which is associated with long-term morbidity.

The rationale for lymphoscintigraphy is to detect the sentinel node so that it can be biopsied. The status of the sentinel node predicts whether nodal metastases are present. Many studies have shown high accuracy for lymphoscintigraphy. Surgeons use a specialized gamma probe in the operating room to help locate the sentinel node. Blue dye may also be used at surgery to identify the sentinel lymph node. Timing for the blue dye is critical because it transits quickly and can flood the field. The combination of both methods may have the highest accuracy.

Filtered ^{99m}Tc-SC is most commonly used for radionuclide sentinel node lymphoscintigraphy in the United States. Various methods of injection are used (e.g., peritumoral, intracutaneous, periareolar). Typically, a total of 0.8 to 1 mCi is injected intracutaneously. Imaging usually is completed within an hour. Lateral and anterior views are needed to localize the sentinel node.

Notes

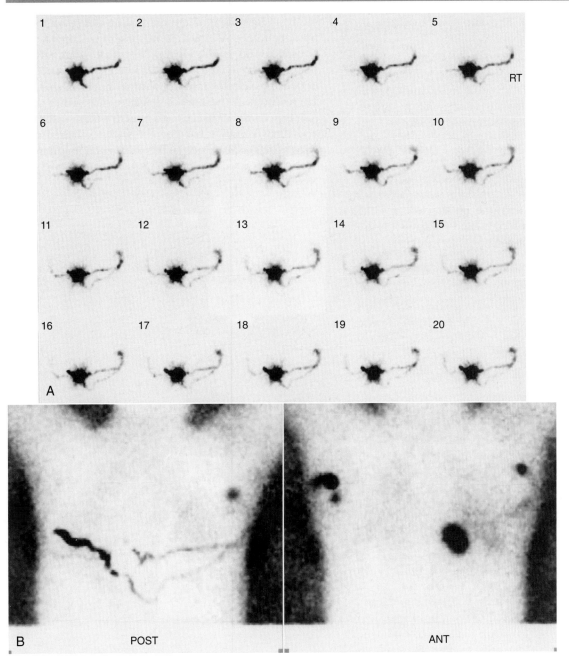

Sentinel node lymphoscintigraphy was performed in a patient with recently diagnosed malignant melanoma in the mid-left posterior thorax. One-minute sequential posterior images (A) are followed by anterior and posterior static images (B). A round lead shield was placed over the injection site on the static posterior images (cold).

1. What is the purpose of melanoma sentinel node lymphoscintigraphy?

2. Describe the study findings. What is the black background in images B?

3. What is the normal drainage of a mid posterior chest or flank lesion?

4. How are patients with melanoma selected for lymphoscintigraphy?

Oncology: Malignant Melanoma, Sentinel Node Lymphoscintigraphy

1. Lymphatic flow can be quite variable and unpredictable regarding which nodal basin the lymphatics will drain to. This is particularly true in the mid-posterior back. In extremities, in-transit nodes may be the sentinel node, which would otherwise be missed.

2. Drainage to the right axilla through two separate lymphatic channels and also lymphatic flow to the left axilla. Nodal uptake in the right axilla is seen on the static posterior view. The anterior view shows two right sentinel nodes and one on the left. A cobalt transmission source placed behind the patient is used to show the body contour.

3. Drainage is unpredictable and may drain to either axillary or inguinal regions.

4. Prognosis is determined by skin lesion depth. Those less than 1 mm are low risk and rarely metastasize; those deeper than 4 mm often metastasize. Patients with intermediate-thickness lesions are referred for preoperative sentinel node lymphoscintigraphy.

References

Berman CG, Choi J, Hersh MR, et al: Melanoma lymphoscintigraphy and lymphatic mapping, *Semin Nucl Med* 30:49–55, 2000.

Scarsbrook AF, Ganeshan A, Bradley KM: Pearls and pitfalls of radionuclide imaging of the lymphatic system. Part 1: sentinel node lymphoscintigraphy in malignant melanoma, *Br J Radiol* 80:132–139, 2007.

Cross-Reference
Nuclear Medicine: THE REQUISITES, 3rd, pp 299–300.

Comment
Regional lymph node sampling is routine clinical practice for the staging of malignant melanoma. Cutaneous melanomas originate from cells located between the dermis and epidermis and drain to the lymphatics in the reticular dermis. Thus, the radiopharmaceutical is best administered with intradermal injection in melanoma patients. As skin melanoma lesions progress, they move deeper into the dermis. Spread from the primary tumor to local lymph nodes occurs before systemic metastases. The pattern of lymphatic drainage is highly variable between patients. In many cases, there is drainage to a solitary regional sentinel node. However, for melanomas located in the midline of the head, neck, and trunk, there may be quite variable drainage. Axillary and femoral regions must be imaged. The current approach is to locate the first lymph node (i.e., the sentinel node) that drains the nodal basin. This sentinel node is located on the lymphoscintigram and marked on the patient's skin preoperatively. At the time of surgery, a gamma probe is used to aid in the localization of the sentinel node that is then removed for pathologic examination. If the node is positive for tumor, the other nodes in that basin are resected. If the node is negative, no further dissection is performed. Because no effective therapy for melanoma exists once it has become widely metastatic, this aggressive surgical approach is now in common use.

Notes

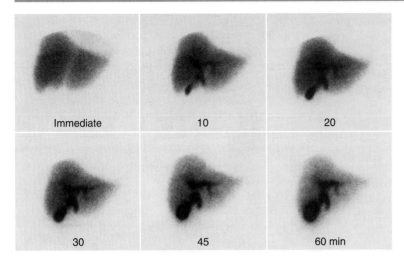

A 43-year-old woman was hospitalized with recent onset of abdominal pain, nausea, and vomiting. She last ate more than 24 hours previously.

1. What are the cholescintigraphic findings?

2. What clinical information would be helpful to correctly interpret the study?

3. What is the differential diagnosis?

4. What would you do next?

Hepatobiliary System: Delayed Biliary-to-Bowel Transit

1. Normal hepatic function, early gallbladder filling, and secretion into biliary ducts; however, no radiotracer clearance from the common duct or biliary-to-bowel transit.

2. Is the patient receiving narcotics? Was sincalide (cholecystokinin octapeptide [CCK-8]) administered before the study?

3. Partial common duct obstruction, functional obstruction caused by sincalide administered before the study, recent narcotic administration, or normal variation.

4. Obtain delayed images at 2 to 3 hours or administer sincalide. The latter would give the answer more promptly.

References

Kim CK, Palestro C, Solomon R, et al: Delayed biliary-to-bowel transit in cholescintigraphy after cholecystokinin treatment, *Radiology* 176:553–556, 1990.

Ziessman HA: Acute cholecystitis, biliary obstruction, biliary extravasation, *Semin Nucl Med* 33:279–295, 2003.

Cross-Reference

Nuclear Medicine: THE REQUISITES, 3rd ed, pp 177–180.

Comment

This study is suspicious for partial common duct obstruction. High-grade obstruction shows hepatic uptake without secretion into the biliary tract (persistent hepatogram) because of the high intrabiliary backpressure. However, with partial common duct obstruction, intraductal pressure is not as high and the ^{99m}Tc-iminodiacetic acid is secreted into the biliary tract but clears poorly into the bowel.

Other causes of delayed biliary-to-bowel transit should be considered in addition to obstruction. In this case, sincalide (Kinevac) was infused before the study to empty the gallbladder because the patient had no oral intake for more than 24 hours. Prestudy sincalide is a common reason for delayed biliary-to-bowel transit. As the gallbladder relaxes after sincalide-stimulated contraction, the resulting negative intravesical filling pressure causes bile to preferentially flow toward the gallbladder rather than through the common duct. Recent opiate administration will cause a pattern of partial biliary obstruction. Opiates should be held for at least 6 hours before the study. Delayed biliary-to-bowel transit is seen with chronic cholecystitis and has been reported in 10%

to 20% of normal subjects. Obtaining delayed images or sincalide infusion can confirm or exclude partial common duct obstruction. The 2.5-minute serum half-life of sincalide allows repeat administration. In a nonobstructed duct, CCK-8 relaxes the sphincter of Oddi and results in prompt biliary-to-bowel transit. Sincalide has a major advantage over delayed imaging in that the answer is known within 30 minutes.

A partial biliary obstruction (e.g., due to cholelithiasis) may show some clearance into the bowel. Biliary clearance does not exclude a partial obstruction. However, the common duct will have poor clearance. Thus, it is important see biliary duct clearance as well as biliary-to-bowel transit to exclude biliary obstruction.

Notes

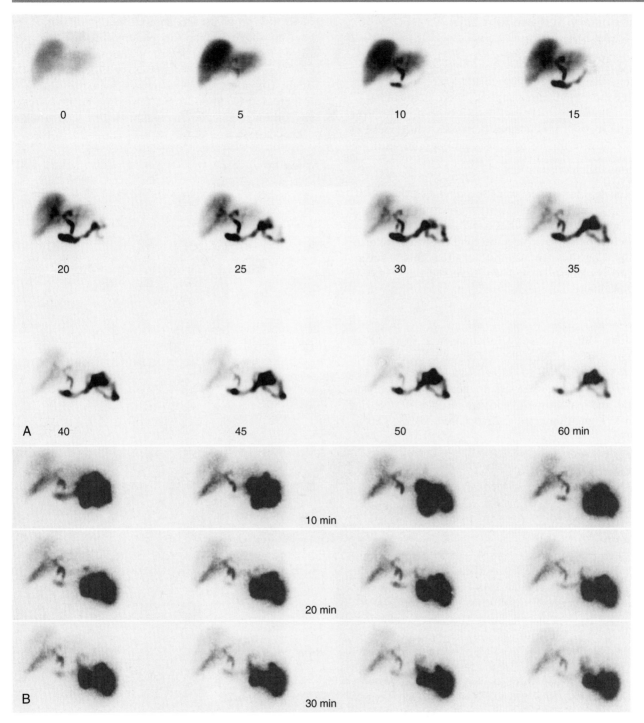

0   5   10   15

20   25   30   35

A   40   45   50   60 min

10 min

20 min

B   30 min

Acute abdominal pain developed in 63-year-old woman today. She has been hospitalized for 9 days after multiple traumatic injuries. She is receiving hyperalimentation. Ultrasonography was normal. A, 60-minute cholescintigraphy. B, Additional 30-minute images after administration of morphine.

1. What preparation should this patient have had before the study?

2. Describe the cholescintigraphic findings before and after morphine.

3. Interpret the study.

4. What additional information can you give the surgeon?

Hepatobiliary System: Rim Sign

1. Sincalide (CCK-8) before the study because of fasting and hyperalimentation.

2. Nonvisualization of the gallbladder after 60 minutes. After morphine administration, there is no filling of the gallbladder. Increased uptake is seen in the liver in the region of the gallbladder fossa, which persists after most of the liver has washed out (rim sign).

3. Acute acalculous cholecystitis.

4. In the setting of concurrent severe illness, there is an increased incidence of false-positive studies for acute cholecystitis. On the other hand, the rim sign is very specific for acute cholecystitis and confirms the diagnosis. The rim sign also indicates that this is severe acute cholecystitis, with an increased likelihood of gallbladder gangrene and perforation.

References

Brachman MB, Tanasescu DE, Ramanna L, et al: Acute gangrenous cholecystitis: radionuclide diagnosis, *Radiology* 151:209–221, 1984.

Meekin GK, Ziessman HA, Klappenbach RS: Prognostic value and pathophysiologic significance of the rim sign in cholescintigraphy, *J Nucl Med* 28:1679–1682, 1987.

Cross-Reference

Nuclear Medicine: THE REQUISITES, 3rd ed, pp 168–174.

Comment

With severe acute cholecystitis, gallbladder inflammation can spread from the inflamed gallbladder wall to the adjacent hepatic parenchyma. In these cases, surgeons note an inflammatory exudate causing adherence of the gallbladder to the adjacent liver. This severe inflammatory reaction is the cause of the rim sign. Because of increased blood flow to the inflamed region, more tracer is delivered and extracted by the hepatocytes with high efficiency. There may also be reduced hepatocyte ability to clear the tracer and possible local obstruction of bile canaliculi due to inflammatory edema. The rim sign is seen in 25% to 35% of patients with acute cholecystitis. Thus, its sensitivity for acute cholecystitis is poor. However, its specificity for acute cholecystitis is very high.

The pathophysiologic progression of acute cholecystitis follows a well-described course. After cystic duct obstruction, there is reduced venous and lymphatic flow, resulting in mucosal congestion and edema, then polymorphonuclear cells infiltrate the gallbladder wall, and, if unchecked, hemorrhage and necrosis occur.

Finally, this progresses to gangrene and perforation. The rim sign suggests that the patient's disease has progressed far along this spectrum. The high specificity of this sign significantly increases confidence that the patient has acute cholecystitis, even in the setting of an increased likelihood for a false-positive study result (e.g., prolonged fasting, hyperalimentation, concomitant serious illness).

Notes

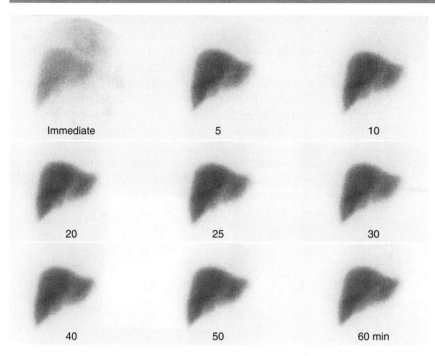

Immediate   5   10

20   25   30

40   50   60 min

A 50-year-old woman has acute onset of abdominal pain of 4 hours' duration. Ultrasonography is normal.

1. What are the cholescintigraphic findings?

2. Is further imaging needed?

3. What is the differential diagnosis?

4. What is the most likely diagnosis?

Hepatobiliary System: High-Grade Biliary Obstruction

1. Good liver function (blood pool clearance by 5 minutes), prompt hepatic uptake, no excretion into the biliary ducts or biliary-to-bowel transit by 60 minutes.

2. Delayed imaging is important if there is evidence of liver dysfunction.

3. High-grade biliary obstruction, cholestatic jaundice, cholangitis, hepatic dysfunction.

4. High-grade biliary obstruction. Cholangitis is usually caused by obstruction and looks similar. Hepatic dysfunction would have delayed blood pool (heart) clearance and high background. If the patient has hepatic dysfunction, delayed imaging is required to separate obstruction from primary liver dysfunction. This is not the clinical picture of cholestatic jaundice (e.g., drug induced). It does not present with pain.

References

Ziessman HA: Acute cholecystitis, biliary obstruction, biliary extravasation, *Semin Nucl Med* 33:279–295, 2003.

Ziessman HA, Zeman RK, Akin EA: Cholescintigraphy: correlation with other hepatobiliary imaging modalities. In: Sandler MP, Coleman RE (eds): *Diagnostic Nuclear Medicine*, 4th ed. Philadelphia: Lippincott Williams & Wilkins, 2003, pp 503–529.

Cross-Reference

Nuclear Medicine: THE REQUISITES, 3rd ed, pp 177–187.

Comment

The pathophysiologic sequence of events in high-grade biliary obstruction progresses in a predictable manner: obstruction, increased intraductal pressure, reduced bile flow, biliary duct dilation, increased cellular permeability, and finally fibrogenesis leading to cirrhosis. The degree of bile duct dilation varies but is directly related to the duration, degree, and cause of obstruction. Dilation is most prevalent in long-standing obstruction, especially when caused by malignancy. Patients with early high-grade, low-grade, or intermittent biliary obstruction may not have dilated ducts. Benign causes of obstruction are less likely to cause significant dilation of the biliary tract. In some cases, ductal dilation may be restricted by edema and scarring as a result of infection or cirrhosis. Once dilated, biliary ducts often remain so even after resolution, for example, after the stone has passed or surgery has relieved the obstruction. Discordance often exists between the physiologic scintigraphic results and the morphologic images of ultrasonography and CT.

Dilation may not become evident until 24 to 72 hours after acute obstruction. Ultrasonography often is the first imaging study in the setting of biliary obstruction. However, in the absence of dilated biliary ducts, cholescintigraphy is indicated. The cholescintigraphic pattern of obstruction becomes manifest soon after the acute event. Cholescintigraphy is required to diagnose or exclude obstruction in patients with previous biliary dilation and suspected acute obstruction. Biliary obstruction may occur without jaundice. Obstruction does not always result in ductal dilation. Dilation can be present without obstruction.

Notes

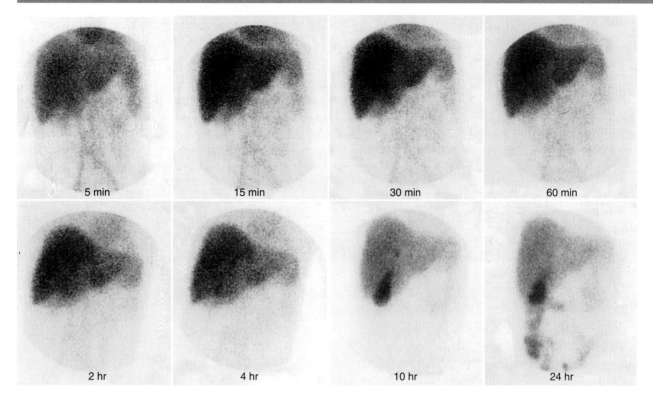

5 min   15 min   30 min   60 min

2 hr   4 hr   10 hr   24 hr

A 50-year-old man with abdominal discomfort and hyperbilirubinemia for several months.

1. Describe the cholescintigraphic findings.

2. What is the differential diagnosis at 60 minutes? At 2 hours?

3. What is the diagnosis at 10 hours?

4. What is your diagnosis at 24 hours?

C A S E 1 1 4

Hepatobiliary System: Hepatic Dysfunction

1. Poor hepatic function with delayed blood pool clearance (heart, great vessels) and background clearance. No secretion into biliary system at 60 minutes. At 2 hours, unchanged; at 10 hours, gallbladder filling is seen; and at 24 hours, there is biliary-to-bowel transit.

2. Biliary obstruction with secondary hepatic insufficiency versus primary hepatic dysfunction.

3. Cystic duct obstruction has been excluded; biliary obstruction is not excluded.

4. Severe hepatic dysfunction. Negative for biliary duct obstruction.

References

Ziessman HA: Acute cholecystitis, biliary obstruction, biliary extravasation, *Semin Nucl Med* 33:279–295, 2003.

Ziessman HA, Zeman RK, Akin EA: Cholescintigraphy: correlation with other hepatobiliary imaging modalities. In: Sandler MP, Coleman RE (eds): *Diagnostic Nuclear Medicine*, 4th ed. Philadelphia: Lippincott Williams & Wilkins, 2003, pp 503–529.

Cross-Reference

Nuclear Medicine: THE REQUISITES, 3rd ed, pp 177–187.

Comment

With recent onset of high-grade biliary obstruction, hepatic function usually remains good. With persistent obstruction, secondary hepatic insufficiency may result. If radiotracer fills the biliary system and transits the common duct into the intestine without evidence of retention, the cause is not obstruction. With partial obstruction, there is retention of activity proximal to the site of obstruction, even though some bowel transit may be seen.

Cholescintigraphy can differentiate primary parenchymal disease from diseases that require surgical intervention (e.g., biliary obstruction). In this case, the liver does not appear small or have a relatively large left lobe as in end-stage cirrhosis. This patient probably has acute or subacute hepatic disease. Patients with hepatic insufficiency do not have abdominal pain, although they may have abdominal discomfort caused by hepatosplenomegaly and ascites.

With normal hepatic function, less than 9% of ^{99m}Tc-disofenin (Hepatolite) is excreted through the kidneys compared with less than 1% for ^{99m}Tc-mebrofenin (Choletec). With increasing hepatic dysfunction, more of the radiotracer is excreted through the kidneys.

^{99m}Tc-mebrofenin is preferable to disofenin with hepatic insufficiency because of its greater hepatic extraction (98% vs. 88%).

Notes

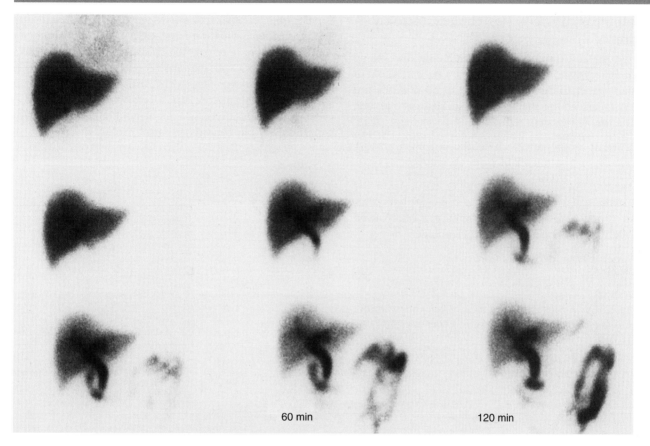

60 min   120 min

A 39-year-old woman has been having recurrent abdominal pain since her cholecystectomy 12 months ago. Ultrasonography findings are normal.

1. Describe the cholescintigraphic findings.

2. What is the differential diagnosis?

3. How is the 120-minute image helpful?

4. Magnetic resonance cholangiopancreatography and endoscopic retrograde cholangiopancreatography showed no stone or stricture. What is the likely diagnosis?

Hepatobiliary System: Postcholecystectomy Syndrome

1. Good hepatic function and prompt bile duct filling and biliary-to-bowel transit. However, retention of biliary tracer in the common duct at 60 minutes and no decrease and probably further increase in bile duct retention at 120 minutes.

2. Recurrent or retained cholelithiasis, inflammatory stricture, and sphincter of Oddi obstruction.

3. If the bile duct cleared well (>50%) between 60 and 120 minutes, this is most likely a nonobstructed dilation. If not, a partial biliary obstruction is likely, even though there is biliary-to-bowel clearance.

4. Sphincter of Oddi dysfunction.

References

Ziessman HA: Acute cholecystitis, biliary obstruction, biliary extravasation, *Semin Nucl Med* 33:279-295, 2003.

Ziessman HA, Zeman RK, Akin EA: Cholescintigraphy: correlation with other hepatobiliary imaging modalities. In: Sandler MP, Coleman RE (eds): *Diagnostic Nuclear Medicine*, 4th ed. Philadelphia: Lippincott Williams & Wilkins, 2003, pp 503-529.

Cross-Reference

Nuclear Medicine: THE REQUISITES, 3rd ed, pp 182-186.

Comment

The postcholecystectomy syndrome describes a group of patients who have recurrent biliary pain after cholecystectomy. The reason may be that they never had cholecystitis, and the diagnosis has not been made. However, the most common causes of recurrent pain after cholecystectomy are residual or recurrent stones. An inflammatory stricture is less common. If the latter is excluded, sphincter of Oddi dysfunction may be the cause.

Sphincter of Oddi dysfunction is essentially a partial biliary obstruction at the level of the sphincter of Oddi. Some are fixed obstructions and others are intermittent (dysfunction). It is thought that the disease becomes symptomatic after cholecystectomy because the gallbladder acts as a pressure relief for transiently elevated biliary pressure. Therapy is usually sphincterotomy.

Ultrasonography and magnetic resonance cholangiopancreatography can confirm biliary dilation and exclude tumor, but they cannot exclude small stones. At some centers, cholescintigraphy is used as a screening test. A normal study excludes partial biliary obstruction, and the diagnostic effort can be turned to nonbiliary causes. If a partial biliary obstruction is suggested on cholescintigraphy, further evaluation is necessary (e.g., cholangiography, endoscopic retrograde cholangiopancreatography). Sphincter of Oddi manometry is sometimes used to confirm sphincter of Oddi obstruction; however, it is performed only at specialized centers, and even in experienced hands, there is a high incidence of morbidity, particularly pancreatitis.

Notes

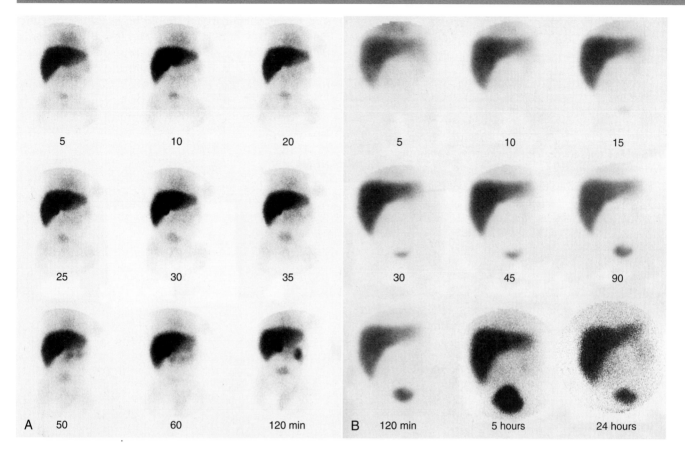

Patients A and B are 4 weeks old, have hyperbilirubinemia, and were referred to rule out biliary atresia.

1. What is the differential diagnosis of hyperbilirubinemia in this age group?

2. What patient preparation is required before the cholescintigraphic study?

3. What are the scintigraphic findings on these studies and your interpretations?

4. What is the accuracy of cholescintigraphy to diagnose biliary atresia?

C A S E 1 1 6

Hepatobiliary System: Biliary Atresia

1. Inflammatory, infectious, and metabolic causes of neonatal hepatitis versus biliary atresia.

2. Phenobarbital 5 mg/kg/day for 3 to 5 days before the study.

3. A, Delayed blood pool clearance (note heart) suggestive of hepatic insufficiency. Biliary clearance at 50 minutes and increasing through 120 minutes. Note the medial edge of the gallbladder. B, Good liver function. No secretion into biliary ducts during the initial 120 minutes or at 5 and 24 hours. Case B is consistent with biliary atresia and case A with neonatal hepatitis.

4. Sensitivity 97%, specificity 82%.

References

Majd M, Reba RC, Altman RP: Effect of phenobarbital on 99mTc-IDA scintigraphy in the evaluation of neonatal jaundice, *Semin Nucl Med* 11:194–199, 1981.

Treves ST, Jones AG, Markisz BA: Liver and spleen. In: *Pediatric Nuclear Medicine,* 3rd ed. New York: Springer, 2007, pp 213–217.

Cross-Reference

Nuclear Medicine: THE REQUISITES, 3rd ed, pp 180–183.

Comment

Neonatal hepatitis and biliary atresia have similar clinical, biochemical, and histologic findings. Early diagnosis is critical because surgery is most successful during the first 3 months of life. The pathologic process of biliary atresia is that of a progressive sclerosing cholangitis of the extrahepatic biliary system. Periportal fibrosis and intrahepatic proliferation of small bile ducts are characteristic. Major biliary ducts are partially or totally absent. Cirrhosis ultimately develops. A surgical Kasai procedure is performed; ultimately, liver transplantation is required. The extrahepatic damaged ducts are removed, and a direct connection is made between the liver and intestines (hepatoportoenterostomy).

Numerous liver diseases mimic biliary atresia. Generally referred to as neonatal hepatitis, they include infectious agents (cytomegalic virus, hepatitis A and B, rubella, toxoplasma) and metabolic defects (α_1-antitrypsin deficiency, inborn errors of metabolism).

Pretreatment with phenobarbital maximizes the test's sensitivity by activating liver excretory enzymes. Although with neonatal hepatitis, the biliary system is patent, ^{99m}Tc-iminodiacetic acid uptake and clearance are delayed because of hepatic insufficiency. Biliary-to-bowel transit is variable but is usually seen by 24 hours.

The serum phenobarbital should be in the therapeutic range. The lack of biliary-to-bowel transit by 24 hours is highly sensitive for biliary atresia. False-positive findings sometimes occur due to severe hepatic dysfunction. A repeat study a few days to a week later can usually confirm the correct diagnosis. Definitive diagnosis is made by transhepatic cholangiography, laparotomy, or laparoscopy.

Notes

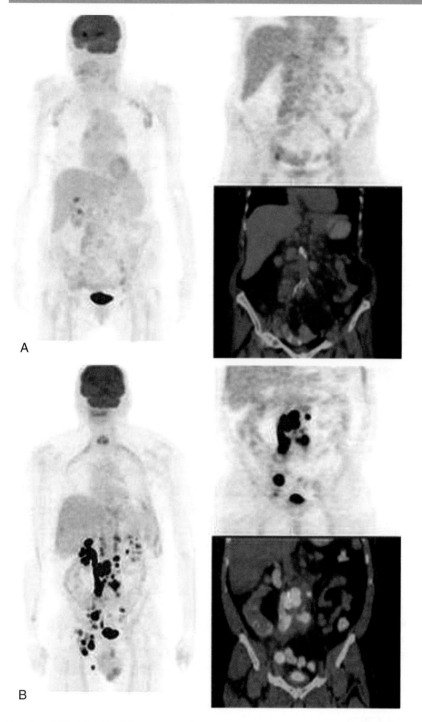

A

B

Staging FDG-PET/CT images of two patients (A and B) with newly diagnosed non-Hodgkin's lymphoma. *Left,* MIP; *right,* coronal FDG-PET (*top*), fused PET/CT (*below*).

1. Describe abnormal uptake in these two patients. Explain the differences in uptake.

2. What are the advantages of FDG/PET compared with CT for staging malignant lymphoma?

3. What response parameters are used to assess therapy effectiveness with FDG-PET?

4. What potentially urgent/emergent finding is seen in one of the two patients?

Oncology: FDG-PET—Non-Hodgkin's Lymphoma

1. A, Mild but extensive increased FDG uptake in axillae and iliac nodes. B, Intense uptake in the abdomen and pelvis, retroperitoneal, internal and external iliac regions. A, Low-grade malignancy. B, High-grade malignancy.

2. CT relies on assessment of lymph node size and morphology to detect malignant involvement. Normal-appearing nodes may harbor malignancy. Enlarged nodes may be inflammatory in origin. FDG uptake can be seen in nodes of normal size and can confirm or exclude pathology in CT enlarged nodes.

3. A reduction in FDG uptake (SUV) from baseline uptake of 25% to 50% suggests a partial response to treatment; reduction of uptake down to background or blood pool suggests a complete response.

4. Retention of tracer in the right kidney pelvis, calices, and ureter suggests urinary outflow obstruction, and in case B was confirmed by Lasix renography.

References

Cheson BD: Staging and evaluation of the patient with lymphoma, *Hematol Oncol Clin North Am* 22:825–837, 2008.

Hutchings M, Barringston SF: PET/CT for therapy response assessment in lymphoma, *J Nucl Med* 50: 21S–30S, 2009.

Cross-Reference

Nuclear Medicine: THE REQUISITES, 3rd ed, pp 333–337.

Comment

Patient A has stage III disease according to the Ann Arbor Staging System with adenopathy above and below the diaphragm. Patient B has disease only below the diaphragm, thus stage II. Neither has evidence of liver, spleen, lung, or bone involvement.

FDG-PET/CT has superior accuracy compared with CT in patients with Hodgkin's and aggressive non-Hodgkin's lymphoma (94% vs. 89%) and changes management (upstaging/downstaging) in 10% to 30%. It can differentiate active residual disease from inactive residual masses with an accuracy of 90% versus 45% for CT. PET has a high negative predictive value, but does not totally exclude the presence of microscopic disease. The negative predictive value of FDG-PET after two to three cycles of chemotherapy is 80% to 100%. Patients with early PET response have a better 5-year event-free survival rate: 89% if PET findings are negative; 59% if minimal uptake on PET; and 16% if PET findings are positive.

Aggressive histologies of non-Hodgkin's lymphoma are intensely FDG avid (e.g., Burkitt lymphoma, diffuse large B-cell lymphoma [patient B]), whereas low-grade tumors (e.g., small lymphocytic lymphoma, peripheral T-cell lymphoma, and follicular lymphoma) generally have less uptake (patient A). FDG avidity should be verified with pretreatment PET exams in patients with non-Hodgkin's lymphoma tumor types known to have lower and variable FDG avidity to allow assessment of response to therapy. False-positive FDG uptake in lymph nodes on PET may occur with infection and inflammation and sarcoidosis. Thymic uptake after therapy is often seen due to physiologic thymic hyperplasia/rebound.

Notes

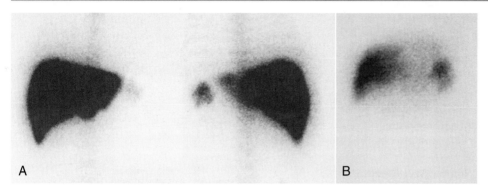

A patient with a history of idiopathic thrombocytopenic purpura and a previous splenectomy. There is clinical evidence of recurrent disease. Anterior, posterior (A) and left lateral (B) views of a radionuclide scan with the image intensity set high.

1. What is the radiopharmaceutical?

2. What is the likely purpose of the study?

3. Could other studies be used to make the same diagnosis?

4. What is your interpretation of the study?

Hepatobiliary System: Splenic Remnant

1. ^{99m}Tc-SC.

2. To detect a splenic remnant, splenosis, or accessory splenic tissue.

3. Heat or chemically damaged ^{99m}Tc-RBC study.

4. Positive for the presence of a splenic remnant.

References

Spencer RP: Spleen imaging. In: Sandler MP, Coleman RE, Wackers FJTh, et al (eds): *Diagnostic Nuclear Medicine*, 3rd ed. Baltimore: Williams & Wilkins, 1996, pp 565–591.

Stewart CA, Sakimura IT, Siegel ME: Scintigraphic demonstration of splenosis, *Clin Nucl Med* 11:161–164, 1986.

Cross-Reference

Nuclear Medicine: THE REQUISITES, 3rd ed, pp 207–209.

Comment

Splenic imaging has a long history in nuclear medicine. This case shows the use of a ^{99m}Tc-SC liver spleen scan to detect a splenic remnant in a patient with a previous splenectomy. ^{99m}Tc-SC is taken up by reticuloendothelial cells in liver (Kupffer cells), splenic tissue, and bone marrow macrophages. This is a very sensitive method for the detection of splenic tissue because of its high uptake. A potential disadvantage of ^{99m}Tc-SC is that if the splenic tissue is adjacent to the liver, it may be difficult to detect small foci of uptake because of the considerable hepatic uptake. SPECT can be helpful in these cases. In most cases, ^{99m}Tc-SC can confirm the diagnosis. However, an alternative method for detecting functioning splenic tissue is to use heat-denatured or chemically damaged ^{99m}Tc-labeled RBCs. This results in good splenic uptake with little or no liver uptake. Splenic tissue can also be seen with an ^{111}In-oxine or ^{99m}Tc-leukocyte scan, but they usually are not used for this purpose. However, this can be a cause of false-positive leukocyte scan finding in a patient suspected of having an infection.

Notes

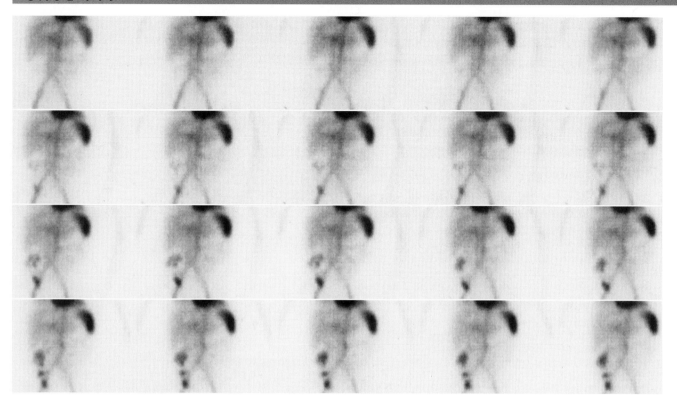

A 70-year-old man who has had a recent onset of rectal bleeding.

1. What radionuclide study is this?

2. Describe the scintigraphic findings.

3. What is the approximate site of bleeding?

4. Provide the differential diagnosis.

Gastrointestinal System: Cecal Gastrointestinal Bleeding, Angiodysplasia

1. ^{99m}Tc-labeled erythrocyte gastrointestinal bleeding study.

2. Initially, no abnormal activity, then focal uptake appearing simultaneously at two sites in the right lower abdomen and increasing in intensity with time and moving antegrade.

3. Cecum and ascending colon.

4. Acute bleeding due to angiodysplasia, diverticula, neoplasm, inflammatory bowel disease, and ischemia. Angiodysplasia was diagnosed by angiography.

References

Howarth DM: The role of nuclear medicine in detection of acute gastrointestinal bleeding, *Semin Nucl Med* 36:133–146, 2006.

Zuckier LS: Acute gastrointestinal bleeding, *Semin Nucl Med* 33:297–311, 2003.

Cross-Reference

Nuclear Medicine: THE REQUISITES, 3rd ed, pp 367–376.

Comment

The radionuclide bleeding scan can determine whether bleeding is active and locate the approximate site of bleeding. In this patient, it was not certain from the images whether there was one or two bleeding sites. Review of the images in a cinematic mode (1 min/frame) confirmed two bleeding sites, subsequently also found on contrast angiography. ^{99m}Tc-RBC scintigraphy is a sensitive method for detecting gastrointestinal hemorrhage. Bleeding rates of 0.1 mL/min can be detected compared with 1 mL/min for contrast angiography. An advantage of RBC scintigraphy is that intermittent bleeding can be identified. Active bleeding must be differentiated from other reasons for ^{99m}Tc-RBC localization (e.g., hemangioma, aneurysms, ectopic kidneys). To diagnose the site of active bleeding, definite criteria must be met: no activity initially, activity increases, and transits in a pattern consistent with intestinal anatomy. Imaging must be continued until the origin is certain (e.g., small vs. large bowel).

Angiodysplasia is a vascular anomaly of the submucosa or mucosa, often multiple, and greater than 0.5 cm in diameter and predominantly found in the right colon. It accounts for 80% of the vascular anomalies of the colon and may coexist with other causes of bleeding. In autopsy series, lesions have been found in 2% of asymptomatic elderly patients. On angiography, the angiodysplasia appears as a tangle of small vessels. Early filling of draining veins may be demonstrated, but extravasation of contrast is not commonly seen.

Notes

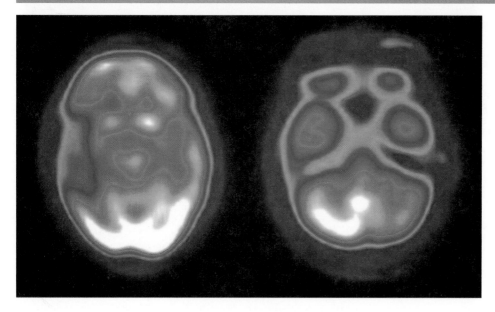

A 71-year-old woman has had acute thrombotic stroke.

1. Which cerebral artery territory displays the area of infarction?

2. Describe the other abnormality seen on these selected ^{18}F-FDG–PET brain slices.

3. What is the term used to describe this pattern of uptake?

4. What else can cause the primary abnormality?

FDG-PET: Crossed Cerebellar Diaschisis

1. Right middle cerebral artery.

2. Asymmetrically decreased FDG uptake in the left cerebellum compared with the right.

3. Crossed cerebellar diaschisis.

4. Tumor, encephalomalacia, status epilepticus, encephalitis, post-surgical.

Reference

Alavi A, Mirot A, Newberg A, et al: Fluorine-18-FDG evaluation of crossed cerebellar diaschisis in head injury, *J Nucl Med* 38:1717–1720, 1997.

Cross-Reference

Nuclear Medicine: THE REQUISITES, 3rd ed, pp 432–434.

Comment

Crossed cerebellar diaschisis refers to an area of decreased uptake in a cerebellar hemisphere contralateral to the supratentorial cerebral area of cortical insult and can be seen very soon after the acute injury. The underlying mechanism of this matched depression of metabolism and blood flow is thought to be a functional disconnection of the cerebropontocerebellar pathways. The pattern of decreased cerebellar uptake is more pronounced the greater the severity of the lesion, but may not be seen in patients with multiple or diffuse brain injuries. The contralateral cerebellar hypoperfusion has been noted in half of the patients with a single focal cerebral insult; however, the ipsilateral cerebellar hypoperfusion is seen in 19% of patients. This finding may be accompanied by clinical cerebellar symptoms, which may be reversible.

In most cases, blood flow closely follows metabolism. Therefore, the pattern of uptake seen on this ^{18}F-FDG–PET study would be expected to be similar on a SPECT perfusion study of the same patient (e.g., ^{99m}Tc-HMPO or ^{99m}Tc-ECD). An exception is during the acute phase of a stroke (3–7 days), when the blood flow may not match the metabolism. The blood flow is preserved in the setting of no metabolism because of failed cerebrovascular autoregulation. Thus, perfusion may be normal even though the FDG-PET study shows hypometabolism. This is referred to as luxury perfusion.

Notes

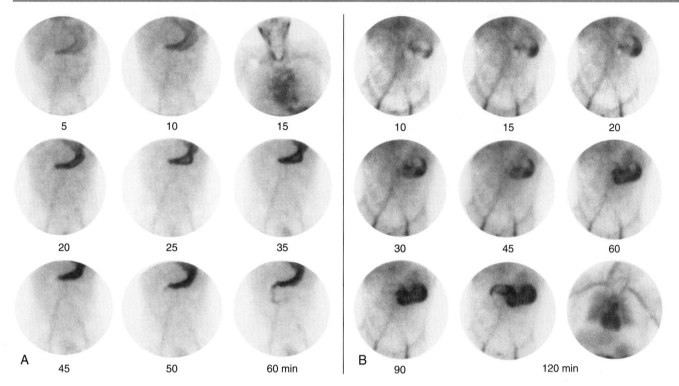

5   10   15   10   15   20

20   25   35   30   45   60

A   45   50   60 min   B   90   120 min

Two patients (A and B) were referred for a radionuclide gastrointestinal bleeding study with ^{99m}Tc-RBCs.

1. Describe the image findings in both studies.

2. Why were the neck/chest images acquired (A, 15 minutes; B, 120 minutes)?

3. Interpret the two studies.

4. What method of ^{99m}Tc-RBC labeling has the highest binding?

Gastrointestinal System: ^{99m}Tc-RBC Study—Gastric Bleeding versus Free Pertechnetate

1. Both patient studies show uptake increasing in the stomach over time and some mild transit into the proximal small bowel.

2. The chest and neck image shows thyroid and salivary uptake in study A (15-minute image) but not in study B (120-minute image). Uptake in the salivary and thyroid gland denotes unbound ^{99m}Tc-pertechnetate caused by poor labeling.

3. A, Negative for gastrointestinal bleeding. Uptake is due to gastric secretion. B, Active bleeding originating from the stomach.

4. In vitro method, UltraTag.

Reference

Srivasta SC, Straub RF: Blood cell labeling with ^{99m}Tc: progress and perspectives, *Semin Nucl Med* 20:41–51, 1990.

Cross-Reference

Nuclear Medicine: THE REQUISITES, 3rd ed, pp 367–373.

Comment

Although the radionuclide bleeding study is usually ordered to diagnose lower gastrointestinal bleeding, upper tract bleeding sites may sometimes be detected. High radiolabeling efficiency is critical for optimum studies and correct interpretation. Free ^{99m}Tc-pertechnetate is taken up by gastric mucosa (mucin cells) and can then move antegrade through the intestines and simulate bleeding. The neck and chest views allow differentiation of the two. With in vitro labeling, free ^{99m}Tc-pertechnetate is uncommon.

Three methods for radiolabeling of the patient's RBCs have been used over the years. The in vivo method is simplest. Stannous pyrophosphate is intravenously injected first, followed 15 minutes later by ^{99m}Tc-pertechnetate. The tin allows the ^{99m}Tc-pertechnetate to bind to the β chain of hemoglobin. This binding occurs in vivo with a labeling efficiency of 75% to 80%. The method is adequate for RVG (MUGA) but not for gastrointestinal bleeding studies. Thus, the modified in vivo method was developed. Stannous pyrophosphate is first intravenously injected, then blood is withdrawn into a syringe containing ^{99m}Tc-sodium pertechnetate; labeling occurs in the syringe over 10 minutes, and then the blood is reinfused. Labeling efficiency is 85% to 90%. The in vitro method is performed totally outside the body and is available in a simple kit form (UltraTag). Labeling efficiency is greater than 97% and is the method of choice.

Notes

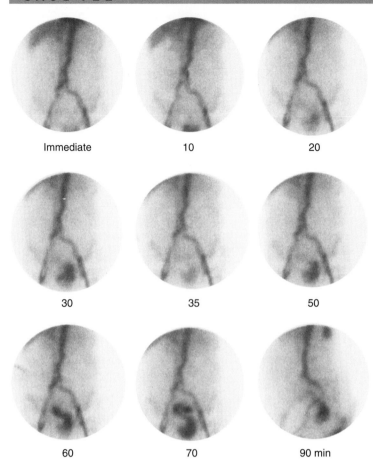

Immediate 10 20

30 35 50

60 70 90 min

A 65-year-old patient has had intermittent rectal bleeding for 2 days.

1. Describe the scintigraphic findings during this 90-minute study.

2. What is the purpose of the oblique/lateral pelvic view (last image)? How is it helpful diagnostically?

3. What is your interpretation of the study?

4. What are the criteria for diagnosing and localizing a bleeding site?

Gastrointestinal System: ^{99m}Tc-RBC Study— Rectal Bleeding

1. Abnormal activity accumulates early in the lower midline pelvis. The activity changes pattern and comes and goes over time.

2. The lateral oblique view helps differentiate activity in the rectum from that in the bladder and penis. In this patient, the activity is in the rectum. No activity is seen in the bladder or genitalia.

3. Active gastrointestinal bleeding. Bleeding originates in the rectum.

4. No activity initially, then activity is seen and increases in amount over time and moves over time intraluminally in a pattern consistent with intestinal anatomy.

References

Howarth DM: The role of nuclear medicine in detection of acute gastrointestinal bleeding, *Semin Nucl Med* 36:133–146, 2006.

Zuckier LS: Acute gastrointestinal bleeding, *Semin Nucl Med* 33:297–311, 2003.

Cross-Reference

Nuclear Medicine: THE REQUISITES, 3rd ed, pp 367–373.

Comment

The radionuclide gastrointestinal bleeding study result is most likely to be positive early in the clinical course (e.g., when the patient arrives in the emergency department or is admitted to the hospital). When the study is ordered after all other evaluation findings are negative and the bleeding has slowed or stopped, the likelihood for localization is poorer. Similarly, the accuracy is not high for chronic slow, intermittent bleeding. Most results of bleeding studies are positive in the first 90 minutes. However, the advantage of radiolabeled RBCs is that delayed imaging can be performed and may occasionally add important diagnostic information. Delayed imaging must be acquired dynamically and the same criteria used for localization. Activity in the left colon at 18 to 24 hours yields no additional information and can be misleading. The radiolabeled blood could have come from anywhere proximal to that site.

Interpretive pitfalls should be considered to provide the referring physician with accurate localization information. This case study demonstrates one. Using anterior views only, a bleeding site in the rectum often cannot be differentiated from activity in the bladder or even the penis blood pool. Lateral images are required. Cinematic display can also aid in the identification of the bleeding site. Potential pitfalls include activity in the genitourinary tract and vascular structures. Many are fixed abnormalities (e.g., aneurysms, varices, hemangioma, ectopic kidney). Others are more problematic (e.g., urinary tract activity, ectopic kidneys).

Notes

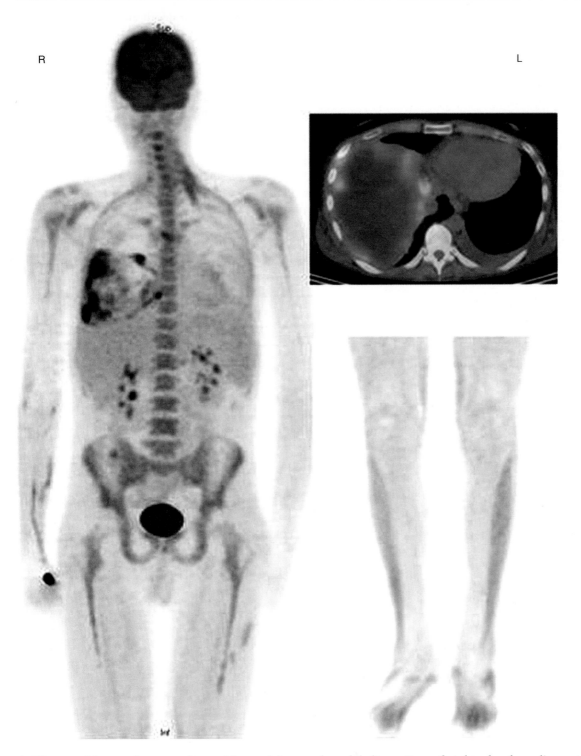

A 30-year-old man 2 years after wide excision and nodal dissection of right cheek malignant melanoma.

1. Describe the FDG-PET findings.

2. In which patients is FDG-PET/CT most useful for staging melanoma?

3. How does FDG-PET compare with CT for the detection of melanomatous disease?

4. What is the likely purpose of imaging the lower extremities in this patient?

C A S E   1 2 3

Oncology: FDG-PET—Malignant Melanoma

1. A large right lung mass with FDG uptake peripherally and central photopenia due to necrosis. The diffusely increased red marrow is likely due to marrow activation secondary to chemotherapy. Focal uptake in the region of the right iliac crest is physiologic, located within overlying bowel. Left thigh uptake is physiologic muscle uptake. Right anterior neck muscle uptake is caused by muscle tension/strain.

2. FDG-PET/CT imaging is most valuable for high-risk patients (primary lesion > 4 mm in depth) for the detection of metastases.

3. PET is more sensitive for the detection of melanomatous lesions in the subcutaneous tissues, nodes, bony skeleton, and abdomen compared with CT. It is less sensitive for micrometastases (e.g., in the lungs).

4. Melanoma is a malignancy that can metastasize to anywhere in the body and often distant from the original site of disease. Ten percent of metastases occur in the skin and subcutaneous tissue. Therefore, for melanoma, the entire body (top of head to soles of feet) is routinely imaged with FDG-PET/CT.

References

Krug B, Crott R, Lonneux M, et al: Role of PET in the initial staging of cutaneous malignant melanoma: systemic review, *Radiology* 249:836–844, 2008.

Segall GM, Swetter SM: *PET and PET/CT Imaging in Melanoma, Positron Emission Tomography*. London: Springer-Verlag, 2006, pp 233–242.

Cross-Reference

Nuclear Medicine: THE REQUISITES, 3rd ed, pp 336–337.

Comment

Malignant melanoma is increasing in incidence around the world and accounts for 3% of all cancers with survival dependent on the stage at the time of diagnosis. FDG uptake is typically quite high with melanoma. FDG-PET/CT imaging is more sensitive than conventional imaging methods for staging high-risk patients, except for the detection of small lung parenchymal lesions on CT and MRI for brain metastases. FDG-PET/CT is particularly useful for the detection of lymph node and deep soft-tissue metastatic disease with a sensitivity approaching 90%.

The prognosis for melanoma is directly related to the millimeter depth of invasion of the primary lesion (Breslow classification) or dermal layer (Clark's level). Melanoma grows vertically in the skin initially, with subsequent spread to regional lymph nodes. Patients with lesions less than 1 mm in depth are at low risk, those with lesions more than 4 mm in depth are high-risk patients. PET/CT is indicated in patients at high risk to determine whether there is regional adenopathy. Regional metastatic adenopathy places the patient in stage III with a less than 10% 10-year survival rate. Sentinel node scintigraphy and biopsy are performed for patients with lesions of 1 to 4 mm at intermediate risk to determine whether regional nodal dissection is indicated. PET/CT may also be useful in patients with intermediate depth lesions (1–4 mm) who have positive sentinel node biopsy results. Restaging of disease is also an approved indication. One study showed a change in management in 49% of melanoma patients when FDG-PET was used.

Notes

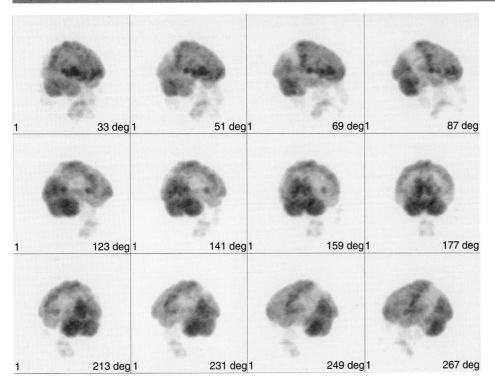

A 55-year-old man has had increasing dementia over the past 10 months.

1. Provide a clinical differential diagnosis for dementia.

2. How can SPECT or FDG-PET aid in this differential diagnosis?

3. Describe the ^{18}F-FDG–PET findings on the reconstructed three-dimensional volume display.

4. What is the likely diagnosis and with what degree of certainty?

C A S E   1 2 4

Central Nervous System: Alzheimer's Disease

1. Common causes include depression, metabolic disorders (hypothyroidism), substance abuse, alcoholism, multi-infarction, AIDS-related, Alzheimer's, Parkinson's, Pick's, Lewy body, and Creutzfeldt-Jacob diseases.

2. Specific patterns can diagnose multi-infarct dementia, Alzheimer's disease, and frontal lobe dementias (e.g., Pick's disease) using ^{99m}Tc-HMPAO/ECD SPECT or FDG-PET.

3. Hypometabolism (decreased FDG uptake) of the posterior parietal and temporal lobes bilaterally and to a lesser extent the frontal lobes. Note persistent metabolism of sensorimotor cortex.

4. Alzheimer's disease; greater than 80% to 90% certainty.

References

Coleman RE: Positron emission tomography diagnosis of Alzheimer's disease, *Neuroimaging Clin N Am* 15:837–846, 2005.

Silverman DH, Mosconi L, Ersoli L, et al: Positron emission tomography scans obtained for the evaluation of cognitive dysfunction, *Semin Nucl Med* 38:251–261, 2008.

Cross-Reference

Nuclear Medicine: THE REQUISITES, 3rd ed, pp 427–432.

Comment

The clinical diagnosis of Alzheimer's disease can be challenging. Reversible causes must be sought. Although so-called presenile dementia occurs in middle-aged patients, most cases of dementia are in the elderly, with an incidence greater than 10% after age 65 and 50% after age 85. Histopathologic changes include abnormal tangles of nerve fibers and degenerative neuritic plaques in the posterior parietotemporal cortex. Frontal lobe involvement also occurs with severe disease.

PET and SPECT can aid in the differential diagnosis in patients with characteristic patterns of disease. The patterns on SPECT and PET are similar. FDG uptake represents glucose metabolism, whereas ^{99m}Tc-HMPAO or -ECD uptake reflects regional cerebral blood flow. The single-photon radiopharmaceuticals are lipophilic and cross the blood–brain barrier. HMPAO is converted to a hydrophilic complex and ECD to a negatively charged complex; both are trapped intracellularly. The typical scintigraphic pattern in Alzheimer's disease is bilateral hypoperfusion/hypometabolism of the posterior parietal and temporal lobes. Sometimes it is asymmetrical, but it always spares the occipital and sensorimotor cortices and subcortical gray matter. A similar distribution can be seen in late Parkinson's dementia and in patients with diffuse Lewy body disease, a degenerative dementia now more widely recognized. Diffuse Lewy body disease usually has decreased occipital uptake as well. The main features are visual hallucinations and fluctuating cognitive decline. Late parkinsonism with dementia may have a pattern similar to that of Alzheimer's disease.

Notes

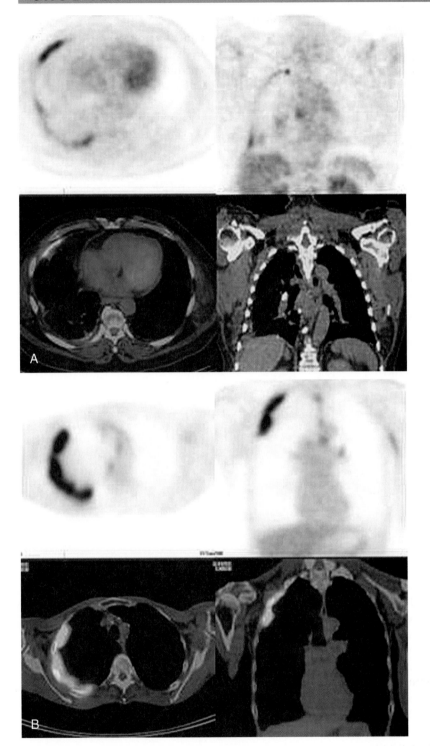

Patients A and B both have lung cancer and were referred for restaging. *Top,* FDG-PET; *bottom,* fused PET/CT; *left,* transverse; and *right,* coronal slices.

1. Describe any abnormal PET/CT findings in the two patients.

2. Provide a differential diagnosis for the findings.

3. What is the significance of FDG uptake in pleural effusions?

4. Explain the difference in the FDG uptake mechanism in patients with malignant versus inflammatory disease.

Oncology: FDG-PET/CT—Mesothelioma

1. Intense FDG uptake along the right lung pleura corresponds to regions of pleural thickening on CT.

2. Mesothelioma (patient B), asbestos-related inflammatory fibrosis, metastases from lung cancer or other primary malignancy, and pleurodesis (patient A).

3. The more FDG uptake in a pleural effusion, the greater the likelihood of malignancy as the etiology.

4. Uptake in tumors is dependent on glucose metabolism and transport into malignant cells. Activated inflammatory cells (neutrophils, macrophages) have increased expression of glucose transporters.

References

Duysinx B, Corhay JL, Larock MP, et al: Prognostic value of metabolic imaging in non-small cell lung cancers with neoplastic pleural effusion, *Nucl Med Commun* 29:982–986, 2008.

Krüger S, Pauls S, Mottaghy FM, et al: Integrated FDG PET-CT imaging improves staging in malignant pleural mesothelioma, *Nuklearmedizin* 46:239–243, 2007.

Cross-Reference

Nuclear Medicine: THE REQUISITES, 3rd ed, pp 485–488.

Comment

As many as 15% of patients presenting with lung cancer have malignant pleural effusions. The presence of increased FDG activity within an effusion, even in patients without definite focal pleural CT abnormalities, predicts the likelihood of malignancy in more than 80%. The presence of an effusion at initial evaluation of non-small cell lung cancer portends a poorer overall 5-year survival rate; in stage IIIB patients with and without malignant effusion, it is 40% and 15%, respectively.

Talc pleurodesis is performed for the treatment of persistent pneumothorax or recurrent pleural effusions, usually due to malignancy. The talc induces inflammation and intense FDG uptake, which can be mistaken for malignancy. The uptake may be focal or diffuse along the pleura; it is most common in dependent locations and the costophrenic angle. The FDG uptake may persist for years.

Mesothelioma arises from the pleural surface and usually presents as a large pleural effusion. Many patients have a history of asbestos exposure. Prognosis is poor, with a mean untreated survival of 4 to 13 months. PET/CT can aid in its diagnosis and staging. Extrapleural pneumonectomy is the treatment of choice for those with resectable malignant mesothelioma, typically 10% to 15% of patients. It is particularly useful in detecting other local or distant disease in patients considered potentially resectable. The addition of FDG-PET to contrast CT can upstage disease in as many as 70% of patients, primarily through the ability of FDG-PET to diagnose metastatic disease and therefore preclude resection.

Notes

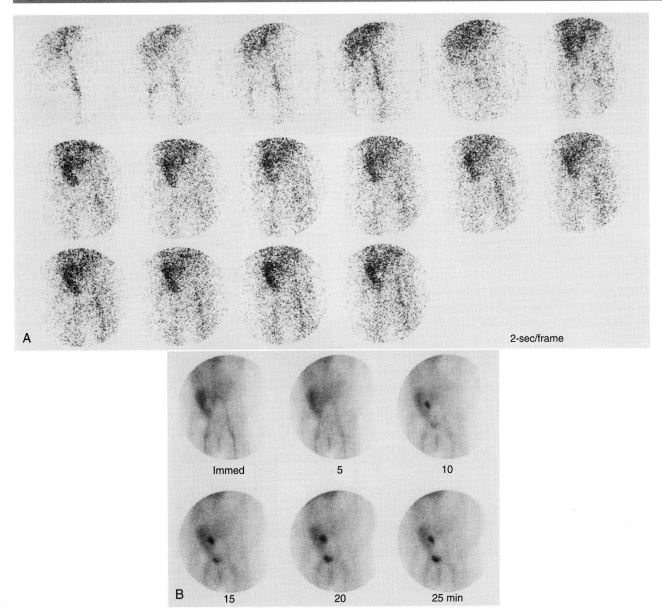

A 25-year-old woman underwent kidney transplantation 7 days earlier. A, 1 sec/frame flow images. B, 25 1-minute dynamic images displayed as 5-minute summed images.

1. What are the scintigraphic findings of this ^{99m}Tc-MAG3 study?

2. What is the most likely diagnosis?

3. What are the usual associated clinical symptoms and findings?

4. What other diagnosis during the first week post-transplantation can be differentiated from this? How?

Genitourinary System: ⁹⁹ᵐTc-MAG3—Acute Renal Transplant Rejection

1. Very delayed and decreased blood flow to the transplant and poor function. Normal perfusion would show flow to the kidney simultaneously with the iliac vessel supplying it.

2. Acute rejection.

3. Fever, transplant tenderness and enlargement, decreased urinary output, and rising serum creatinine level.

4. ATN is the most common cause of renal dysfunction the first week post-transplantation. Blood flow on the renal scan is typically normal.

References

Boubaker A, Prior JO, Meuwly JY, Bischof-Delaloye A: Radionuclide investigations of the urinary tract in the era of multimodality imaging, *J Nucl Med* 47:1819–1836, 2006.

Choyke PL, Becker JA, Ziessman HA: Imaging the transplanted kidney. In: Pollack HM, McClennan BL (eds): *Clinical Urology*, 2nd ed. Philadelphia: WB Saunders, 2000, pp 3091–3118.

Cross-Reference

Nuclear Medicine: THE REQUISITES, 3rd ed, pp 239–252.

Comment

Acute rejection is a cell-mediated process. Sensitized lymphocytes migrate to the graft and destroy the cells of the graft without the participation of humoral antibodies. Chronic rejection is mediated by an antibody-induced injury to the endothelial and interstitial cells, which suggests a humoral mechanism. Histologic changes include arterial narrowing, which progresses to eventual complete obliteration of the lumen, and glomerular lesions.

Acute allograft rejection is a clinical diagnosis. Patients have typical symptoms and findings as described previously. Imaging studies are performed to ensure adequate blood flow and viability, to differentiate it from ATN, and to rule out obstruction. Renal scintigraphy can be used to follow the clinical course to confirm response to therapy. Scintigraphy demonstrates blood flow at the capillary level.

The typical scintigraphic findings of acute rejection of decreased blood flow and poor function are seen in this study. Although acute rejection of the renal allograft often begins 5 to 7 days after transplantation, it may occur weeks or months later. Accelerated acute rejection begins the first week after transplantation in patients who have received previous transplants or have received multiple blood transfusions before transplantation that have sensitized their immune systems. Acute rejection usually is reversible with appropriate therapy, steroids, and immunotherapy. Conversely, chronic rejection progresses slowly over months and years and is unresponsive to therapy. ATN occurs usually early in the first week of transplantation and resolves over 1 or 2 weeks. Scintigraphy reveals good blood flow but poor function.

Notes

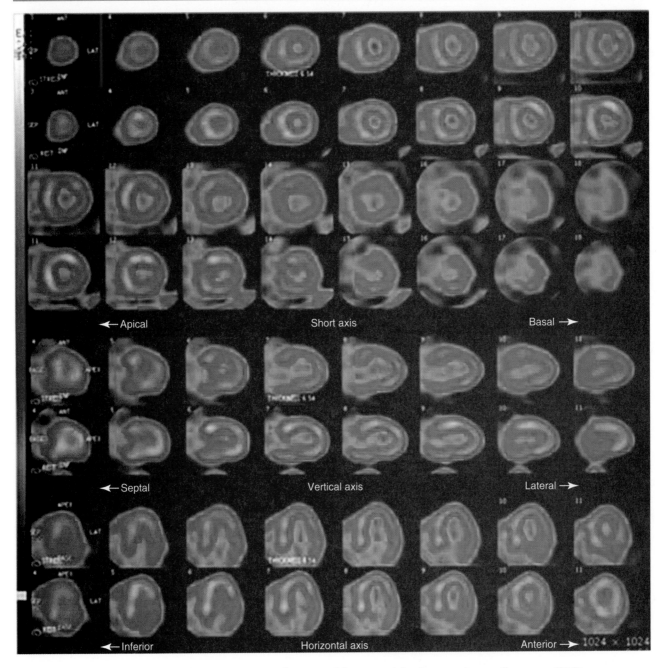

←— Apical Short axis Basal —→

←— Septal Vertical axis Lateral —→

←— Inferior Horizontal axis Anterior —→

Stress rest myocardial perfusion study in a 68-year-old man with chest pain to diagnose CAD.

1. Which radiopharmaceuticals are used for PET myocardial perfusion imaging? What are their advantages and disadvantages?

2. Describe the perfusion pattern at rest and stress and interpret the study.

3. What method of stress is used for PET myocardial perfusion imaging?

4. Is attenuation correction necessary for clinical PET cardiac perfusion imaging?

Cardiovascular System: Rest/Stress Rubidium-82 (^{82}Rb)–PET Myocardial Perfusion Imaging—Ischemia and Infarction

1. ^{82}Rb is most commonly used because it is produced on-site in a strontium-82 (^{82}Sr)-^{82}Rb generator. ^{13}N-NH$_3$ is used at locations with an on-site cyclotron; it has a very short half-life ($t_{1/2}$ = 10 minutes). ^{15}O-H$_2$O also requires an on-site cyclotron ($t_{1/2}$ = 2 minutes) and is limited to research purposes.

2. At stress, a large region of severely decreased perfusion in the anterior/distal lateral myocardial walls, which is markedly improved at rest, diagnostic of ischemia. Also, a large area of moderately decreased perfusion in the mid-to-basal lateral wall, mostly fixed, consistent with myocardial infarction, peri-infarct ischemia.

3. Pharmacologic stress with a coronary vasodilator (adenosine, dipyridamole, regadenoson) or adrenergic stress (dobutamine) with imaging during peak pharmacologic action compared with resting study. The PET radiotracers have too short a half-life for exercise stress.

4. Attenuation correction is mandatory and usually done using the CT data from the hybrid PET/CT scan.

References

Mayo JR, Leipsic JA: Radiation dose in cardiac CT, *AJR Am J Roentgenol* 192:646–653, 2009.

Nandalur KR, Dwamena BA, Choudhri AF, et al: Diagnostic performance of positron emission tomography in the detection of coronary artery disease: a meta-analysis, *Acad Radiol* 15:444–451, 2008.

Cross-Reference

Nuclear Medicine: THE REQUISITES, 3rd ed, pp 485–488.

Comment

^{82}Rb has a mean path length of 2.6 mm compared with 0.7 mm for ^{13}N and 1.1 mm for ^{15}O. The longer path length of ^{82}Rb and its high emission energy (maximum energy, 3.35 MeV) result in reduced resolution compared with ^{13}N-NH$_3$. However, ^{82}Rb images are superior to SPECT images. Most protocols involve imaging the patient at rest, followed by pharmacologic stress and imaging without moving the patient from the table. PET perfusion agent is injected and imaged during peak stress, allowing the detection of transient stress-induced wall motion abnormalities. This is in contrast to SPECT imaging, which is obtained 20 to 35 minutes after stress, and thus significant stunning is required to detect stress-induced wall motion abnormalities. Differences in the LVEF at rest and stress with PET correlate with the severity of CAD, even in the absence of detectable perfusion abnormalities.

The sensitivity and specificity of PET for the detection of CAD are reported to be 91% and 90%, respectively, compared with 89% and 76%, respectively, for SPECT. Perfusion studies with ^{82}Rb typically deliver only 4 to 7 mSv of radiation to the patient, given the short physical $t_{1/2}$ of ^{82}Rb (75 seconds). The CT component of cardiac PET/CT studies may result in an additional 8 to 20 mSv if coronary CT angiography is done or as much as 5 to 8 mSv when the CT is performed for attenuation correction only. CT radiation dose may be minimized by acquiring a single CT image used for attenuation correction of both rest and stress images rather than a CT for each acquisition, prospective ECG-triggering with step-and-shoot CT acquisition, ECG-dependent x-ray tube current modulation, and attenuation-dependent tube current modulation.

Notes

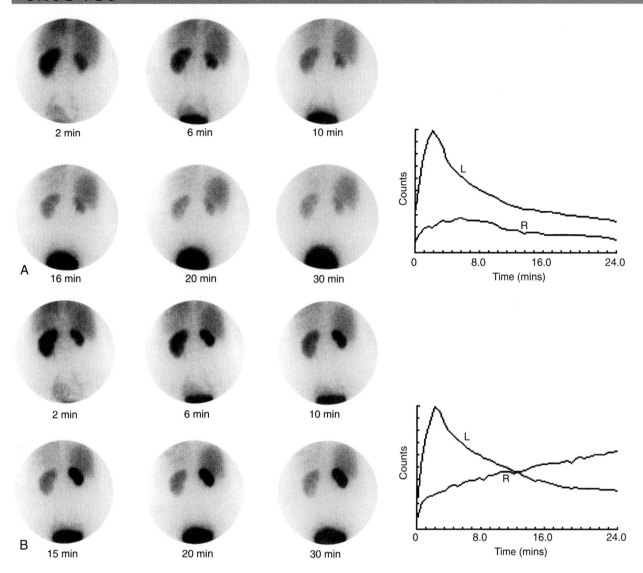

A 30-year-old man has poorly controlled and accelerating hypertension. Baseline study without captopril (A) and ^{99m}Tc-MAG3 renal studies with captopril (B) are shown.

1. What is the rationale and physiologic mechanism for the captopril renal study?

2. What are the scintigraphic and time-activity curve findings and diagnosis?

3. Could ^{99m}Tc-DPTA have been used instead?

4. What is the accuracy of captopril renography?

Genitourinary System: Captopril Renography

1. With renal artery stenosis, glomerular perfusion and glomerular filtration rate (GFR) decrease. Renin is released from the juxtaglomerular apparatus and converts angiotensin I to angiotensin II, which causes vasoconstriction of the glomerular efferent arterioles, increasing filtration pressure and maintaining the GFR. Captopril is an angiotensin-converting enzyme inhibitor that blocks conversion of angiotensin I to II, resulting in a decrease in the GFR.

2. The right kidney is small but with good function. With captopril, cortical retention persists, consistent with renin-dependent renovascular hypertension of the right kidney. This is confirmed by the renal cortical time-activity curves.

3. Yes. The accuracy of ^{131}I-hippuran, ^{99m}Tc-DTPA, and ^{99m}Tc-MAG3 are similar.

4. Sensitivity, 90%; specificity, 95%. Sensitivity is reduced if the patient has been on long-term angiotensin-converting enzyme inhibitor therapy or has renal insufficiency.

References

Fine EJ: Diuretic renography and angiotensin converting enzyme inhibitor renography, *Radiol Clin North Am* 39:979–996, 2001.

Taylor A: Radionuclide renography: a personal approach, *Semin Nucl Med* 29:102–127, 1999.

Cross-Reference

Nuclear Medicine: THE REQUISITES, 3rd ed, pp 336–340.

Comment

Renal artery stenosis refers to anatomic narrowing. Renovascular hypertension is the pathophysiologic result in some patients. Many patients with stenosis do not have renin-dependent hypertension, and their hypertension will not be cured by surgical or angioplastic intervention. Captopril renography is a functional test that allows selection of patients with renovascular hypertension who will likely respond to therapy aimed at the stenosis. Intravenous enalapril can be used as an alternative to oral captopril; the advantage is a shorter test with no need to wait for enteric absorption, as with captopril. The angiotensin-converting enzyme inhibitor and baseline studies can be performed the same day. Diagnosis depends on seeing cortical function and deriving accurate time-activity curves. Both could be obscured or erroneous in the presence of renal pelvocalyceal retention; thus, a diuretic can be given with the radiotracer.

The MAG3 finding in renin-dependent renovascular hypertension is persistent cortical retention as a result of delayed urine flow in the renal tubules on the affected side, as seen in this case. Delayed uptake can be seen with ^{99m}Tc-DTPA and ^{131}I-hippuran, but often cannot be seen with MAG3. Bilateral renovascular hypertension is rare. When it occurs, it frequently is asymmetrical. A symmetrical response would suggest other factors (e.g., dehydration).

Notes

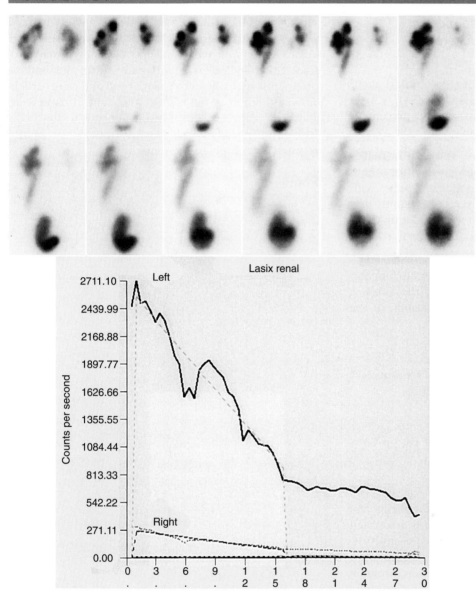

A 7-year-old patient has hydronephrosis demonstrated on ultrasonography. Lasix was administered at the beginning of the study immediately after radiopharmaceutical injection.

1. List the preferred radiopharmaceutical(s) for this study.

2. Why would or would not a renal cortical agent be appropriate?

3. Describe the findings.

4. List the differential diagnosis and most likely diagnosis.

Genitourinary System: Furosemide Renography—Primary Megaureter

1. ^{99m}Tc-MAG3 or ^{99m}Tc-DTPA.

2. No, the majority of uptake of a renal cortical agent (e.g., ^{99m}Tc-dimercaptosuccinic acid [DMSA]) is fixed to the proximal tubules. Twenty-five percent is excreted by glomerular filtration.

3. Prompt uptake by both kidneys. The right is smaller and clears rapidly. The left kidney has an initial central photopenic region likely due to a dilated pelvis with cold urine. The radiotracer is excreted promptly into a prominent left ureter and into the bladder by visual and quantitative assessment.

4. Dilated nonobstructed hydroureteronephrosis. Possible causes: VUR, corrected ureteral vesicle junction obstruction, and primary megaureter; the latter is more likely based on the prominent dilation of the distal ureter.

Reference

Piepsz A, Ham HR: Pediatric applications of renal nuclear medicine, *Semin Nucl Med* 36:16–35, 2006.

Cross-Reference

Nuclear Medicine: THE REQUISITES, 3rd ed, pp 234–239.

Comment

Primary megaureter is unilateral in 75% of patients and usually is discovered incidentally. It often is associated with urinary tract infection or urolithiasis. Because ureteral reflux is a possible cause of ureteral dilation, a contrast or radionuclide voiding cystourethrogram should be obtained to distinguish the entities. Generally, primary megaureter leads to a massive dilation of the lower third of the ureter, although the entire ureter may become dilated; the calyces generally maintain a normal appearance. Occasionally, it is associated with another congenital abnormality, megacalycosis, in which the calices are increased in number. Megacalyces are often squared, which can be mistaken for obstruction. Therefore, when megaureter and megacalycosis coexist, it is important to distinguish this from chronic ureteral obstruction by analyzing the number of calices and their shape on iodinated contrast studies.

^{99m}Tc-MAG3, a tubular agent, has a higher renal extraction fraction (60%) than ^{99m}Tc-DTPA (20%), a glomerular agent. Thus, MAG3 is the preferable agent in patients with renal insufficiency. The timing of diuretic infusion varies. At different centers, it is administered at the beginning of the study with the radiotracer or as the pelvis fills (15-20 minutes), or at the beginning of a second acquisition after the initial routine renogram, with 20 minutes of additional imaging. All these techniques work well when the methodology is standardized. Good hydration is important. Many institutions place a urinary catheter to ensure good drainage, particularly in children. A full bladder can cause backpressure and slow emptying. Renal insufficiency is a cause of a false-positive study result because the kidney cannot respond adequately to the diuretic.

Notes

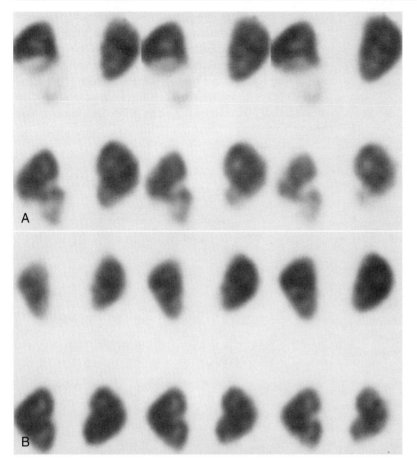

A 6-year-old girl had a recent urinary tract infection. A, ^{99m}Tc-DMSA SPECT sequential coronal long-axis slices are shown. B, Repeat study 6 months later.

1. What is the mechanism of uptake of ^{99m}Tc-DMSA?

2. What are the most common indications for a ^{99m}Tc-DMSA study?

3. What are the scintigraphic SPECT findings and what is the diagnosis? What would have been the diagnosis if the second study (B) looked similar to the first study (A)?

4. What is the clinical importance of differentiating upper and lower tract infections?

Genitourinary System: ^{99m}Tc-DMSA SPECT and Pyelonephritis

1. Forty percent to 50% of ^{99m}Tc-DMSA binds to functioning proximal cortical renal tubules.

2. Diagnosis of acute pyelonephritis or cortical scarring.

3. Decreased uptake in the lower half of the right kidney on initial imaging (A). Repeat SPECT (B) shows normalization of uptake. The diagnosis for the first study is acute pyelonephritis; if it had not improved, the diagnosis would be cortical scarring.

4. ^{99m}Tc-DMSA is the best predictor of renal sequelae. Identification of pyelonephritis or scarring will often result in long-term antibiotic prophylaxis.

References

Brenner M, Bonta D, Eslamy H, Ziessman HA: Comparison of 99mTc-DMSA dual-head SPECT versus high-resolution parallel-hole planar imaging for the detection of renal cortical defects, *AJR Am J Roentgenol* 193:333–337, 2009.

Ziessman HA, Majd M: Importance of methodology on ^{99m}Tc-DMSA scintigraphic image quality: Imaging pilot study for RIVUR (randomized intervention for children with vesicoureteral reflux) multicenter investigation. *J Urol* 182:272–279, 2009.

Cross-Reference

Nuclear Medicine: THE REQUISITES, 3rd ed, pp 222–226, 254–255.

Comment

^{99m}Tc-DMSA renal scintigraphy is the most sensitive imaging modality for the detection of renal infection or scarring. The advantage of ^{99m}Tc-DMSA over ^{99m}Tc-MAG3 is that DMSA produces high-resolution cortical images without the presence of overlying collecting system activity. Only 25% of DMSA is cleared by the bladder via glomerular filtration and this occurs early; most binds to the proximal renal tubules of the renal cortex. Delayed imaging at approximately 2 hours allows adequate time for urinary clearance except in patients with obstruction or severe VUR. Both planar imaging and SPECT imaging have good accuracy.

In many cases, infection can be differentiated from scarring. With scarring, the kidney is contracted with abnormal configuration and volume loss. Acute pyelonephritis typically has regions of decreased uptake but normal contour and some visualization of the cortex. Diffuse involvement is less common. In some cases, it is not so clear cut, and follow-up imaging in 3 to 6 months can clarify this.

With planar imaging, a pinhole collimator is sometimes used, particularly for children, for magnification and improved resolution. However, many hospitals use a parallel-hole collimator, with good results. SPECT usually requires sedation of younger children. A follow-up study to differentiate infection from scar should be conducted 3 to 6 months later, allowing time for adequate antibiotic therapy and infection resolution.

Notes

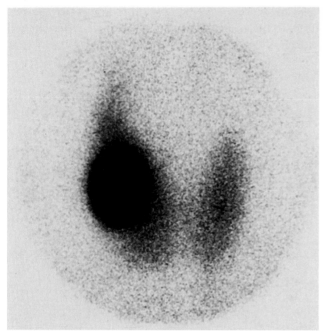
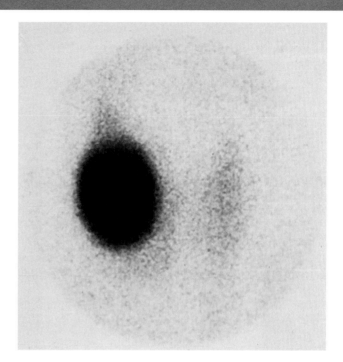
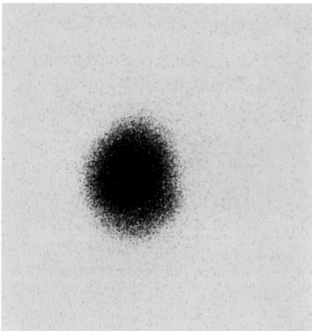

A 39-year-old woman has a 3-year history of thyrotoxicosis. ^{123}I thyroid scans were obtained each year (*shown from left to right*). She has not been treated because she had been asymptomatic until the time of the third scan.

1. Describe the scintigraphic findings.

2. Provide the cause of the thyrotoxicosis.

3. What treatment options are appropriate for this patient?

4. What would you expect the radioactive iodine thyroid uptake to be?

Endocrine System: ^{123}I—Toxic Autonomous Thyroid Nodule

1. Hot nodule in the mid-right lobe of the thyroid with increasing suppression of the remaining gland with each successive year.

2. Toxic autonomous thyroid nodule.

3. Radioactive ^{131}I is the usual method of treatment. Surgery is occasionally done.

4. RAIU is often normal with a single toxic nodule RAIU, but it may be moderately elevated.

References

Freitas JE: Therapeutic options in the management of toxic and nontoxic nodular goiter, *Semin Nucl Med* 30:88-97, 2000.

Sarkar SD: Benign thyroid disease: what is the role of nuclear medicine? *Semin Nucl Med* 36:185-193, 2006.

Cross-Reference

Nuclear Medicine: THE REQUISITES, 3rd ed, pp 88-94.

Comment

The patient in this case had subclinical thyrotoxicosis at the time of the first two scans (i.e., suppressed TSH and normal thyroxine). Because she had no symptoms, she would not accept surgery or radioactive iodine therapy until she developed symptoms by the time of the third scan. Nodules larger than 2.5 cm usually produce clinical symptoms. A "hot nodule" is defined as a palpable or sonographically confirmed nodule with increased uptake on a ^{123}I scan and suppression of the remaining gland. The increased thyroxine/triiodothyronine suppresses TSH and ^{123}I uptake in the nonautonomous portion of the gland. Occasionally, a region on a thyroid scan may appear focally hot, but the remainder of the gland is not suppressed. This can be caused by a small autonomous nodule producing insufficient thyroxine/triiodothyronine to suppress TSH or be due to hyperplastic nonautonomous tissue with relatively better function than other portions of the gland, sometimes seen in resolving thyroiditis.

The advantage of ^{131}I therapy for toxic nodule disease is that it is taken up preferentially by the nodule, with very little taken up by the normal suppressed gland. After therapy, the hyperfunctioning nodule becomes nonfunctional and the remaining gland, no longer suppressed, usually functions normally. Typically, 20 to 25 mCi of ^{131}I is given for therapy because autonomous nodules are more resistant to therapy than Graves' disease. After treatment of a single hot nodule, hypothyroidism is very uncommon, in contrast to Graves' disease, because the remaining gland receives little β radiation.

Notes

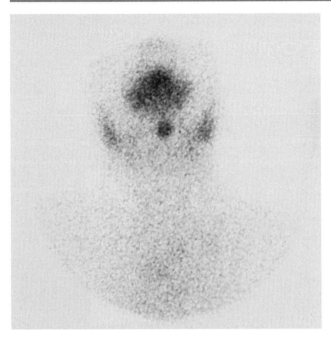

A 2-year-old child has an upper neck mass and hypothyroidism. A ^{99m}Tc-pertechnetate thyroid scan was performed.

1. What is the mechanism of ^{99m}Tc-pertechnetate and ^{123}I-sodium iodide uptake?

2. What is the advantage of ^{99m}Tc-pertechnetate over ^{123}I in this patient?

3. Describe the scintigraphic findings.

4. What is the diagnosis?

Endocrine System: ^{99m}Tc-Pertechnetate Scan—Sublingual Thyroid

1. ^{99m}Tc-pertechnetate is taken up (trapped) by thyroid follicular cells similar to iodine but not organified. ^{123}I is both trapped and organified.

2. Lower radiation exposure to the young patient.

3. Focal uptake at the base of the tongue, immediately below activity in the mouth (saliva). No thyroid tissue is seen in the neck. Parotid glands are seen bilaterally.

4. Sublingual thyroid.

References

Kalan A, Tariq M: Lingual thyroid: clinical evaluation and comprehensive management, *Ear Nose Throat J* 78:340-349, 1999.

Rahbar R, Yoon MJ, Connolly LP, et al: Lingual thyroid in children: a rare clinical entity, *Laryngoscope* 118:1174-1179, 2008.

Cross-Reference

Nuclear Medicine: THE REQUISITES, 3rd ed, pp 93-94.

Comment

Lingual thyroid is the term applied to ectopic thyroid tissue located at the base of the tongue midline. This is a rare anomaly resulting from failure of the embryonic gland anlage to descend, occurring between 3 and 7 weeks of embryologic development. Thyroid tissue may be located in any position along this thyroglossal tract. The lingual thyroid is the only functioning thyroid tissue in 70% of cases. Hypothyroidism occurs in as many as 33% of patients because the ectopic tissue often is hypofunctional. Other symptoms include dysphagia, dysphonia, dyspnea, and hemorrhage. Rare thyroid carcinomas may arise.

Lingual thyroids have two primary clinical pictures. One group consists of infants and young children whose hypothyroidism is detected on routine screening. The differential diagnosis of congenital hypothyroidism includes an absent gland, an ectopic gland (usually lingual), or an inborn error of metabolism causing goiter. These patients often fail to thrive and have mental retardation if thyroid hormone replacement is not initiated early in life. A second group of patients present with dysphagia and oropharyngeal obstruction before or during puberty.

^{99m}Tc-pertechnetate scans avoid the need for diagnostic biopsy with the attendant risks of intractable hemorrhage and acute thyrotoxicosis. Suppression with thyroid hormone often is the treatment of choice, although surgery sometimes is necessary for symptomatic patients.

Notes

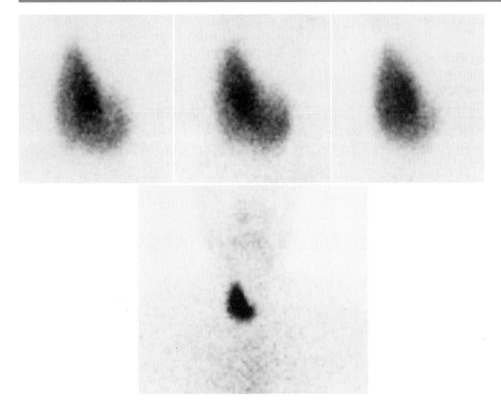

A thyroid scan performed in a 36-year-old patient with clinical thyrotoxicosis.

1. Describe the scintigraphic findings.

2. Describe the scan evidence that supports the reported clinical diagnosis of thyrotoxicosis.

3. What is the differential diagnosis regarding the left lobe?

4. The right lobe is two times normal size by examination. The left lobe is not palpable, no nodules are felt, and no scars are present. What is the most likely diagnosis?

Endocrine System: Thyroid Left Lobe Agenesis—Graves' Disease

1. Uniform uptake in a bulbous-appearing right lobe without focal areas of increased or decreased uptake. No activity in the expected location of the left lobe or elsewhere in the neck or upper chest.

2. The uniform activity in the right lobe is considerably more intense than in the salivary glands or other background, indirect evidence of an elevated uptake in the absence of intrinsic salivary gland disease.

3. Previous surgical excision, replacement by hypofunctioning adenoma or carcinoma, suppression by autonomously functioning adenoma on the right, agenesis of the left lobe with Graves' disease of the solitary right lobe.

4. Graves' disease with agenesis of the left lobe.

Reference

Mittra ES, Niederkohr RD, Rodriquez C, et al: Uncommon causes of thyrotoxicosis, *J Nucl Med* 49:265–278, 2008.

Cross-Reference

Nuclear Medicine: THE REQUISITES, 3rd ed, pp 88–93.

Comment

Common causes of hyperthyroidism include Graves' disease (diffuse toxic goiter), toxic multinodular gland, solitary toxic adenoma, and subacute and painless thyroiditis. Less common are iatrogenic ingestion of thyroid hormone, iodine-induced hyperthyroidism (e.g., secondary to contrast), and ectopic disease (e.g., struma ovarii).

Thyroid development begins early in embryonic life between the second and third weeks and is completed by the 11th week. Embryologic descent occurs, which can leave remnants of thyroid tissue anywhere along the course of the thyroglossal duct. During descent, interaction with the developing brachial pouches occurs, which may explain the occasional existence of ectopic thyroid tissue in the larynx, esophagus, lateral neck, mediastinum, and pericardium. Morphologic features and size of the normal adult thyroid vary. Asymmetry is common. Agenesis can be complete or unilateral. Hemiagenesis is more common on the left.

^{99m}Tc-pertechnetate is commonly used in children for thyroid imaging because of its low radiation dose and good image quality due to its higher administered dose (adult dose of ^{123}I is 300 μCi compared with 3 to 5 mCi of ^{99m}Tc). ^{99m}Tc uptake can be quantified at 15 to 20 minutes after injection (normal, 0.3–3%); however, iodine uptakes are better standardized and usually calculated at 4 and 24 hours (normal, 10–30%).

Notes

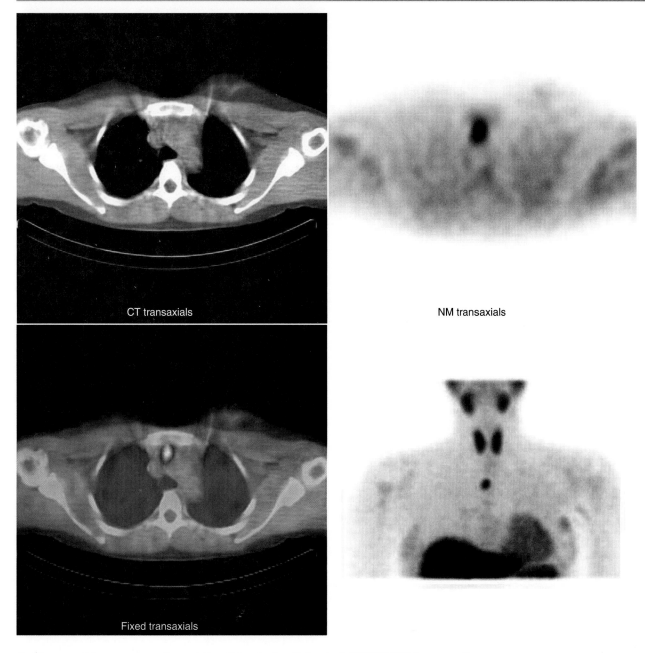

CT transaxials

NM transaxials

Fixed transaxials

A 45-year-old woman referred for this study. Selected SPECT/CT images shown.

1. What is the radiopharmaceutical and study?

2. Describe the scintigraphic findings.

3. What is the differential diagnosis for these findings?

4. What is the likely diagnosis in this clinical setting?

Endocrine System: ^{99m}Tc-Sestamibi SPECT/CT, Mediastinal Parathyroid Adenoma

1. Parathyroid scan with ^{99m}Tc-sestamibi. This is the same agent used for myocardial perfusion studies. Note the heart.

2. Focal abnormal midline uptake in the mediastinum, anterior and just superior to the aortic arch. Because the thyroid has intense uptake, this must be an image acquired soon after injection, usually 5 to 15 minutes.

3. Various benign or malignant neoplasms.

4. Mediastinal parathyroid adenoma.

References

Eslamy HK, Ziessman HA: Parathyroid scintigraphy in patients with primary hyperparathyroidism: 99mTc sestamibi SPECT and SPECT/CT, *Radiographics* 28:1461–1476, 2008.

Nichols KJ, Tomas MB, Tronco GG, et al: Preoperative parathyroid scintigraphic lesion localization: accuracy of various types of readings, *Radiology* 248:221–232, 2008.

Cross-Reference

Nuclear Medicine: THE REQUISITES, 3rd ed, pp 101–105.

Comment

Parathyroid adenomas usually are solitary. The parathyroid glands are derived from the pharyngeal pouches. Most persons have four glands: two superior and two inferior ones located close to the thyroid. Only 3% of parathyroid adenomas are found in the mediastinum. Those in the anterior mediastinum are derived from inferior glands; those in the posterior mediastinum are superior glands. Occasionally, adenomas are found high in the neck; thus, oblique imaging encompassing the upper neck can be helpful.

Mediastinal parathyroid adenomas are easily seen on ^{99m}Tc-sestamibi scans because of the low background activity, unlike the thyroid bed. Although computer subtraction of the thyroid can be helpful in the neck, it is not necessary in the chest. SPECT/CT nicely localizes this mediastinal parathyroid adenoma, which would be difficult to do with planar imaging or even SPECT alone. A two-phase study is commonly performed; however, in the setting of hyperparathyroidism, this study is diagnostic.

^{99m}Tc-sestamibi and ^{99m}Tc-tetrofosmin are nonspecific tumor-imaging agents taken up by a variety of benign and malignant neoplasms. However, in the setting of persistent hyperparathyroidism after neck dissection, focal uptake in the mediastinum is likely to be the culprit parathyroid adenoma. SPECT and SPECT/CT is increasingly used to better localize the gland in the anterior posterior plane.

Notes

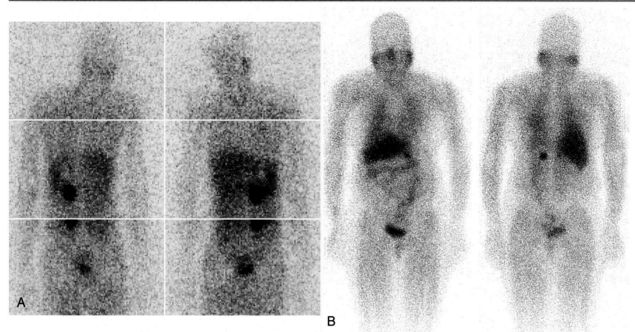

A

B

Two patients (A and B) with histories of poorly controlled hypertension and elevated catecholamine levels.

1. What are the radiopharmaceuticals?

2. What is the mechanism of uptake?

3. What is the diagnosis? What is the accuracy of this study?

4. What other diseases take up this radiopharmaceutical?

Endocrine System: MIBG—Pheochromocytoma

1. A, ^{131}I-MIBG. B, ^{123}I-MIBG. ^{123}I-MIBG is now commercially available and is preferable to ^{131}I-MIBG because of its lower radiation dose and superior image quality.

2. Localization occurs through the norepinephrine reuptake mechanism. It localizes intracellularly and in catecholamine storage vesicles in presynaptic adrenergic nerve endings and the cells of the adrenal medulla.

3. Sensitivity, 90%; specificity, 95%, for the detection of pheochromocytomas.

4. Various neuroendocrine tumors take up the radiopharmaceutical: neuroblastoma (90%), carcinoid (50%), and medullary carcinoma of the thyroid (25%).

Reference

Wiseman GA, Pacak K, O'Dorisio MS, et al: Usefulness of 123I-MIBG scintigraphy in the evaluation of patients with known or suspected primary or metastatic pheochromocytoma or paraganglioma: results from a prospective multicenter trial, *J Nucl Med* 50:1448–1454, 2009.

Cross-Reference

Nuclear Medicine: THE REQUISITES, 3rd ed, pp 109–112.

Comment

As can be seen, ^{123}I-MIBG has superior image quality compared with ^{131}I-MIBG; however, MIBG has such a high target-to-background ratio that diagnostically they are usually similar, although there are reports of patients with negative findings on ^{131}I-MIBG scans and positive findings on ^{123}I-MIBG scans. A major advantage is the lower radiation dose to the patient and the better image quality with SPECT.

MIBG has a molecular structure similar to the neurotransmitter catecholamine, norepinephrine, and the ganglionic blocking drug guanethidine. Numerous drugs may interfere with uptake of ^{123}I- or ^{131}I-MIBG, and they must be discontinued before the study. These include reserpine, tricyclic antidepressants, labetalol, and both α- and β-blockers. The patient's thyroid must be blocked with supersaturated potassium iodide to prevent free radioiodine uptake.

Radiolabeled MIBG is not a screening test for pheochromocytoma. The diagnosis must first be made clinically with elevated serum or urinary catecholamine levels. The role of MIBG is in the localization of the tumor. The majority of pheochromocytomas are single, sporadic, and localized in the adrenal gland. MIBG can be particularly valuable for localizing the 10% of pheochromocytomas that are extra-adrenal and occur at various locations from the base of the skull to the pelvis where frequently they are not detected by conventional imaging. Ten percent of pheochromocytomas are multifocal and 10% are malignant. The most common sites of metastases are the skeleton, lymph nodes, lung, and peritoneum.

Notes

Challenge

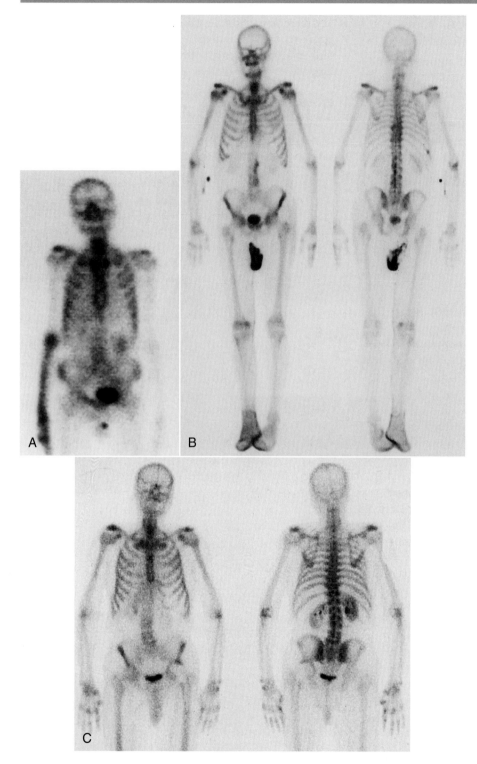

Bone scans of patients A, B, and C.

1. Describe the bone scan findings in the three cases.

2. Explain the findings.

3. Name the physical principle that is involved in patient C.

4. Name the most likely type of material involved in patient C.

Skeletal System: Arterial Injection, Boot Artifact, Photopenic Attenuation Artifact

1. A, Increased distribution in the right upper extremity from the elbow through the hands. B, Uptake outside bone in both feet and ankles, right greater than left. Urinary contamination of the scrotum. C, Photopenia of a portion of the right mid-humerus on the posterior view only. Additional photopenia produced by a left hip prosthesis.

2. A, Intra-arterial injection. B, Urinary contamination of socks ("boot artifact"). C, Attenuation artifacts of a right humerus and hip prosthesis.

3. Attenuation of photons.

4. Metal.

References

Chandra R: *Nuclear Medicine Physics; the Basics*, 5th ed. Baltimore: Williams & Wilkins, 1998, pp 128, 154.

Ryo UY, Alavi A, Collier BD, et al: *Atlas of Nuclear Medicine Artifacts and Variants*, 2nd ed. Chicago: Year Book, 1990.

Cross-Reference

Nuclear Medicine: THE REQUISITES, 3rd ed, pp 13-15, 113-116.

Comment

Given that the majority of bone abnormalities appear as "hot" lesions, through experience, imagers are conditioned to "look for" and therefore "see" lesions that demonstrate increased activity. Photopenic lesions on bone scans can be overlooked easily if one does not specifically check to see that all the expected structures are demonstrated. In patient C, once the finding is "seen" and noted not to be present on the anterior view, artifacts should be considered. Because the finding is photopenic with normal bone uptake in this region on the anterior view, some material must be between the bone and the posterior detector to account for the reduction in photons reaching the detector. Attenuation is removal of photons from a radiation flux because of absorption. The materials that block or absorb gamma rays are the same as those that block x-rays; therefore, metal is the most likely, although barium and calcium also cause attenuation. The technologist confirmed that a metal strip left by maintenance personnel had been found on the imaging table when the patient left. The most common cold artifacts are metal on clothing, coins in the pocket, and metal medallions on the chest.

An intra-arterial injection is very uncommon and occurs inadvertently. The technologist was not aware of it or did not want to admit it, but the pattern is characteristic and tells the story. The "boot" artifact is a more common finding and is seen in patients with urinary incontinence. Invariably other evidence of urinary contamination is seen on the scan.

Notes

Two patients (A and B) referred with low back pain to rule out metastases from their primary tumor. Selected coronal, sagittal, transaxial slices, and MIP images from ^{99m}Tc-MDP SPECT are shown.

1. Describe the scintigraphic SPECT findings in studies A and B.

2. Give the likely diagnosis in both patients.

3. Why is diagnostic accuracy of lumbar spine for SPECT higher than for planar imaging?

4. How can bone SPECT be clinically helpful in diagnosing the cause of pain in a patient 1 year after spinal surgery?

Skeletal System: Increased Specificity with Bone Scan Lumbar SPECT

1. A, Uptake in the region of the L4 right pedicle, extending to the vertebral body. B, Uptake in the region of the L2 facet joints bilaterally, right greater than left.

2. A, Metastatic tumor. B, Articular facet osteoarthritis.

3. SPECT improves the target-to-background ratio by removing overlying activity from adjacent slices and allows three-dimensional display and localization.

4. One year after surgery, a healed fusion has no more than minimally increased activity, whereas a pseudoarthrosis shows active bony repair with increased activity.

References

Horger M, Bares R: The role of single photo emission computed tomography in benign and malignant bone disease, *Semin Nucl Med* 36:286–294, 2006.

Van der Wall H, Fogelman I: Scintigraphy of benign bone disease, *Semin Musculoskelet Radiol* 11:281–300, 2007.

Cross-Reference

Nuclear Medicine: THE REQUISITES, 3rd ed, pp 52–62.

Comment

Bone scans are very sensitive for the detection of osseous disease. However, the specificity and thus the etiology of the uptake are often not certain. Benign and malignant uptake can appear similar. Specificity often can be improved by noting the distribution of the abnormal uptake (e.g., metastases are typically random and fractures are often in adjacent ribs). Spine disease can be particularly problematic because of overlapping activity of the anterior and posterior elements. Ascertaining whether the increased focal spine uptake is in the pedicle, body, or posterior elements can improve the diagnostic specificity and aid in the differential diagnosis. Malignant lesions involve the pedicle and may extend into the vertebral body. Articular facet osteoarthritis, a common cause of bone scan abnormalities, typically involves the posterior elements of the vertebral body. Posterior oblique views can sometimes be helpful in making this distinction.

The three-dimensional display of SPECT permits differentiation between the vertebral body, pedicle, and posterior element uptake. Thus, SPECT often can confirm or exclude malignant disease. Newer hybrid SPECT/CT systems offer the potential to further improve specificity. Although increased uptake is the rule, cold lesions caused by lytic or destructive lesions are not rare with malignant disease and may not always be obvious on two-dimensional planar images because of overlying activity.

Notes

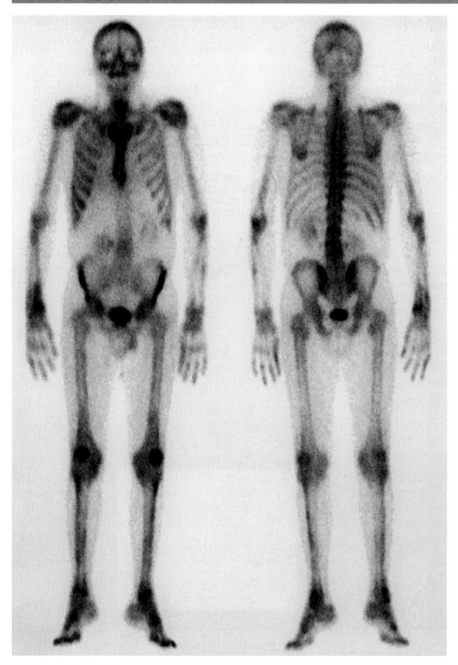

This patient was referred for bone scan because of bone and joint pain.

1. Describe the scintigraphic bone scan findings.

2. Describe any soft-tissue findings. What is the likely cause?

3. What other imaging study should be ordered?

4. What is the likely diagnosis and cause for this scan pattern?

Skeletal System: Pulmonary Hypertrophic Osteoarthropathy

1. Diffuse increased uptake in the upper and lower extremities and in the periarticular regions of the elbow, wrist, and ankle joint, predominantly periosteal in pattern. There is uptake in the seventh right rib anteriorly and the right ulna.

2. Diffuse uptake in the right thorax. The most common cause is malignant pleural effusion. Note that the right kidney appears ptotic.

3. Chest x-ray.

4. Hypertrophic pulmonary osteoarthropathy. Bronchogenic carcinoma of the lung.

Reference

Silberstein EB, Elgazzar AH, Fernandez-Ulloa M, et al: Skeletal scintigraphy in non-neoplastic osseous disorders. In: Henkin RE (ed): *Nuclear Medicine*. St. Louis: Mosby, 1996, pp 1185–1186.

Cross-Reference

Nuclear Medicine: THE REQUISITES, 3rd ed, pp 126, 130–132.

Comment

Hypertrophic osteoarthropathy is characterized clinically by the presence of periostitis causing bone pain, arthralgia, and clubbing of the fingers and toes. The characteristic radiographic and scintigraphic changes usually precede the development of clinical symptoms and signs. The hypertrophic changes regress after successful therapy of the underlying disease.

The bone scan changes of hypertrophic pulmonary osteoarthropathy are evident before radiographic changes. The pattern consists of generally increased activity in long bones and increased activity in the periarticular regions of the long bones, phalanges, scapulae, and clavicles. Pericortical striping along the medial and lateral aspects of the lower extremities (railroad tracking) is characteristic.

The pathophysiologic process of hypertrophic pulmonary osteoarthropathy is poorly understood. It is seen in a large number of benign and malignant conditions of the chest and abdomen. Thoracic benign and malignant tumors are the most common; most are bronchogenic carcinoma. Other less common causes of hypertrophic osteoarthropathy include mesothelioma, pulmonary metastases, bronchiectasis, and lung abscess. In children, it has been reported with asthma, cystic fibrosis, bronchiectasis, mediastinal disease (Hodgkin's disease), cardiovascular disease (cyanotic heart disease, bacterial endocarditis), and gastrointestinal disease (regional enteritis, ulcerative colitis, congenital biliary atresia).

Notes

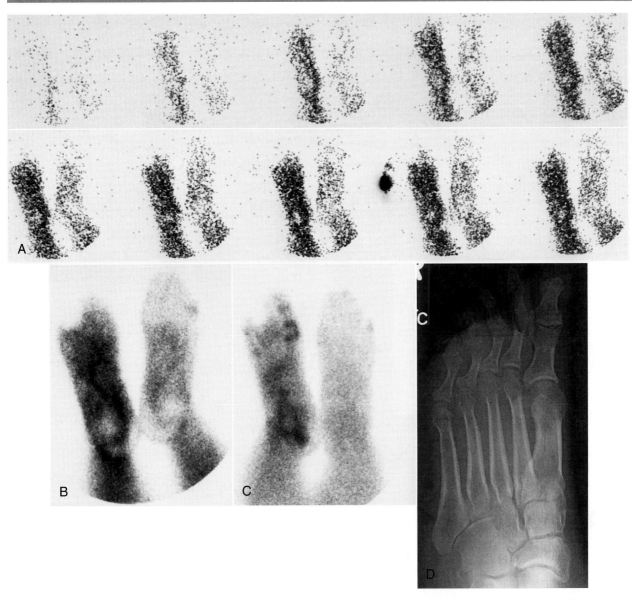

A patient with diabetes mellitus was referred with cellulitis of the right lower leg to rule out osteomyelitis. Plantar views shown: blood flow (A), blood pool (B), delayed uptake (C), radiograph (D).

1. Discuss the advantage of a three-phase bone scan compared with the delayed phase only.

2. Describe the scintigraphic bone scan findings.

3. Provide the differential diagnosis.

4. What is the most likely diagnosis?

Skeletal System: Cellulitis, Osteomyelitis, Gangrene of the Toes

1. Blood flow/pool images increase the diagnostic specificity and narrow the differential diagnosis.

2. Diffuse increased blood flow and blood pool to the foot and ankle of the right lower extremity. No blood flow, pool, or uptake of the right third and fourth toes. Mild increase uptake in all bones on the delayed image, slightly worse at the first metatarsophalangeal joint.

3. Vascular insufficiency, previous surgery, acute osteomyelitis, frostbite, replacement by tumor, artifact.

4. Cellulitis, arterial insufficiency and gangrene of the third and fourth toes, reactive changes of first metatarsophalangeal joint due to degenerative disease.

Reference
Palestro CJ, Love C: Nuclear medicine and diabetic foot infections, *Semin Nucl Med* 39:52–65, 2009.

Cross-Reference
Nuclear Medicine: THE REQUISITES, 3rd ed, pp 147–153.

Comment
Artifacts such as a lead shield or metal object causing attenuation should be excluded as a cause of nonvisualization. With nonvisualization of bony structures, the radiologist should consider previous surgery, which can be confirmed easily by history, physical inspection, or radiography. In this case, amputation is excluded by the radiograph showing all digits. An adequate vascular supply is required for delivery of the radiopharmaceutical and its subsequent deposition. Nonvisualization of the third and fourth toes indicates absent flow, which could result from acute or chronic arterial insufficiency or venous occlusion. In a patient with diabetes, chronic arterial insufficiency is the most likely cause. Acute photopenic osteomyelitis occurs more commonly in children.

A three-phase bone scan can provide additional important diagnostic information on vascular status of the limb or digit and on the degree of active bone remodeling. Osteomyelitis is classically three-phase positive with increased flow, blood pool, and delayed uptake at the site of osteomyelitis. The sensitivity of this finding is high; however, the specificity is less so. Fractures, tumors, and Charcot's joint may produce a three-phase positive pattern. A radiolabeled leukocyte study often is needed to confirm the diagnosis in nonvirgin bone.

Rarely, acute osteomyelitis in children may show abnormalities on the early phases of the bone scan with a normal delayed phase if imaging is performed early after onset.

Notes

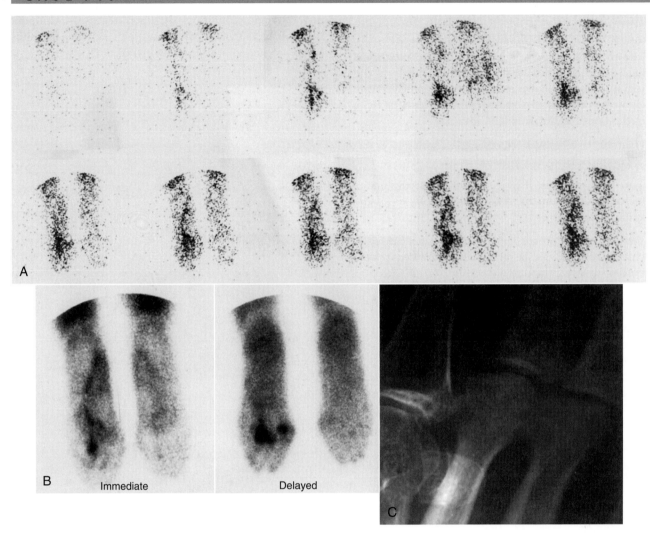

A

B   Immediate   Delayed

C

This patient was referred for foot pain.

1. Describe the abnormalities on the three-phase bone scan. A, Blood flow study. B, Immediate and delayed plantar views.

2. Provide the differential diagnosis.

3. Given the radiograph (C), name the entity. List at least three other sites subject to the same process.

4. List at least three conditions associated with this entity.

Skeletal System: Avascular Necrosis of Metatarsal Head (Freiberg's Disease)

1. The three-phase bone scan demonstrates abnormal increased blood flow and blood pool activity in the region of the second and third metatarsal heads. The delayed bone phase demonstrates increased activity in the bones in the same distribution.

2. Fracture, osteotomy, osteomyelitis, primary or secondary neoplasm, avascular necrosis.

3. Avascular necrosis. Tarsal navicular, carpal lunate, femoral head, humeral head, ring apophyses of the spine, tibial tubercle.

4. Trauma, hypercortisolism, collagen vascular disease, chronic renal disease, aspirin, sickle cell disease, alcoholism, dysbaric conditions.

References

Groshar D, Gorenberg M, Ben-Haim S, et al: Lower extremity scintigraphy: the foot and ankle, *Semin Nucl Med* 28:62–67, 1998.

Manaster BJ, May DA, Disler DB: *Musculoskeletal Imaging: The Requisites*, 3rd ed. St. Louis: Mosby, 2007, pp 346–350.

Cross-Reference

Nuclear Medicine: THE REQUISITES, 3rd ed, pp 142–147.

Comment

This patient's bone scan is an example of Freiberg's disease, one of the osteochondroses, a heterogeneous group of disorders that radiographically display the features of increased density and fragmentation, with or without flattening of the epiphysis or apophysis, as seen on the radiograph involving the third and, to a lesser extent, the second metatarsal heads. The causes include osteonecrosis, trauma, and normal variation.

Avascular necrosis, osteonecrosis, and *ischemic necrosis* are terms applied to the results of inadequate blood flow to bone. Compared with other portions of the bone, the epiphyseal ends of long bones are predisposed because they have relatively limited arterial and venous pathways, which are even more pronounced while growth plates are present. Typically, the epiphysis is supplied by a single artery, which increases risk. When the dominant blood supply is compromised, severe ischemia and, if prolonged, necrosis, occur. Mechanisms of vascular compromise include obstruction, compression, and disruption. Causes or associated conditions include trauma, hypercortisolism, chronic renal disease, aspirin, collagen vascular disease, sickle cell disease, alcoholism, and dysbaric conditions (Caisson disease). Although osteonecrosis can occur at any joint surface, the sites listed are the most frequently involved.

Notes

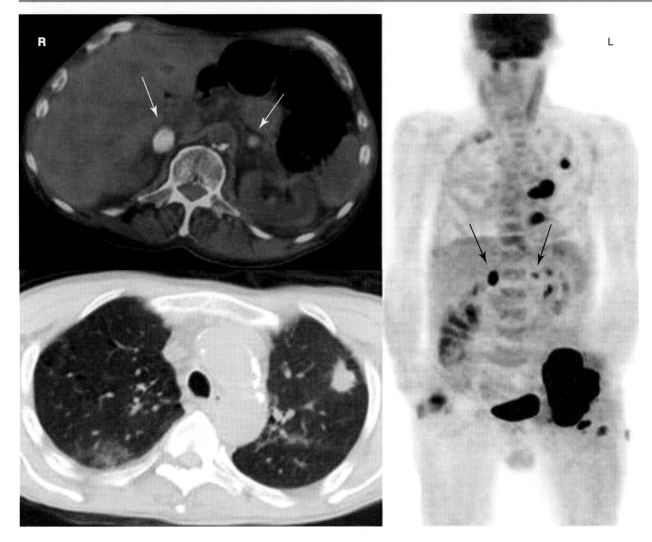

A 65-year-old man with metastatic lung cancer. *Upper left,* FDG fused PET/CT abdominal image; *lower left,* chest CT; *right,* MIP image.

1. What is the most likely cause for the abnormal FDG uptake in the left chest region?

2. What is the most likely cause for the FDG uptake in the mid-abdomen (*arrows*)?

3. What PET/CT criteria would indicate malignancy in this area (*arrows*)?

4. What are the most common malignancies that metastasize to this region?

Oncology: FDG-PET/CT—Lung Cancer and Adrenal Metastases

1. The focal uptake in the left upper chest region correlates with the left upper lobe spiculated primary lung malignancy with evidence of FDG uptake and likely metastasis to the left hilum.

2. The abnormal FDG-PET focal uptake in the right upper abdomen is bilateral adrenal gland metastatic disease.

3. If FDG uptake is greater than in the liver, malignant involvement is likely.

4. Lung, gastrointestinal, breast, melanoma, kidney, and pancreas.

References

Blake MA, Slattery JMA, Kalra MK, et al: Adrenal lesions: characterization with fused PET/CT image in patients with proved or suspected malignancy—initial experience, *Radiology* 238:970–977, 2006.

Yun M, Kim W, Alnafisi N, et al: F-18-FDG PET in characterizing adrenal lesions detected on CT or MRI, *J Nucl Med* 42:1795–1799, 2001.

Comment

Incidentally discovered adrenal masses in patients with no history of malignancy are rarely metastatic. An adrenal mass detected in a patient with cancer has an approximately 30% probability of being malignant. Conventional CT with and without intravenous contrast cannot usually differentiate adrenal metastases from benign nonhyperfunctioning adenomas, but more specific CT protocols, with delayed washout images, and MRI with T2-weighted imaging improves diagnostic differentiation.

Benign causes of FDG uptake include adrenal adenomas, pheochromocytoma, and adrenal cortical hyperplasia. Adrenal malignancy diagnosed by FDG-PET is reported to have a sensitivity of 99%, specificity of 92%, and diagnostic accuracy of 94% when using a maximum SUV cutoff of 3.1. Specificity is further increased when using combined FDG-PET/CT. Causes of false-negative findings on FDG-PET in malignant adrenal gland tumors include the presence of hemorrhage or necrosis, small size (lesions < 1 cm), and lack of FDG avidity of the primary tumor (e.g., bronchoalveolar lung carcinoma and neuroendocrine tumors). FDG-PET imaging is most useful when other imaging modalities such as CT and MRI have indeterminate findings regarding adrenal lesions. If discordant findings between anatomic and metabolic PET imaging remain, biopsy may be necessary.

Notes

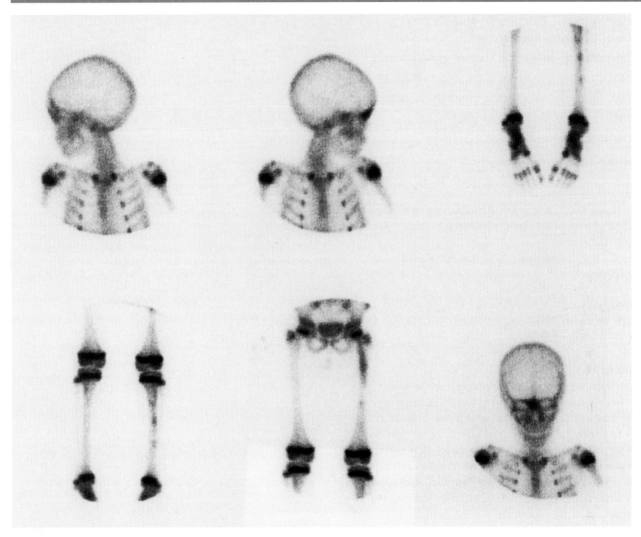

A 5-year-old child has precocious puberty and bone pain.

1. Name two findings that might be seen when examining this patient.

2. Describe the scan findings.

3. What bone disease is most likely?

4. What syndrome does this patient have?

Skeletal System: Fibrous Dysplasia, McCune-Albright Syndrome

1. Pigmented café-au-lait skin lesions, gynecomastia.

2. Abnormal uptake is seen in the frontal bone, left femur, and left tibia, with a nonuniform pattern of uptake in the long bones.

3. Polyostotic fibrous dysplasia.

4. McCune-Albright syndrome.

References

Ma JJ, Kang BK, Treves ST: Pediatric musculoskeletal nuclear medicine, *Semin Musculoskelet Radiol* 11:322–324, 2007.

Nadel HR: Bone scan update, *Semin Nucl Med* 37:322–329, 2007.

Cross-Reference

Nuclear Medicine: THE REQUISITES, 3rd ed, pp 132–133, 138.

Comment

Fibrous dysplasia is a developmental abnormality that results in localized proliferation of fibroblasts that replace normal cancellous bone. The abnormal fibrous tissue results in a trabecular pattern of immature woven bone, the radiographic density of which varies depending on the amount of bone present. The condition may be monostotic, monomelic, or polyostotic. The disease begins in childhood and may be seen in infants. Pathologic fracture of the abnormally weak bone is the most frequent complication.

Scintigraphy is helpful in determining the activity and distinguishing monostotic from polyostotic disease. The majority of lesions in fibrous dysplasia are tracer avid on ^{99m}Tc-MDP bone scans. Seven percent to 14% of lesions have uptake equivalent to that of normal bone; however, the remainder show supranormal uptake.

Localized abnormal pigmentation, café-au-lait spots, are present in approximately one third of patients with polyostotic disease. These skin lesions have an irregular outline ("coast of Maine") in contrast to the smoothly marginated ("coast of California") pigmented lesions seen in neurofibromatosis. Several endocrine manifestations can be seen in these patients. Hyperthyroidism may occur in as many as 5% of patients. Sexual precocity occurs in as many as 30% of women with polyostotic disease, is rare in men, and is referred to as McCune-Albright syndrome.

Notes

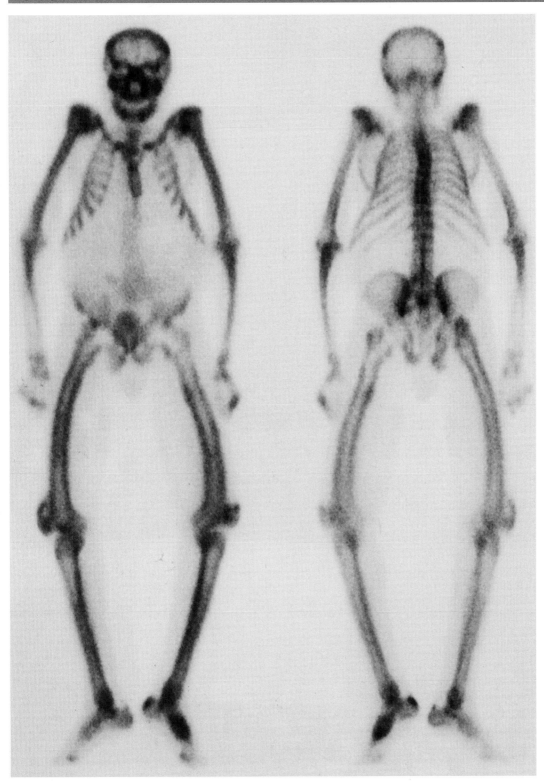

1. Describe the bone scan skeletal abnormalities.

2. Provide the differential diagnoses for the bone abnormalities.

3. Describe the ancillary nonbone abnormalities.

4. Provide the most likely diagnosis.

Skeletal System: Renal Osteodystrophy

1. Increased cortical radiotracer activity in the long bones of the upper and lower extremities. "Railroad tracking" and bowing of the femurs. Bilateral hip prostheses.

2. Hypertrophic osteoarthropathy, vitamin A intoxication, fluorosis, renal osteodystrophy, thyroid acropachy, melorheostosis.

3. High bone-to-soft tissue uptake ratio. Renal nonvisualization. Minimal bladder activity. Additional history: patient is undergoing dialysis after a failed kidney transplant.

4. The scan is characteristic of renal osteodystrophy. Previous hip replacements for avascular necrosis caused by steroid therapy related to kidney transplant.

Reference

Ryan PJ, Fogelman I: Bone scintigraphy in metabolic bone disease, *Semin Nucl Med* 27:291–305, 1997.

Cross-Reference

Nuclear Medicine: THE REQUISITES, 3rd ed, pp 131–133, 139–142.

Comment

Renal osteodystrophy occurs in patients with chronic renal failure resulting from abnormal vitamin D metabolism and secondary hyperparathyroidism. The former occurs because the kidney is the site of conversion of inactive 25-hydroxyvitamin D to the active form 1,25-dihydroxyvitamin D. Secondary hyperparathyroidism occurs because phosphate retention depresses serum calcium levels, prompting an increase in parathyroid hormone levels. Often, radiographs show evidence of rickets, osteomalacia, or secondary hyperparathyroidism. Osteosclerosis is seen more often in secondary than in primary hyperparathyroidism, predominantly in the axial skeleton.

The term *superscan* signifies a bone scan that appears to be of excellent quality because of the high target-to-soft tissue ratio with minimal or no evidence of urinary activity. Patient factors unrelated to the skeleton can result in a "beautiful" bone scan (e.g., enhanced renal clearance because of imaging delay longer than usual, good hydration and renal function, and little soft tissue). The differential for superscan includes renal osteodystrophy, diffuse skeletal metastases, myelofibrosis, fluorosis, mastocytosis, and pyknodysostosis and overlaps the gamut for diffuse osteosclerosis with that of some normal well-conditioned athletes. However, this patient's bone scan is clearly not normal and very characteristic of renal osteodystrophy. Characteristic increased uptake in renal osteodystrophy is commonly seen throughout the calvaria and mandible, costochondral junctions (beading), axial skeletal, and sternum (tie sign).

Notes

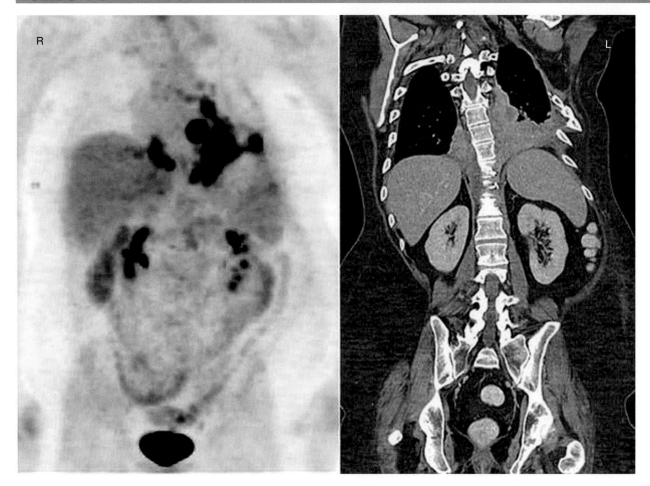

A 17-year-old patient with increased FDG uptake in the bilateral chest corresponding to soft-tissue masses on CT.

1. What is the differential diagnosis for the FDG-avid masses?

2. Is there any evidence of distant metastatic disease?

3. How is the FDG-PET study helpful in this case?

4. What is the likely treatment plan based on the image findings?

Oncology: FDG-PET/CT—Ewing's Sarcoma

1. Lymphoma, sarcoma, neuroblastoma, rhabdomyo-sarcoma. This patient had biopsy-proven Ewing's sarcoma arising from bilateral ribs.

2. No. There is no evidence of distant metastases on these images.

3. The PET study confirmed that tumor was confined to the chest without distant disease, thus directing management decisions.

4. The usual treatment is systemic chemotherapy in combination with local control (e.g., radiation therapy or surgery).

References

Iwamoto Y: Diagnosis and treatment of Ewing's sarcoma, *Jpn Clin Oncol* 37:79–89, 2006.

Volker T, Denecke T, Steffen I, et al: Positron emission tomography for staging of pediatric sarcoma patients: results of a prospective multicenter trial, *J Clin Oncol* 25:5435–5441, 2007.

Cross-Reference

Nuclear Medicine: THE REQUISITES, 3rd ed, p 344.

Comment

Ewing's sarcoma is the second most common malignant skeletal tumor in children and adolescents and typically arises from an intramedullary location with bony expansion/destruction and surrounding soft-tissue involvement. Patients typically present with monostotic disease, unlike in this patient who has bilateral rib involvement.

Plain film is considered the initial imaging strategy to evaluate for periosteal reaction or tumor osteolysis from primary sarcomatous tumor. However, MRI is routinely performed for staging and surgical planning purposes because it can also evaluate the extent of soft-tissue involvement and also be used for monitoring of therapy.

FDG-PET/CT as a whole-body imaging approach and its quantitative capability has been shown to be a useful adjunct to other imaging methods in sarcoma patients. It provides additional information such as the presence of metastatic disease and has an impact on therapy planning and monitoring. FDG-PET/CT is superior to other imaging modalities for the detection of bony metastatic disease with a sensitivity of 88% compared with 37% for conventional imaging modalities. Higher grade sarcomatous disease typically has greater accumulation of FDG and therefore higher SUV. High-grade sarcomas also tend to accumulate FDG at faster rates than those of lower grades. This has been shown to correlate with increased cellularity and mitotic activity as well as glucose utilization of the tissue.

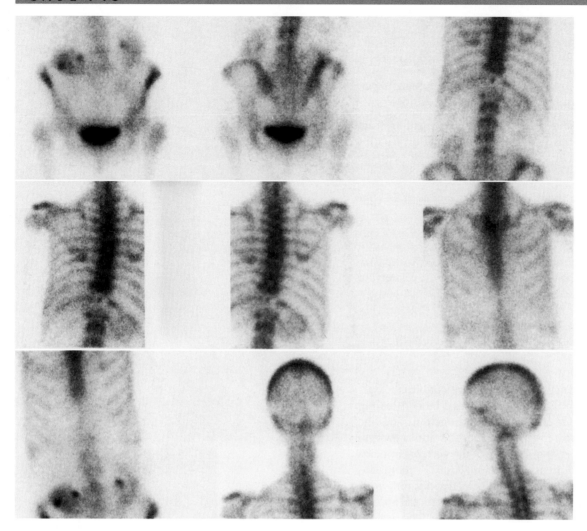

The patient was referred for back pain.

1. Describe the bone findings.

2. Describe any other nonosseous findings.

3. Provide the differential diagnosis for the bone abnormality.

4. List three possible primary neoplasms that might cause this finding.

Skeletal System: Metastasis to Bone (Photopenic) and Adrenal Gland

1. Photopenia of a low thoracic vertebra, probably T11.

2. Ptotic kidneys, abnormal soft-tissue uptake seen between the posterior right 11th and 12th ribs.

3. Primary or metastatic neoplasm, attenuation from external or internal source (e.g., buckle on back of clothing, metallic orthopedic hardware, or previous vertebroplasty).

4. Breast, colon, lung; neuroblastoma in a child, but clearly this patient is an adult.

Reference

Silberstein EB, McAfee JG, Spasoff AP: *Diagnostic Patterns in Nuclear Medicine*. Reston, VA: Society of Nuclear Medicine, 1998, p 207.

Cross-Reference

Nuclear Medicine: THE REQUISITES, 3rd ed, p 124.

Comment

The differential diagnosis for a solitary cold lesion on a bone scan is long, but can be shortened by considering the pattern of the abnormality, its location, and the patient's age. On careful inspection, the spinous process is visible, whereas the remainder of the vertebra appears photopenic. Benign or malignant primary neoplasms such as hemangioma, brown tumor of hyperparathyroidism, and myeloma/plasmacytoma could have this appearance. Metastases that result in primarily lytic lesions (e.g., thyroid and renal) should be considered. However, more often photopenic lesions in adults are caused by common malignancies, such as breast or lung. The majority of metastases from breast or lung scintigraphically show increased activity or occasionally photopenic centers with "hot" margins, but some appear photopenic, as in this case. The lung cancer metastasis to the right adrenal gland shows abnormal soft-tissue uptake. Other examples in this text illustrate bone scan radiotracer uptake in soft tissue. Liver metastases are another example of uncommon, but not rare, uptake by a bone tracer.

Both kidneys are noted to be ptotic and located near the iliac crests on the anterior and posterior views of the abdomen. If one failed to note this, the finding in the right posterior flank could easily be overlooked. The bone scan was obtained with the patient standing. Ptosis rather than ectopia can be confirmed by imaging the patient in the supine position.

Notes

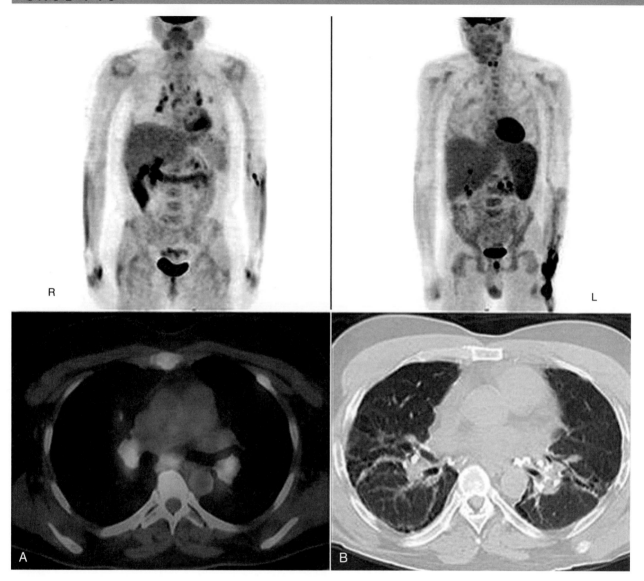

R

L

A

B

Patients A and B both presented with persistent cough and an abnormal chest x-ray.

1. Describe abnormal findings in patient A. Provide a differential diagnosis.

2. Describe any abnormal findings in patient B.

3. What is the most likely diagnosis for these patients?

4. What is the cause of the abnormal ^{18}F-FDG uptake in both of these patients?

Inflammatory Disease: FDG-PET/CT—Sarcoidosis

1. Bilateral hilar FDG uptake and adenopathy. Primary considerations would be sarcoidosis and lymphoma.

2. Bilateral enlarged calcified hilar nodes. Infiltrative changes in the lungs bilaterally on CT with FDG uptake. Splenomegaly with increased FDG uptake.

3. Sarcoidosis.

4. FDG uptake occurs with infection and inflammation. Mechanism is uptake by T lymphocytes, mononuclear phagocytes, and noncaseating epithelioid granulomas. All utilize glucose.

References

Deepak D, Shah A: Thoracic sarcoidosis: the spectrum of roentgenologic appearances, *Ind J Radiol Imaging* 11:191-198, 2001.

Prabhakar HB, Rabinowitz CB, Gibbons FK, et al: Imaging features of sarcoidosis on MDCT, FDG PET, and PET/CT, *AJR Am J Roentgenol* 190:S1-S6, 2008.

Cross-Reference

Nuclear Medicine: THE REQUISITES, 3rd ed, pp 414-418.

Comment

Enlarged nodes, as seen in this case, are not considered active disease unless they have FDG uptake above the adjacent mediastinal blood pool activity. Mildly and symmetrically increased uptake can be seen in this region with other inflammatory processes such as granulomatous disease and reactive lymph nodes. With granulomatous disease, there may be associated calcification on CT.

In sarcoidosis, the hilar nodes on CT are typically enlarged and sometimes called "potato nodes." Nodes typically involved are in the hilar, tracheobronchial, and paratracheal distribution and may have calcification bilaterally in long-standing sarcoidosis. The CT for patient B has lung parenchymal involvement of sarcoid. In 25% to 50% of patients, this infiltrative pattern is seen with or without hilar nodal involvement and most commonly involves central regions and particularly the upper lobes. Fibrous bands and cystic radiolucencies may be seen in advanced disease.

Sarcoidosis can coexist in patients with malignant disease. The increased FDG uptake of sarcoid could be misinterpreted as metastatic disease. Both may have intense uptake with high SUVs. The typical pattern of sarcoid is helpful in discriminating between the two, but not totally reliable.

^{67}Ga citrate has been used to evaluate patients with suspected or known sarcoidosis. Early disease may demonstrate bilateral hilar and paratracheal nodal uptake and may be referred to as the lambda sign. Uptake may also be seen in the lung parenchyma with or without associated nodal uptake.

Notes

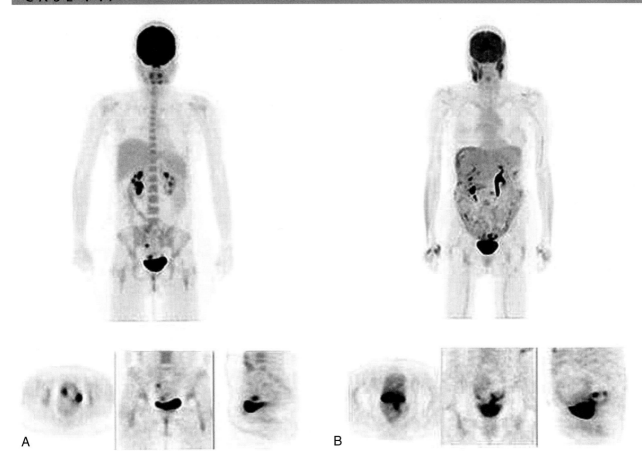

A

B

A, A 28-year-old woman with breast cancer. B, A 45-year-old woman with ovarian carcinoma. Both patients were referred for restaging. ^{18}F-FDG-PET images (MIP, transverse, coronal, sagittal).

1. Describe the different uptake pattern in the pelvis of patient A compared with patient B. What are the likely causes?

2. List potential false negatives and false positives for malignancy on PET imaging of the female pelvis.

3. What maneuvers or imaging alternatives can aid in the differentiation of perivesicular uptake?

4. What is the primary clinical benefit of FDG-PET in ovarian carcinoma?

Oncology: FDG-PET/CT—Ovarian Carcinoma, Female Pelvis

1. A, Two foci of FDG uptake superior and to the right of the bladder, likely physiologic in the uterus and right ovary. History and sonography could confirm. B, Diffuse uptake throughout the peritoneum, extending around liver and above/posterior to bladder, suggestive of peritoneal metastases.

2. False negatives: malignancy can be misinterpreted as physiologic (e.g., intravesical urine, mucinous adenocarcinoma, cystadenocarcinoma). False positives: corpus luteum cyst, cystadenoma, dermoid cyst, diverticulitis, leiomyoma, adenoma, fibroma, thecoma, adenomyoma, ureteral retention, endometriosis.

3. Additional imaging of the pelvis after voiding, dual-phase imaging (e.g., at both 1 and 2-3 hours), ingestion of water before voiding near the end of the uptake phase to dilute urine FDG activity, furosemide.

4. Detection of recurrent disease in patients with elevated serum markers (CA125, CA19-9) and negative or indeterminate conventional imaging (i.e., CT). In this setting, FDG-PET is 90% sensitive and 86% specific compared with conventional imaging, which is 68% sensitive and 58% specific.

References

Fanti S, Nanni C, Ambrosini V, et al: PET in genitourinary tract cancers, *Q J Nucl Med Mol Imaging* 51(3):260–271, 2007.

Schwarz JK, Grigsby PW, Dehdashti F, Delbeke D: The role of 18F-FDG PET in assessing therapy response in cancer of the cervix and ovaries, *J Nucl Med* 50(Suppl 1):64S–73S, 2009.

Cross-Reference

Nuclear Medicine: THE REQUISITES, 3rd ed, pp 341–344.

Comment

Normal intense FDG uptake may be seen in the ovaries and uterus during the late follicular/early luteal menstrual phase. Postmenopausal patients can have mild physiologic uterine uptake because the endometrium is more quiescent than atrophic, especially early in menopause. More than mild uptake requires workup.

The most common gynecologic cancer is endometrial, usually occurring in postmenopausal women. FDG-PET/CT is valuable in preoperative staging by identifying additional sites of lymph node and distant organ metastases. FDG-PET/CT has an accuracy of 94% for the detection of nodal disease and changes management in 30%. In ovarian cancer, FDG-PET/CT has superior accuracy compared with CT in preoperative disease assessment (87% vs. 53%). It is also cost-effective for detecting recurrent ovarian cancer and assessing response to therapy.

With cancer of the uterine cervix, determination of lymph node status at diagnosis is crucial. Even in patients with FIGO stage IB disease (confined to the cervix), those with positive nodal involvement have a poorer overall survival rate than those without (45–55% vs. 85–95%). PET performs well compared with MRI with a positive predictive value of 90% for detecting metastatic lymph nodes during staging compared with 64% by MRI. In addition, patients with therapeutic response to chemotherapy and/or radiotherapy as determined by FDG-PET have a better 5-year survival rate compared with those who do not respond or progress through therapy (80% vs. 32%).

Notes

Immediate   60 min   90 min

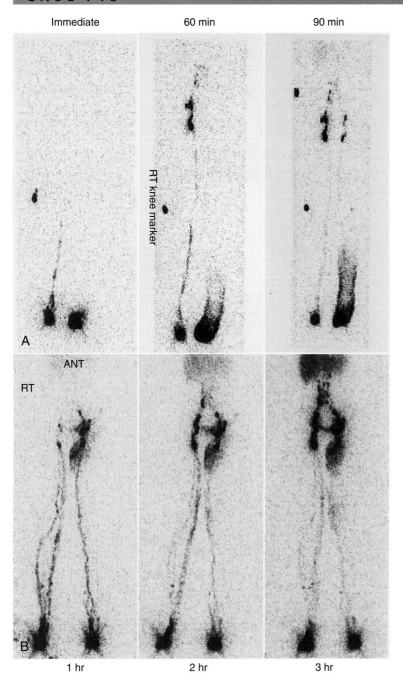

RT knee marker

A

ANT

RT

B

1 hr   2 hr   3 hr

Patient A is a 50-year-old woman with recurrent cellulitis and chronic edema of the left lower extremity. Patient B is a 60-year-old man with swelling in the left upper thigh for several months after femoral artery surgery. Both patients had radionuclide lymphoscintigraphy.

1. What radiopharmaceutical is most commonly used in the United States for lymphoscintigraphy?

2. What is the differential diagnosis of chronic lower extremity edema if systemic disease (e.g., cardiac, hepatic, renal) has been excluded?

3. Describe the lymphoscintigraphic pattern in these two patients.

4. What are the diagnoses?

Musculoskeletal System: Lymphoscintigraphy of the Lower Extremities

1. Filtered ^{99m}Tc-SC.

2. Chronic venous insufficiency and lymphedema, primary or secondary.

3. A, Normal deep lymphatic flow to femoral and inguinal nodes on the right. Dermal backflow pattern on the distal left lower extremity. B, Abnormal focal accumulation in the medial left thigh. One superficial collateral lymphatic vessel on the right.

4. A, Lymphatic obstruction of left lower extremity. B, Left leg: lymphatic leak with extravasation becoming a lymphocele; right leg: normal scintigram (asymptomatic).

References

Pui MH, Yueh TC: Lymphoscintigraphy in chyluria, chyloperitoneum and chylothorax, *J Nucl Med* 39:1292–1296, 1998.

Scarsbrook AF, Ganeshan A, Bradley KM: Pearls and pitfalls of radionuclide imaging of the lymphatic system. Part 2: evaluation of extremity lymphoedema, *Br J Radiol* 80:219–226, 2007.

Cross-Reference

Nuclear Medicine: THE REQUISITES, 3rd ed, pp 299–300.

Comment

Lymphedema usually is progressive. Early in the disease, edema predominates; later, chronic soft-tissue inflammation and ultimately irreversible fibrosis result. Lymphedema can be a primary condition (aplasia, hypoplasia, lymphangiectasia), but most commonly is secondary (infection, inflammation, trauma, malignancy, surgical or radiation therapy). Venous and lymphatic causes may coexist. Lymphedema usually is diagnosed on a clinical basis; imaging studies can confirm or exclude lymphatic obstruction. Contrast lymphangiography is technically difficult to perform; especially in this patient group; it does not allow functional assessment of lymph flow and may produce lymphadenitis.

Radionuclide lymphoscintigraphy demonstrates the physiology of lymphatic flow. Radiolabeled colloid particles are injected subcutaneously in the web spaces of the second and third toes. In patients without lymphatic disease, lymphoscintigraphy shows lymph flowing along the medial aspect of the leg to lymph nodes in the groin, pelvis, and para-aortic region. Abnormal patterns of obstruction include no or delayed flow, collateral vessel flow, dermal backflow because of obstructed or non-functioning lymph channels with interstitial dermal lymph transport (A), extravasation into lymphoceles or fistulae (B), and lymphangiectasia.

Lymphoscintigraphy is also used to diagnose, confirm, and localize chyluria, chyloperitoneum, and chylothorax.

Notes

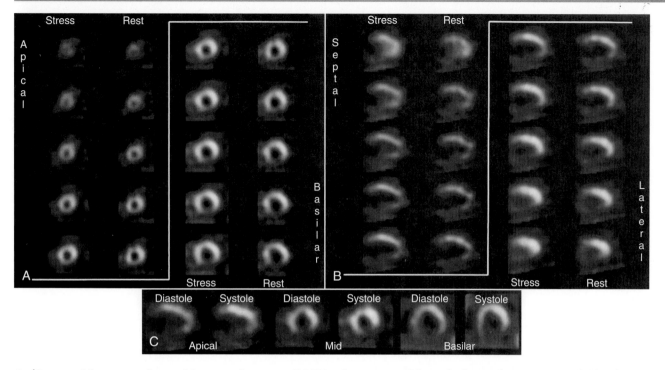

A 48-year-old woman has a history of severe COPD, shortness of breath, bronchospasm, and claudication. SPECT perfusion images (A, short axis; B, vertical long axis; C, select gated poststress SPECT images). The LVEF is 20%.

1. What is the appropriate stress technique for this patient? Why?

2. What potential problems may occur with this method?

3. Describe the SPECT image findings.

4. What is the mechanism of cardiac uptake for ^{99m}Tc-sestamibi and ^{99m}Tc-tetrofosmin?

Cardiovascular System: Dobutamine Stress

1. Dobutamine stress. Claudication precludes exercise stress. Patients with bronchospasm cannot be given coronary vasodilators (e.g., dipyridamole, adenosine, or regadenoson).

2. Side effects, including angina, occur commonly and many patients cannot tolerate the required dose.

3. Severe fixed inferior defect with absent wall thickening. Mild fixed anteroseptal perfusion defect with reduced wall thickening. Dilated left ventricular cavity. No reversibility. Myocardial thickening and wall motion signify viable myocardium.

4. Sestamibi is an isonitrile monovalent cation, diffuses passively from the blood into myocardial cells because of its lipophilicity, and then localizes in the mitochondria. Tetrofosmin, a diphosphene, has a similar mechanism.

Reference

Botvinich EH: Current methods of pharmacologic stress testing and the potential advantages of new agents, *J Nucl Med Technol* 37:14–25, 2009.

Cross-Reference

Nuclear Medicine: THE REQUISITES, 3rd ed, pp 461–466.

Comment

Dobutamine is a synthetic catecholamine that acts on α- and β-adrenergic receptors (inotropic and chronotropic). It indirectly increases coronary blood flow by increasing myocardial oxygen demand (increased heart rate, systolic blood pressure, contractility), thus, resulting in dilation of coronary arteries. The protocol for administering intravenous dobutamine involves infusion of increasingly higher dose rates up to a maximum of 40 μg/kg/min under constant ECG monitoring. Because of its short half-life, side effects can be managed by discontinuing the infusion.

Typical candidates for dobutamine are those who cannot exercise because of arthritis, peripheral vascular disease, or lower extremity weakness and cannot be given adenosine or dipyridamole because of bronchospastic pulmonary disease (COPD, asthma). Dobutamine also can be used in patients in whom xanthine-containing medications or foods were not discontinued before the appointment for adenosine or dipyridamole stress testing. Patients with low systolic blood pressure also may be candidates because blood pressure tends to increase with dobutamine rather than decrease with adenosine and dipyridamole. Relative contraindications to dobutamine are recent myocardial infarction or unstable angina, significant left ventricular outflow obstruction, atrial tachyarrhythmias, ventricular tachycardia, uncontrolled severe hypertension, aortic dissections, or aneurysms.

Notes

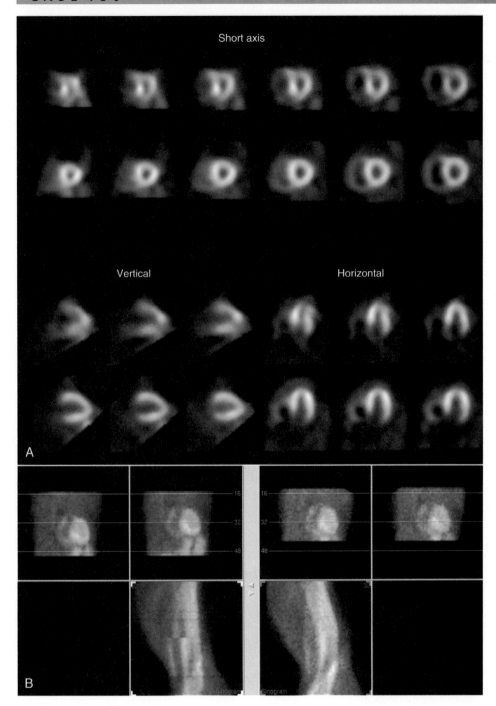

A, Two exercise myocardial SPECT perfusion studies are shown: the patient's initial stress acquisition (*top*) and a repeat study (*bottom*). B, Sinograms for the first (*left*) and second (*right*) scans.

1. Describe the purpose of the sinogram.

2. Describe the findings based on the SPECT images (A) and sinograms (B).

3. List other techniques in addition to the sinogram that can be used for a similar purpose.

4. What is the explanation for the difference in the two sets of images and sonograms?

Cardiovascular System: Patient Movement Artifact

1. To evaluate for patient motion by reviewing the unprocessed projection images in a form that makes motion easily detected.

2. A, The first study (*top*) shows an abnormal configuration of the anterior wall; the repeat study (*bottom*) is normal. B, The initial sinogram shows a discontinuity or break; the second is normal.

3. Review SPECT unprocessed projection data image by image or in cinematic display.

4. Artifact caused by patient motion.

Reference

DePuey EG: Artifacts in SPECT myocardial perfusion imaging. In: DePuey EG, Garcia EV, Berman DS (eds): *Cardiac SPECT Imaging*, 2nd ed. Philadelphia: Lippincott Williams & Wilkins, 2001, pp 232–262.

Cross-Reference

Nuclear Medicine: THE REQUISITES, 3rd ed, p 467.

Comment

An artifact should be considered when the myocardium appears irregular in shape and contour. Linear rays of activity (comet tails) are present in the initial study, strongly suggestive of motion, but are not seen on the repeat study. One should also consider center of rotation error as a mechanism for the artifact. Sinograms are constructed by stacking all raw projection unprocessed images of a single cross-sectional slice (plane indicated by the horizontal line crossing the cardiac projection images in the top row of part B). The first sinogram shows an abnormal sharp stepoff or discontinuity; the second shows a normal, smooth-curving appearance.

The unprocessed projection images from the SPECT acquisition should be inspected before image reconstruction. As seen in this study, motion can severely degrade the quality of the SPECT scan. Patient movement resulting in displacement greater than two pixels often produces significant artifacts. Some gamma camera–computer systems offer motion correction software that can be used to adjust for horizontal or vertical motion of the patient. However, this algorithm cannot correct for off-plane motion. When possible, imaging should be repeated if significant patient motion has occurred.

Routine gamma camera quality-control procedures are even more critical for SPECT than for planar imaging. Factors determining image quality include center of rotation, pixel size, uniformity, spatial resolution and linearity, detector head alignment, and head matching if a multihead camera is used.

Notes

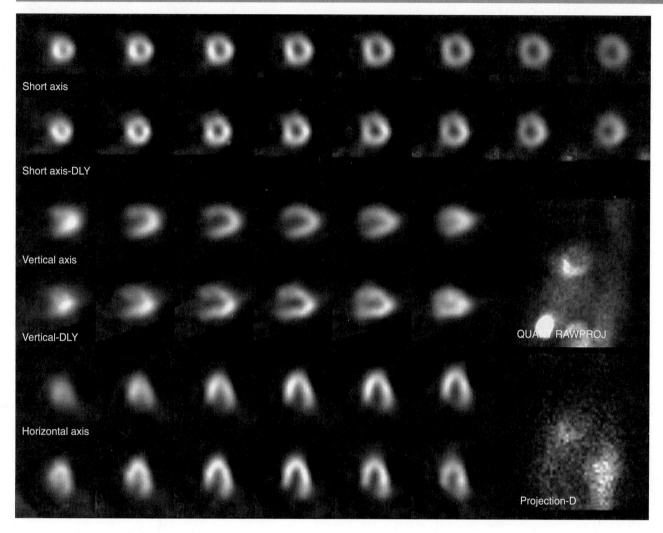

Short axis

Short axis-DLY

Vertical axis

Vertical-DLY

QUANT RAWPROJ

Horizontal axis

Projection-D

Stress and rest SPECT myocardial perfusion cross-sectional images and a left lateral single unprocessed projection image from a cine loop (*lower right*) are shown.

1. Describe the SPECT cross-sectional image findings.

2. Describe any additional information available from the cine loop stress and rest projection images.

3. List the differential diagnosis.

4. List the advantages of adding ECG synchronization (gating) to SPECT myocardial perfusion imaging.

Cardiovascular System: Breast Attenuation

1. Mild fixed defect in the anterior wall.

2. Projection images: decreased uptake in the upper half of the heart in a curvilinear configuration that is similar on both stress and rest studies.

3. Breast attenuation, anterior wall myocardial scar (infarction).

4. Assessment of regional wall motion, wall thickening, and ejection fraction.

Reference

DePuey EG: Artifacts in SPECT myocardial perfusion imaging. In: DePuey EG, Garcia EV, Berman DS (eds): *Cardiac SPECT Imaging*, 2nd ed. Philadelphia: Lippincott Williams & Wilkins, 2001, pp 232–262.

Cross-Reference

Nuclear Medicine: THE REQUISITES, 3rd ed, pp 469–471.

Comment

Breast tissue often causes attenuation of photons arising from the heart, reducing the number of counts available for image reconstruction in that region. This can lead to spurious defects varying in location depending on the breast position at the time of imaging. Breast attenuation defects most commonly occur in the anterior and antero-lateral walls but also are seen in the anteroseptal and lateral walls, depending on the location, density, and mobility of breast tissue. Breast attenuation would be expected to appear as a "fixed" defect; however, with a change in breast position between the stress and rest images, a stress-rest pattern can be seen that may mimic ischemia. Unprocessed acquisition projection image data should be reviewed to confirm the presence of attenuation and determine whether the breast has changed position between stress and rest.

Various interventions have been used to minimize attenuation, including the use of a breast binder to flatten and hold the breasts in the same position for the stress and rest scans or imaging the patient with the bra on to ensure similar positioning on both studies. Others image with the bra off, contending that gravity will flatten the breast (decreasing its thickness and attenuation). No method eliminates the problem. Gated SPECT can help to differentiate attenuation effects from myocardial infarction in patients with fixed defects. Attenuation correction programs are now widely available and can be helpful in selected cases. Infarcts show abnormal motion and thickening; attenuation defects have normal function.

Note the large focal hot spot seen on the stress projection image caused by gallbladder filling. Both ^{99m}Tc-sestamibi and ^{99m}Tc-tetrofosmin have hepatobiliary clearance.

Notes

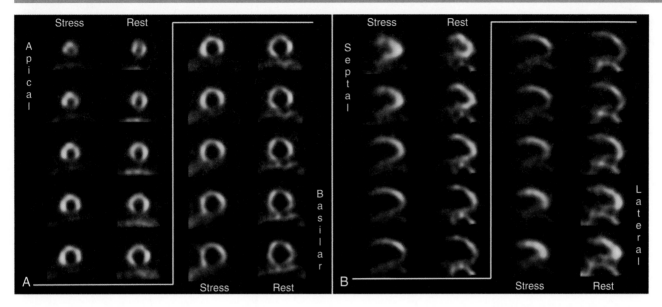

Dipyridamole (Persantine) sestamibi SPECT myocardial perfusion study. Short-axis (A) and vertical long-axis (B) images are shown.

1. List foods and medications that counteract the pharmacologic effect of dipyridamole.

2. Describe the optimal timing of radiotracer injection with respect to dipyridamole administration and management of dipyridamole side effects.

3. Describe the SPECT image findings.

4. List maneuvers to deal with the problem of abdominal (liver and intestinal) activity.

Cardiovascular System: Dipyridamole, Inferior Ischemia, Overlying Bowel Activity

1. Coffee, tea, caffeine-containing soft drinks or foods such as chocolate, theophylline, and aminophylline. Even some so-called caffeine-free products can be culprits.

2. Dipyridamole is infused for over 4 minutes. Radiotracer is given 3 to 4 minutes after completion of the infusion. Side effects can be reversed with intravenous aminophylline.

3. Mild-moderate severity fixed defect of the anterior wall. Severe fixed defect involving the entire inferior wall, a small area of mild reversibility in the inferoapical region. Dilated left ventricle.

4. Perform delayed SPECT to allow additional hepatic clearance or movement of bowel activity, have the patient drink water, or both.

References

DePuey EG: Artifacts in SPECT myocardial perfusion imaging. In: DePuey EG, Garcia EV (eds): *Cardiac SPECT Imaging*, 2nd ed. Philadelphia: Lippincott Williams & Wilkins, 2001, pp 232–262.

Rehm PK, Atkins FB, Ziessman HA, et al: Frequency of extracardiac activity and its effect on Tc-99m sestamibi cardiac SPECT interpretation, *Nucl Med Commun* 17:851–856, 1996.

Cross-Reference

Nuclear Medicine: THE REQUISITES, 3rd ed, pp 461–466.

Comment

The radiopharmaceutical is injected at peak dipyridamole effect, which occurs 3 to 4 minutes after completion of infusion. Relative contraindications to dipyridamole and adenosine include asthma or bronchospastic pulmonary disease, hypotension, severe bradycardia, and heart block greater than first degree. Adverse effects can be treated with intravenous injection of 125 to 250 mg aminophylline. Because dipyridamole's duration of action is longer than that of aminophylline, a subsequent injection of aminophylline may be necessary if side effects recur. Side effects with adenosine require only cessation of the infusion because of its short duration of action.

Extracardiac subdiaphragmatic activity can cause interpretation difficulties, whether related to a persistent hepatogram or hepatobiliary clearance of ^{99m}Tc perfusion agents into the intestines. Abdominal activity is common on rest or vasodilator stress studies because of increased splanchnic distribution compared with exercise stress studies. With exercise, splanchnic flow is diverted to the muscles. In this study case, curvilinear activity is noted adjacent to the inferior wall, but the area of the ischemia can be seen separate from bowel activity. However, at times, extracardiac activity may overlie the inferior wall or cause significant scatter, making it difficult or impossible to evaluate that portion of the myocardium. Repeat imaging after drinking fluids and some delay can be helpful on occasion.

Notes

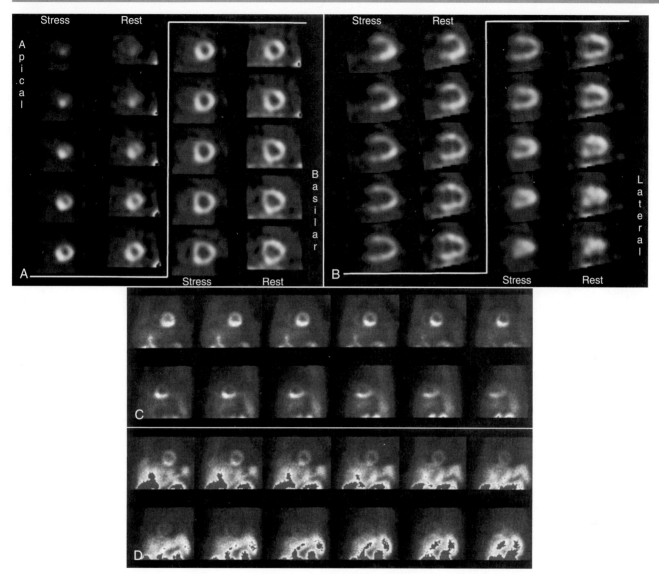

A 45-year-old woman has chest pain and hypercholesterolemia. Short-axis (A) and vertical long-axis (B) SPECT stress myocardial perfusion images, and sequential unprocessed projection images from the stress (C) and rest (D) scans.

1. Describe the SPECT cross-sectional perfusion image findings.

2. List three reasons to review the raw data projection images.

3. Compare the two sets of projection images.

4. What is the most likely diagnosis?

Cardiovascular System: Attenuation and Change of Breast Position

1. Partially reversible perfusion defect in the apical-anteroseptal wall. Mild fixed defect in the inferolateral wall. Dilated left ventricle.

2. To detect patient motion, attenuation/scatter, or camera malfunction.

3. Decreased radiotracer in the upper portions of the myocardium that appears different in location and degree on the stress and rest projection images.

4. Position-dependent breast artifact. Concomitant ischemia may or may not be present.

Reference

DePuey EG: Artifacts in SPECT myocardial perfusion imaging. In DePuey EG, Garcia EV (eds): *Cardiac SPECT Imaging*, 2nd ed. Philadelphia: Lippincott Williams & Wilkins, 2001, pp 232–262.

Cross-Reference

Nuclear Medicine: THE REQUISITES, 3rd ed, pp. 469–471.

Comment

Attenuation artifacts most commonly occur in the anterior and lateral walls and less often in the anteroseptal wall, depending on location, size, density, and mobility of breast tissue. The apparent reduced uptake in the superior portion of the heart on the stress projection images is different in the two studies, extending considerably more inferiorly at rest. Breast attenuation would be expected to be a fixed defect; however, a change in breast position between stress and rest can mimic ischemia. Thus, this stress-rest perfusion pattern could be caused by changing attenuation alone or may be caused by ischemia and breast movement. A standardized protocol improves the likelihood that the breasts are in the same position for both studies (e.g., both with or both without bra or binding).

An increased incidence of false-positive results of stress SPECT myocardial perfusion studies occurs in young women. This case illustrates one reason. Another is predicted by Bayes' theorem. Patient groups with a low pretest probability of disease have an increased false-positive rate, whereas those with a high pretest likelihood have an increased false-negative rate. Thus, the best diagnostic use of this study for CAD diagnosis is to select patients at intermediate risk. Young women with few risk factors have a low likelihood of disease. A similar problem occurs with other screening tests (e.g., HIV). Screening patients at increased risk results in relatively few false-positive results; however, mass screening results in more false-positive than true-positive results. Myocardial perfusion studies are performed not only for diagnosis but, importantly, also for risk stratification and prognosis in patients with known disease.

Notes

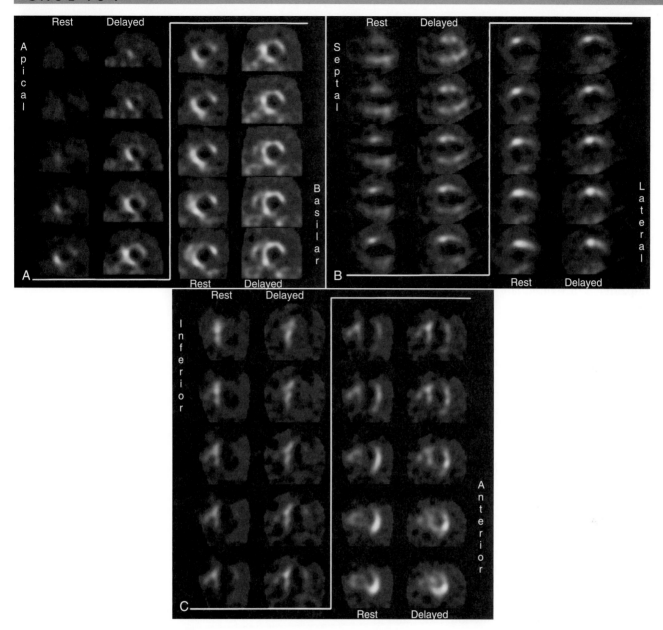

A 62-year-old man with known CAD had fixed perfusion defects with no reversibility on a ^{99m}Tc perfusion SPECT study at another hospital. This is a rest-rest ^{201}Tl SPECT study. A, short axis; B, vertical long axis; C, horizontal long axis.

1. Describe the SPECT findings on the initial rest and the 4-hour delayed rest study.

2. What is the clinical significance of these findings?

3. Based on the available evidence, should revascularization be considered?

4. What is hibernating myocardium?

313

Cardiovascular System: ^{201}Tl Viability Study

1. Initial rest images show extensive defects: (1) the anterior wall extending to the apex, septum, and anterolateral wall and (2) the inferolateral wall extending to the inferior and lateral regions. Delayed rest images show some improvement in perfusion in the anterior wall extending to the apex and septum (see short-axis slices) and anterolateral region (see long axis slices).

2. There is viable myocardium in the left anterior descending artery distribution.

3. Yes.

4. Chronic ischemic myocardium in which both blood flow and function (contractility) are reduced. Although hibernating myocardium is viable, the impairment of wall motion mimics infarction.

References

Canty JM Jr, Fallavollita JA: Chronic hibernation and chronic stunning: a continuum, *J Nucl Cardiol* 7:509–527, 2000.

Schelbert HR: Merits and limitations of radionuclide approaches to viability and future developments, *J Nucl Cardiol* 1(2 Pt 2):S86–S96, 1994.

Cross-Reference

Nuclear Medicine: THE REQUISITES, 3rd ed, p 477–480.

Comment

Distinguishing chronically ischemic (hibernating myocardium) from scarred myocardium is important for clinical management. Depending on the extent of hibernation, revascularization may improve cardiac function as manifested by improvement in wall motion, LVEF, and long-term outcome. Patients with viable myocardium have better survival from revascularization than from medical management. Those with infarction do not benefit from revascularization and may be candidates for cardiac transplantation similar to patients with nonischemic cardiomyopathies.

Rest-rest ^{201}Tl imaging is an alternative to ^{18}F-FDG-PET imaging. Improved ^{201}Tl uptake on delayed images is indicative of myocardial viability and the likelihood of improvement after revascularization. Reinjection of ^{201}Tl and subsequent imaging is an alternative to the 4-hour delayed imaging method. *Stunned* myocardium refers to myocardium that is reperfused after occlusion, either through spontaneous recanalization or commonly after angioplasty. Blood flow is normal or even increased with stunning, but wall motion is decreased because of the severe ischemic event. This stunned myocardium usually regains function with time, usually a few weeks.

Notes

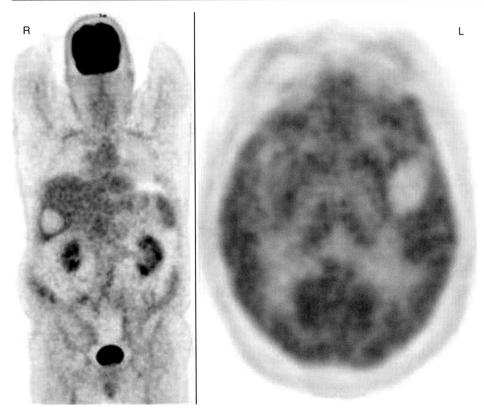

R

L

1. Describe the pattern of FDG uptake in the liver and brain in these two different patients.

2. What diagnoses might demonstrate this pattern of uptake?

3. Describe the typical pattern of FDG uptake in an abscess.

4. What would the pattern of FDG uptake look like for a liver hemangioma?

Inflammatory Disease: FDG-PET—Brain and Liver Abscesses

1. There are round cold or photopenic areas in the right lobe of the liver and in the left brain.

2. Causes of hypometabolism or photopenic areas include cysts, necrotic tumor, hematoma, seroma, abscess, stroke, regions of previous irradiation. Both cases were due to pyogenic abscess formation.

3. Characteristically, abscesses have a central cold focus with surrounding rim of increased uptake on FDG-PET imaging that represents the wall of the abscess exhibiting an inflammatory response. This rim may be thin.

4. Hemangiomas on FDG-PET imaging tend to have isointense uptake (similar to surrounding liver background activity) and are typically not hypermetabolic.

References

Kaim AH, Weber B, Kurrer MO, et al: Autoradiographic quantification of F-18-FDG uptake in experimental soft-tissue abscesses in rats, *Radiology* 223:446-451, 2002.

Lin E, Alavi A: *PET and PET/CT: A Clinical Guide*. New York: Thieme, 2006, pp 78–80.

Okazumi S, Isono K, Enomoto K, et al: Evaluation of liver tumors using fluorine-18-fluorodeoxyglucose PET: characterization of tumor and assessment of effect of treatment, *J Nucl Med* 33:333–339, 1992.

Cross-Reference

Nuclear Medicine: THE REQUISITES, 3rd ed, p 396.

Comment

The central "cold" area in abscesses is thought to be due to central liquefaction/necrosis, which does not have associated inflammation or uptake. Three distinct phases of abscess formation and associated FDG uptake have been described. During the acute phase, there is a photopenic center with surrounding peripheral uptake due to an inflammatory neutrophil infiltrate. Next is an early chronic phase, again with central necrosis and peripheral uptake due a mixed cellular infiltrate of granulocytes and macrophages with an SUV of 5.32 ± 2.30. The final late chronic infection phase has a prominent layer of peripheral macrophages around central necrosis and fibroblast-enriched granulation tissue. The peripheral FDG uptake in the late phase is due to the macrophages and not the granulation tissue. Thus, all phases demonstrate ringlike uptake.

Not only tumor, but also inflammatory lesions, can demonstrate increased FDG uptake, which is related to GLUT expression. Both have high expression of GLUT-1 and GLUT-3; however, GLUT-1 expression is higher in tumor than inflammatory cells and, therefore, FDG uptake is generally higher in tumor than in inflammation and infection. Dual time-point imaging has been used to separate inflammatory uptake from malignant uptake. Reports have found continuing uptake in tumor but not with inflammation. Some reports have not found this pattern consistent enough to separate infection and tumor with a high degree of certainty.

Notes

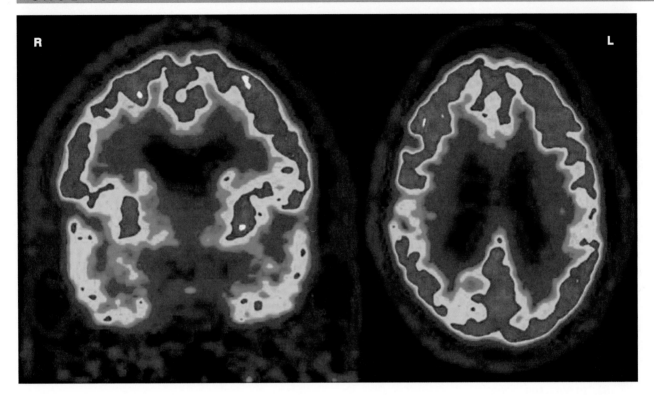

^{18}F-FDG selected brain images of a 72-year-old man with memory loss that has worsened over the past year.

1. Describe the pattern of brain uptake on these selected images.

2. What is the most likely diagnosis?

3. What would be the expected histopathology?

4. What other patterns of uptake would suggest an alternative diagnosis?

FDG-PET: Alzheimer's Dementia

1. Bilateral parietotemporal lobe hypometabolism. The frontal and posterior lobe regions show normal uptake.

2. This pattern of FDG uptake is characteristic of Alzheimer's disease, although it is not always so completely symmetrical. Frontal brain hypometabolism can be seen in advanced disease.

3. The hypometabolic regions correspond on histopathology to areas of abnormal nerve fiber tangles and degenerative neuritic plaques.

4. Lewy body dementia has a pattern similar to that of Alzheimer's disease except that it also involves the occipital lobes. Decreased metabolism in the frontal and temporal lobes suggests a frontotemporal dementia (e.g., Pick's disease).

References

Mosconi L, Tsui WH, Herholz K, et al: Multicenter standardized F-18-FDG PET diagnosis of mild cognitive impairment, Alzheimer's disease, and other dementias, *J Nucl Med* 49:390–398, 2008.

Silverman DH, Small GW, Chang CY, et al: Positron emission tomography in evaluation of dementia: regional brain metabolism and long-term outcome, *JAMA* 286:2120–2127, 2001.

Cross-Reference

Nuclear Medicine: THE REQUISITES, 3rd ed, pp 427–432.

Comment

Alzheimer's disease is the most common cause of dementia. Its incidence is said to be greater than 10% in those older than age 65 and 50% for those older than age 80. There is a strong genetic link. The APOE-ε4 allele is associated with an increased risk of the disease. Clinically, it can be difficult to differentiate Alzheimer's disease from other causes of dementia. SPECT and PET can diagnose Alzheimer's disease earlier than clinical criteria or MRI, and FDG-PET has somewhat higher accuracy than SPECT brain perfusion agents, with reported sensitivity and specificity of 94% and 73%, respectively. In addition to Alzheimer's disease, other causes of dementia can be diagnosed that have characteristic patterns of regional cerebral blood flow with SPECT and cerebral glucose metabolism with FDG-PET. These patterns of reduced blood flow/metabolism can be generally characterized as posterior (Alzheimer's, diffuse Lewy body disease), frontotemporal (Pick's disease), or vascular (multi-infarct). A well-accepted role for FDG-PET is in the differentiation of Alzheimer's disease and frontotemporal dementia.

There are a number of molecular imaging PET tracers in development to aid in the diagnosis of Alzheimer's disease. These tracers include those able to detect β-amyloid plaques, serotonin receptors, norepinephrine transporters, dopamine receptors, and acetylcholinesterase. Amyloid is invariably present in the brains of patients with Alzheimer's disease. As amyloid is invariably present in the brains of patients with Alzheimer's disease, a number of radiopharmaceutical companies are developing amyloid radiotracers.

Notes

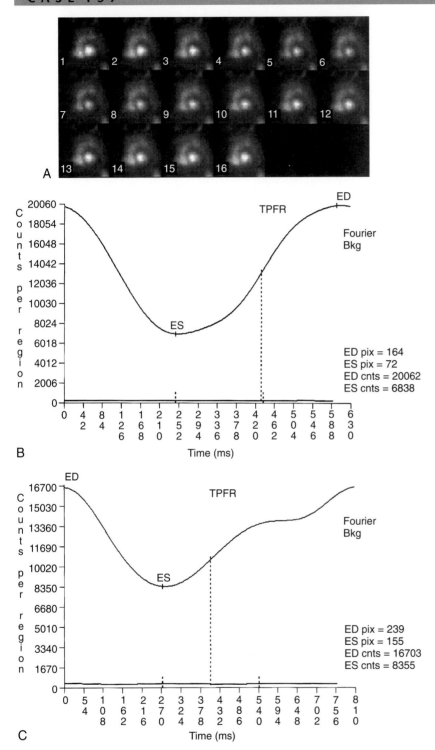

A patient with malignant lymphoma received doxorubicin (Adriamycin). RVG or MUGA performed at time of initial diagnosis reported a 60% LVEF. A, Follow-up RVG with all 16 image frames and left ventricular time-activity curves before (B) and after (C) therapy.

1. Discuss sequential images and the time activity curves.

2. What is the likely diagnosis?

3. List features that should be included in reporting RVG or MUGA studies.

4. List three reasons why RVG is preferred over echocardiography for monitoring left ventricular function.

Cardiovascular System:
Doxorubicin Toxicity

1. Sequential images (A) show a normal LVEF. The ventricle appears slightly dilated. End-systole is image number 7. Time-activity curves show counts for each of 16 frames of the gated acquisition. Study B is normal. Study C shows deterioration from baseline with a slower, broad diastolic up slope and decreased stroke volume (end-systolic volume minus end-diastolic volume). This suggests ventricular dysfunction with deterioration compared with baseline. The post-therapy LVEF was 50%.

2. Doxorubicin toxicity.

3. Qualitative assessment of cardiac chambers and great vessels in terms of size and relationships, regional wall motion based on review of cinematic display, and quantitative analysis (LVEF).

4. Echocardiography is operator dependent, relies on visual estimates of the LVEF, and may not be technically feasible in as many as 30% of patients because of poor acoustic window. RVG is relatively free of operator-dependent factors and is reproducible within an institution and across institutions.

References

Borges-Neto S, Coleman RE: Radionuclide ventricular function analysis, *Radiol Clin North Am* 31:817–830, 1993.

Germano G, Borer JS, Berman DS: Myocardial function assessment by nuclear techniques. In: *Atlas of Nuclear Cardiology*, 2nd ed. Philadelphia: Current Medicine, 2006, pp 115–131.

Cross-Reference

Nuclear Medicine: THE REQUISITES, 3rd ed, pp 490–503.

Comment

Doxorubicin chemotherapy is associated with a risk of cardiotoxicity and cardiomyopathy. While doxorubicin cardiotoxicity rarely occurs with cumulative doses less than 400 mg/m^2, doses in excess of 550 mg/m^2 result in cardiotoxicity in approximately one third of patients. However, some patients can tolerate considerably higher doses. The latter patients should have their LVEF measured both before and during each treatment. A decrease in LVEF suggests drug-related cardiotoxicity. Doxorubicin usually is withheld from patients with baseline LVEFs less than 30%. The drug usually is discontinued if the LVEF decreases by more than 10% below a pretreatment level of 50%. Functional recovery of cardiotoxicity after cessation of doxorubicin therapy is poor. Monitoring of potential drug cardiotoxicity is now the most common indication for RVG. Cardiac biopsy is an invasive alternative to RVG to determine cardiotoxicity.

^{99m}Tc-radiolabeled red blood cells are used for RVG or MUGA (multigated acquisition). The high count rate from the labeled RBCs allows for accurate quantification. Division of the R-R cycle into 16 frames allows for high temporal resolution, allowing precise localization of end-systole and end-diastole. With myocardial perfusion imaging with ^{99m}Tc-sestamibi, the counts are in the myocardium and therefore considerably fewer than with radiolabeled RBCs in the ventricular cavity; thus, 8 frames are usually obtained, with some loss in temporal resolution.

Notes

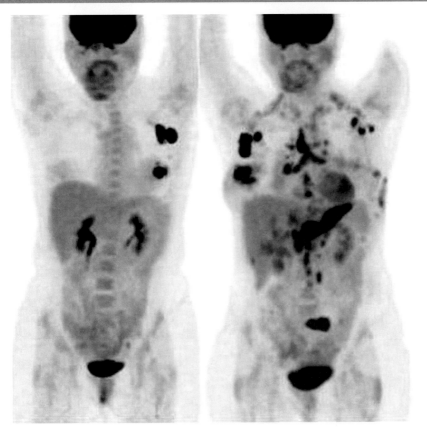

A 44-year-old woman with estrogen receptor–negative and progesterone receptor–positive left breast ductal carcinoma, clinical stage T1N1MX. *Left,* ^{18}F-FDG MIP image pre-therapy; *right,* follow-up MIP image 13 months after left mastectomy, left axillary node dissection, neoadjuvant therapy, and left chest wall irradiation.

1. What was the likely clinical indication for the ^{18}FDG-PET studies in this patient?

2. Describe the changes that have taken place between the two imaging studies.

3. What is the current role of FDG-PET imaging for breast cancer?

4. Name some limitations of FDG-PET imaging in patients with breast cancer.

Oncology: FDG-PET—Breast Cancer

1. Initial study for staging of advanced breast cancer. Follow-up scan was requested because of suspicion of recurrent and metastatic disease suggested by physical examination and increasing serum cancer markers.

2. Disease was initially limited to the left breast and left axillary lymph nodes. On the follow-up study, there is evidence of progression with metastatic disease to the right breast and axilla, mediastinum, hila, lungs, left chest wall skin surface, liver, and abdominal lymph nodes.

3. Initial staging, restaging, therapy monitoring, and detecting recurrent disease. The whole-body approach is useful for assessing the presence or extent of systemic disease.

4. FDG uptake in primary breast cancer (particularly lobular carcinoma) is typically lower than that in other cancers. Primary breast lesions are often smaller than 1 cm, making PET sensitivity for detection poor. Axillary nodal sensitivity is only 75% to 85%. False-negative results may occur in osteoblastic metastatic bone disease.

References

Uematsu T, Yuen S, Yukisawa S, et al: Comparison of FDG PET and SPECT for detection of bone metastases in breast cancer, *AJR Am J Roentgenol* 184:1266–1273, 2005.

Von Schulthess GK, Schmid DT: *Molecular Anatomic Imaging: PET and SPECT-CT Integrated Modality Imaging*. Philadelphia: Lippincott Williams & Wilkins, 2007, pp 393–408.

Yap CS, Seltzer MA, Schiepers C: Impact of whole-body F-18-FDG PET on staging and managing patients with breast cancer: the referring physician's perspective, *J Nucl Med* 42:1334–1337, 2001.

Cross-Reference

Nuclear Medicine: THE REQUISITES, 3rd ed, pp 337–341.

Comment

Bone scans detect the osteoblastic effects of breast cancer and overall are more sensitive than FDG-PET for the detection of most breast cancer metastases. Purely lytic lesions are rare in breast cancer, but are better detected with FDG-PET. Osteoblastic or sclerotic lesions are relatively acellular with a smaller volume of viable cancer cells and have a lower glycolytic rate, thus the lower sensitivity for FDG-PET.

The role of FDG-PET is primarily for staging patients with advanced disease, monitoring response to therapy, restaging, and detecting recurrent disease. FDG-PET is particularly useful for detecting distant metastases.

FDG uptake is higher in ductal carcinomas compared with lobular carcinomas, in higher grade tumors, and in those with high levels of *p53* expression. FDG-PET is better at detecting distant metastases in the liver and chest compared with conventional imaging modalities. Data suggest that there can be a major impact or change in management for breast cancer patients based on PET findings, with a trend toward better cost-effectiveness. Initial reports of positron emission dedicated mammography suggest improved detection and diagnosis of primary breast cancer and guidance of biopsy.

Notes

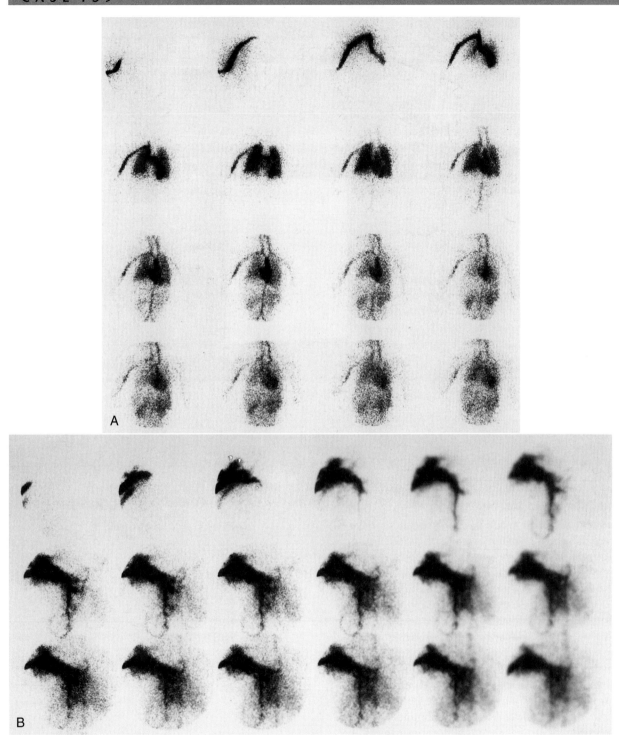

Two patients (A and B) have radionuclide blood flow imaging after right upper extremity injection.

1. Describe the route of the radiotracer in patient A. Give an interpretation.

2. What are the image findings and interpretation of patient B?

3. What radiopharmaceuticals could be used for this study?

4. What is the framing rate (seconds/frame) and minimum injected dose required to obtain a good flow study?

Cardiovascular System: Superior Vena Cava Obstruction

1. Subclavian vein, superior vena cava, right ventricle, lungs, left ventricle, carotids, aorta. Normal blood flow.

2. Superior vena cava obstruction with collateral flow over the anterior chest.

3. Any ^{99m}Tc radiopharmaceutical. All that is needed is enough activity for a good arterial flow study. ^{99m}Tc-DTPA is often used because it is cleared rapidly by the kidneys and can be repeated if necessary.

4. 1 to 3 seconds/frame; 5 mCi or greater.

Reference

Mishkin FS, Freeman LM: Miscellaneous applications of radionuclide imaging. In: Freeman LM (ed): *Freeman and Johnson's Clinical Radionuclide Imaging*, 3rd ed. Philadelphia: WB Saunders, 1984, pp 1400–1419.

Cross-Reference

Nuclear Medicine: THE REQUISITES, 3rd ed, pp 205–207.

Comment

Radionuclide flow studies can be a rapid, easily performed method for the evaluation of the patency of venous access lines. Rapid acquisition images provide a sensitive means for detecting obstruction of axillary, subclavian, or innominate veins. This is particularly important in modern medicine when patients frequently have central venous access lines for infusion of various therapeutic drugs that increase the risk of thrombosis. A good bolus is necessary to maximize the diagnostic information of the flow sequence. Although resolution is poor compared with a contrast study, this noninvasive radionuclide angiogram can provide valuable diagnostic information. With superior vena cava obstruction, a radiotracer will likely take the route of venous collaterals (e.g., chest wall to umbilical vein to left portal vein and sometimes focal uptake in the region of the quadrate lobe). This has been seen with ^{99m}Tc-SC, FDG-PET, and MAA lung scan.

Radionuclide blood flow studies are commonly used to study a variety of arterial and venous abnormalities. A vascular sequence is performed routinely for three-phase bone scans to diagnose osteomyelitis or to estimate the age of a fracture. Flow studies are performed in association with renography to assess renal arterial blood flow (e.g., to diagnose renal artery stenosis, acute transplant rejection, kidney viability). With a gastrointestinal bleeding study, occasionally the site of increased vascularity can be detected from the flow study when there is no evidence of active bleeding (e.g., angiodysplasia). With HIDA imaging, increased blood flow sometimes can be seen in the region of the gallbladder fossa with acute cholecystitis. Sometimes there are unexpected findings pointing to another diagnosis, for example, an intra-abdominal infection or tumor.

Notes

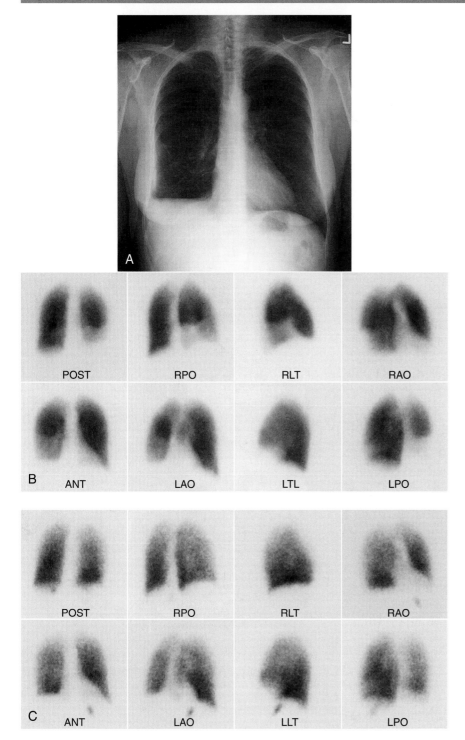

A 62-year-old patient with right-sided chest discomfort and shortness of breath. A, Posteroanterior chest radiograph; B, perfusion; C, ventilation.

1. Describe the ventilation perfusion image findings and chest x-ray.

2. Interpret the study. Give your reasoning.

3. What is the probability of pulmonary embolus in this patient?

4. What are the two most common chest x-ray findings in patients with pulmonary emboli?

Pulmonary System: High Probability of Pulmonary Embolus

1. Decreased perfusion in the right lower lobe except for the superior segment. Near-normal ventilation. A small right pleural effusion is noted on the chest x-ray.

2. Intermediate probability of pulmonary embolus. Mismatch between perfusion and ventilation in all basal segments. However, there is also a pleural effusion.

3. Greater than 80%.

4. Normal and atelectasis. These are also the most common radiographic findings in studies of patients determined by angiography not to have emboli.

References

Freeman LM, Stein EG, Sprayregen S, et al: The current and continuing important role of ventilation perfusion scintigraphy in evaluating patients with suspected pulmonary embolism, *Semin Nucl Med* 38:432–440, 2008.

Freitas JE, Sarosi MG, Nagle CC, et al: Modified PIOPED criteria used in clinical practice, *J Nucl Med* 36:1573–1578, 1995.

Cross-Reference

Nuclear Medicine: THE REQUISITES, 3rd ed, pp 522–532.

Comment

The large, multi-segmental mismatch in the right lower lobe represents a high probability of pulmonary embolus by PIOPED criteria. The perfusion defect is considerably larger than the pleural effusion, which is another criterion for high probability. However, the PIOPED criteria should be used cautiously. The chest radiograph is obtained with maximal inspiration. The lung scan image is acquired during tidal breathing. Thus, the heart is more horizontal on the lung scan than the radiograph, and the lung fields appear smaller on the lung scan than the radiograph. In this case, the perfusion defect is definitely larger than the radiographic finding. No significant ventilatory defects are apparent. On the other hand, it is unusual for multiple pulmonary emboli to involve only one portion of the lung. A patient with a high-probability scan has a greater than 80% probability of pulmonary embolus. Thus, 20% have something else as the cause. In a case with a unilateral lung perfusion abnormality or regional one like this, another cause should be considered. The most common alterative diagnosis with a high probability scan is lung cancer. A mediastinal tumor can preferentially occlude the pulmonary vessels, which are easily compressible in contrast to the more rigid bronchi.

Old emboli with persistent mismatches are another common cause of a false-positive study for acute pulmonary embolus when no previous study is available for comparison. Vasculitis is a less common cause.

Fewer than half of patients determined to have pulmonary embolus have a high-probability scan. The majority of patients with pulmonary emboli have an intermediate-probability scan. Thus, it is not sensitive for the diagnosis of pulmonary embolus, but it is fairly specific. However, this emphasizes that intermediate probability does not exclude pulmonary embolus.

Notes

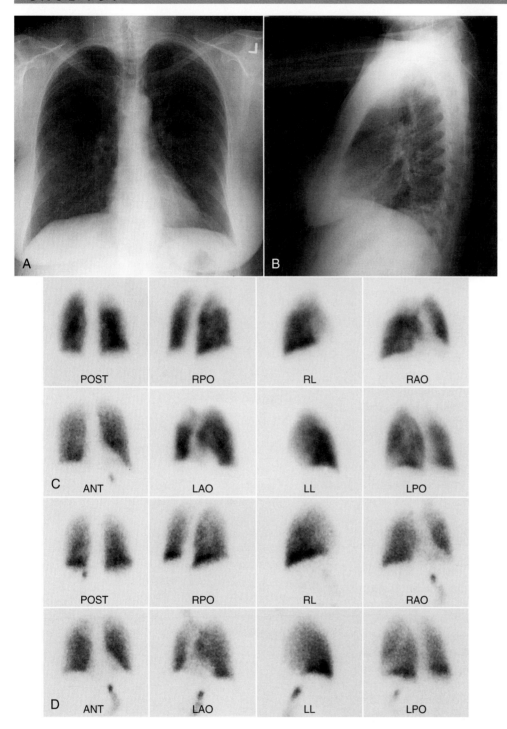

A 59-year-old patient with COPD reports right-sided chest discomfort and shortness of breath. A, Postero-anterior chest radiograph; B, lateral chest radiograph; C, perfusion; D, ventilation.

1. Describe the ventilation-perfusion image findings.

2. Interpret the study.

3. What is a stripe sign and what is its significance?

4. What is the physiologic basis of a stripe sign?

Pulmonary System: Low Probability and the Stripe Sign

1. Decreased perfusion in the right upper lobe (apical and anterior segments). Stripe sign in the region of the posterior segment of the right upper lobe. Ventilation is also reduced, although not as prominently.

2. Two matched segments with a clear chest x-ray is low probability.

3. Its presence signifies perfused lung tissue between a perfusion defect and the adjacent pleural surface and, thus, pulmonary embolus as the etiology for abnormal perfusion.

4. Usually a manifestation of airway obstruction. The sign has been correlated with CT and PET showing spared perfusion of the cortex of the lung in asthma and emphysema.

References

Freitas JE, Sarosi MG, Nagle CC, et al: Modified PIOPED criteria used in clinical practice, *J Nucl Med* 36:1573–1578, 1995.

Sostman HD, Gottschalk A: Prospective validation of the stripe sign in ventilation-perfusion scintigraphy, *Radiology* 184:455–459, 1992.

Cross-Reference

Nuclear Medicine: THE REQUISITES, 3rd ed, pp 508–534.

Comment

The natural history of pulmonary embolism is clot fragmentation in the right side of the heart, which induces multivessel segmental embolization of the pulmonary vasculature with preservation of segmental ventilation. Most emboli occur in the lower lobes and have a random distribution. Evidence against pulmonary embolus in this case is the fact that the abnormal perfusion is limited to adjacent upper lobe segments. Thus, even though this finding of ventilation perfusion mismatch might indicate a high-probability scan by established criteria, this pattern is atypical. Published data also have suggested that the specificity for pulmonary embolus is maximized in patients with cardiopulmonary disease if three segmental mismatches are present. Thus, it would not be incorrect to classify this study as indeterminate or intermediate probability. If one thought that these two segments were mismatched, this would not make it high probability. Mismatches limited to the upper lobes are usually not pulmonary emboli and most would classify it as intermediate or even low probability.

The stripe sign is seen in approximately 5% of ventilation-perfusion studies. To be defined as a stripe sign, the finding needs only to be seen in one projection. It is an ancillary sign that helps lower the probability from intermediate to low probability. The stripe sign only is useful for evaluating the segment in question. The sign is not totally specific for nonembolic causation. It also can be seen in areas of reperfused lung previously obstructed by emboli. If one were not totally convinced in this case that the perfusion and ventilation were matched, the stripe sign would increase one's certainty.

Notes

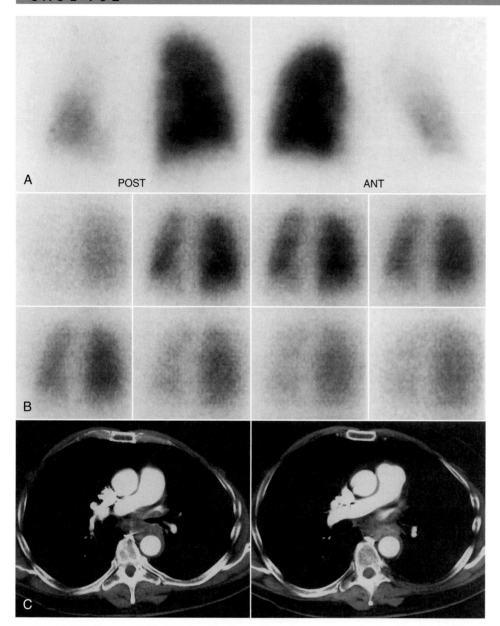

Patient reports a recent increase in shortness of breath. Chest x-ray (not shown) was negative.

1. Describe the scintigraphic findings for perfusion, anterior and posterior only (A), ^{133}Xe washin-washout ventilation image sequence (B), and CT scan (C).

2. What pulmonary embolus probability category would you assign?

3. Provide the differential diagnosis.

4. Chest CT was performed to further evaluate the symptoms. What is the most likely diagnosis?

Pulmonary System: Unilateral Matched Ventilation-Perfusion Abnormality

1. Perfusion images: global decreased perfusion to the entire left lung. ^{133}Xe ventilation images: decreased and delayed ventilation of the entire left lung with no significant air trapping.

2. Low probability.

3. Hilar mass (lung cancer or adenopathy), severe unilateral parenchymal lung disease, Swyer-James syndrome, hypoplastic pulmonary artery, previous shunt for congenital heart disease.

4. Lung cancer.

Reference

Freeman LM, Stein EG, Sprayregen S, et al: The current and continuing important role of ventilation perfusion scintigraphy in evaluating patients with suspected pulmonary embolism, *Semin Nucl Med* 38:432–440, 2008.

Cross-Reference

Nuclear Medicine: THE REQUISITES, 3rd ed, pp 515–534.

Comment

Lung cancer and hilar adenopathy can result in perfusion defects disproportionate to ventilation. This is the most common cause for a false-positive high-probability ventilation-perfusion study. A high-probability ventilation-perfusion scan has an 80% positive predictive value for pulmonary embolus. The other 20% must have another cause. The majority of false positives are related to hilar masses. A proximal pulmonary embolus may manifest as a unilateral, whole-lung mismatch; however, the latter should always raise the question of tumor. The mass abuts hilar structures. The thin-walled vessels (veins and arteries) are relatively compressible compared with the thick-walled bronchi; thus, ventilation is relatively preserved compared with perfusion. A good posteroanterior and lateral chest radiograph usually narrows the differential, and if not, the question can be resolved by CT. Pathologic study is needed to confirm the correct diagnosis.

Swyer-James syndrome, a variant of postinfectious obliterative bronchiolitis, shares some common radiographic features with congenital unilateral absence of the pulmonary artery, including a small lung manifested by cardiac and mediastinal shift, absence of pulmonary arterial shadow, elevation of the hemidiaphragm, and a decrease in the size of pulmonary vessels on the affected side with oligemia. Swyer-James syndrome, caused by bronchiolitis, is associated with air trapping, which can be documented by an expiration radiograph or a ^{133}Xe ventilation scan.

Notes

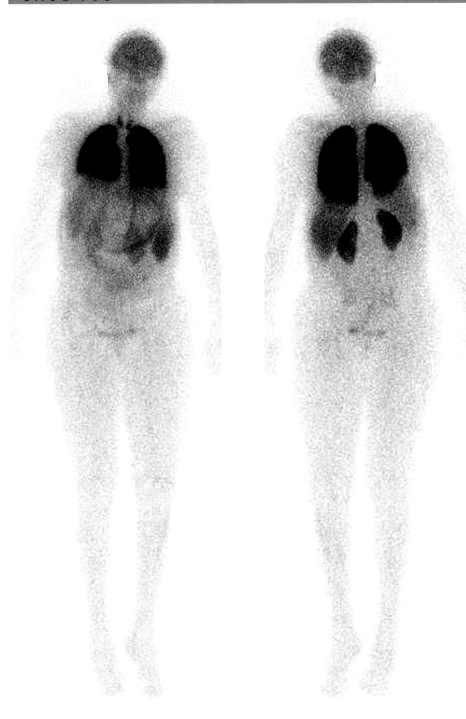

A 41-year-old woman has a history of cirrhosis and recently increasing symptoms of shortness of breath and hypoxia.

1. What is the radiopharmaceutical?

2. Describe the scintigraphic findings.

3. What is your interpretation and diagnosis?

4. What are relative contraindications to this study?

Pulmonary System: Right-to-Left Shunt, Hepatopulmonary Syndrome

1. ^{99m}Tc-MAA.

2. Uptake in the lungs, brain, liver, spleen, and kidneys.

3. Right-to-left shunt. The MAA particles are larger than capillary size. When given intravenously, they occlude the first arteriolar-capillary bed that they reach, normally the lungs. With a right-to-left shunt, some will bypass the lungs and be delivered systemically in proportion to the size of the shunt. Hepatopulmonary syndrome.

4. Relative contraindications include pregnancy, severe pulmonary hypertension, and right-to-left shunt. However, there are no absolute contraindications. The number of particles is reduced in these patients.

Reference

Rodriquez-Roisin R, Krowka MJ: Hepatopulmonary syndrome—a liver-induced lung vascular disorder, *N Engl J Med* 358:2378–2387, 2008.

Cross-Reference

Nuclear Medicine: THE REQUISITES, 3rd ed, pp 515–519.

Comment

This study was requested to look for a right-to-left shunt in a patient with hepatopulmonary syndrome. Brain uptake is diagnostic of a right-to-left shunt. Visualization of the thyroid and kidneys could be due to free pertechnetate. However, the presence of free pertechnate does not explain the other findings. The percentage of right-to-left shunt can be calculated. In this case, it was 20%. The hepatopulmonary syndrome is characterized by a defect in arterial oxygenation induced by pulmonary vascular dilation in the setting of liver disease. More commonly, right-to-left shunts are diagnosed in patients with congenital heart disease.

Particle size range of ^{99m}Tc-MAA is 10 to 90 μm (mean, 30–40 μm). Capillary size is 7 μm. The particles occlude only 1/1000 to 1/10,000 of the arteriolar capillary bed. Pulmonary infarction does not occur because of the dual circulation of the lungs and the nature of the particles. The particles are malleable, cause partial occlusions, and break down rapidly into smaller particles that pass through the lungs. The direct injection of ^{99m}Tc-MAA particles into the carotid artery has been done during investigation in humans to map cerebral perfusion without serious adverse effect. However, in a patient with known severe pulmonary hypertension or a right-to-left shunt, the usual approach would be to reduce the number of ^{99m}Tc-MAA particles. A minimum of 60,000 particles is required to provide adequate uniformity, and 100,000 or more are usually recommended. A perfusion study generally has 300,000 to 400,000 particles. To maximize the count rate with a reduced number of particles, a high-specific activity ^{99m}Tc is required for radiolabeling.

Notes

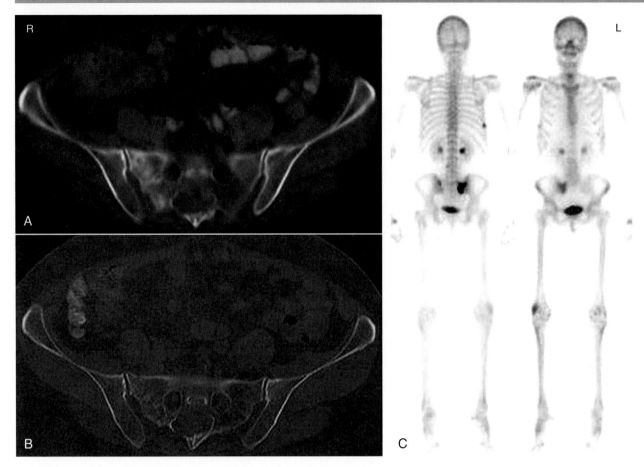

A 69-year-old woman with breast cancer has a recent onset of low back pain. ^{18}F-FDG-PET/CT fused images (A) and CT (B). Posterior and anterior whole-body bone scan (C).

1. Describe the abnormality on the FDG-PET/CT (A) and bone scan (C).

2. Describe the abnormality on the CT scan (B). Correlate it with image A.

3. What is the diagnosis? What is the pathophysiology?

4. What PET radiotracer can be used in a manner similar to a bone scan?

Inflammatory Disease: FDG-PET/CT—Sacral Stress Fracture

1. FDG uptake involving the right sacral ala (A). This corresponds to the intense, abnormal increased uptake in the right sacral region on the bone scan (C).

2. On CT (B), there is an ill-defined sclerotic line in the right sacrum with fracture in the same area as uptake of FDG and bone scan radiotracer.

3. Unilateral sacral insufficiency fracture, a stress fracture.

4. ^{18}F-sodium fluoride (^{18}F-NaF).

References

Even-Sapir E, Metser U, Flusser G, et al: Assessment of malignant skeletal disease: initial experience with F-18-fluoride PET/CT and comparison between F-18-fluoride PET and F-18-fluoride PET/CT, *J Nucl Med* 45:272–278, 2004.

Fujii M, Abe K, Hayashi K, et al: Honda sign and variants in patients suspected of having a sacral insufficiency fracture, *Clin Nucl Med* 30:165–169, 2005.

Cross-Reference

Nuclear Medicine: THE REQUISITES, 3rd ed, pp 138–139.

Comment

Stress fractures often occur due to a significant change in the level of activity or with repetitive activity causing an imbalance between bone resorption and replacement. Prompt diagnosis allows for a reduction in activity before complete fracture occurs and thereby lessens the time required for healing. Sacral insufficiency fractures are most common in women older than 60 years of age with osteoporosis.

This case illustrates the nonspecificity of FDG. It is taken up not only by tumor, but also inflammation and healing. Without the CT correlation, focal FDG uptake might be mistaken for tumor.

The classic pattern of uptake on a bone scan is that of a "butterfly" or H shape (i.e., bilateral sacral alae). The sensitivity and positive predictive value of this pattern on bone scintigraphy for sacral insufficiency fracture is 96% and 92%, respectively. However, other patterns have been described (e.g., horizontal linear sacral uptake or even curvilinear uptake in an intermittent pattern [dot-dot-dot sign]). Sacral insufficiency fractures can be identified on a bone scan before becoming evident on plain film and the same is probably true for FDG-PET.

The mechanism of ^{18}F-NaF skeletal uptake is similar to that of ^{99m}Tc-labeled diphosphonates: blood flow and osteoblastic activity. Uptake is seen in both osteolytic and osteoblastic lesions, whereas with ^{99m}Tc bone scintigraphy, lytic disease is sometimes difficult to identify. ^{18}F-NaF can detect minimal osteoblastic activity in predominantly lytic lesions. In addition, there is improved spatial resolution and lesion contrast with ^{18}F-fluoride skeletal imaging. One disadvantage of ^{18}F-NaF bone imaging is the difficulty in differentiating between benign and malignant disease. When integrated with CT, diagnostic accuracy is improved.

Notes

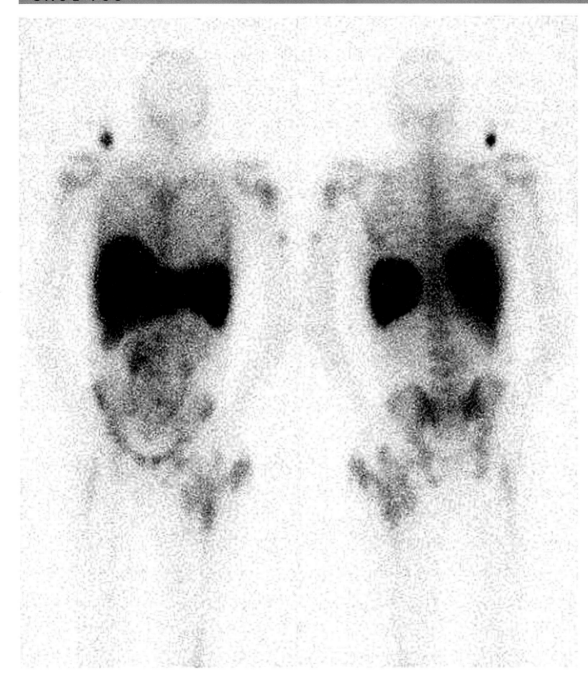

A 20-year-old man sustained multiple gunshot wounds of the extremities and abdomen. He has had a prolonged hospital stay for infectious and orthopedic complications. This study was ordered because of persistent fever.

1. Which radiopharmaceutical was used?

2. What is the photopeak(s) of the radionuclide used? What is its half-life?

3. Which organ receives the highest radiation absorbed dose? Estimate the dose.

4. Describe any abnormal findings and give your interpretation of this scan.

Inflammatory Disease: ^{111}In-Oxine Leukocytes, Peritonitis, Fractures

1. ^{111}In-oxine leukocytes.

2. 173 and 247 keV. Physical half-life is 77 hours.

3. Spleen, approximately 15 to 20 rad in adults.

4. Abnormal increased inhomogeneous uptake throughout the peritoneum, diffuse irregular uptake in soft tissue in the left hip region, probable proximal femur uptake, left proximal humerus uptake. The uptake in the left humerus was due to fracture. There was soft-tissue infection around the left hip and fracture of the proximal femur. Uptake with the abdomen was due to peritonitis. The hot spot above the right shoulder is a marker for the right side.

References

Bleeker-Rovers CP, van der Meer JW, Owen WJ: Fever of unknown origin, *Semin Nucl Med* 39:81–87, 2009.

Oyen JG, Boerman OC, Corstens FHM: Radiolabeled agents for the localization of infection and inflammation. In: Ell PJ, Gambhir SS (eds): *Nuclear Medicine*. Edinburgh: Churchhill Livingstone, 2006.

Cross-Reference

Nuclear Medicine: THE REQUISITES, 3rd ed, pp 412–418.

Comment

Choosing the appropriate infection-seeking radiopharmaceutical in a particular clinical setting requires weighing of the advantages and disadvantages of each. [67]Ga detects tumor and infection; therefore, it can be useful for patients with fever of unknown origin. ^{18}F-FDG is increasingly used for this purpose. Radiolabeled leukocytes are preferable if infection localization is the clinical question. Radiolabeled leukocytes require cell labeling, at least a 2-hour procedure and have the potential problem of blood-borne disease. ^{99m}Tc-HMPAO leukocytes provide better image quality because of the ^{99m}Tc radiolabel and larger administered dose, but have the disadvantage of clearance through the kidneys and biliary system, interfering with intra-abdominal visualization. Abdominal imaging by 1 to 2 hours, before intra-abdominal clearance, circumvents this problem. For intra-abdominal infection, ^{111}In-oxine leukocytes are preferable because they are not cleared intra-abdominally. Otherwise, the distribution is similar to that of the spleen, liver, and bone marrow. Image quality is lower with ^{111}In-oxine because of the lower administered dose (500 µCi vs. 10 mCi for ^{99m}Tc-HMPAO), higher energy photopeaks (173, 247 keV), and the need for a medium-energy collimator. Images are usually obtained at 24 hours.

[111]In-oxine diffuses through the neutrophil cell membrane. Intracellularly, it dissociates and the ^{111}In binds to intracellular proteins; oxine diffuses back out of the cell. In addition to labeling leukocytes (granulocytes, lymphocytes, monocytes), erythrocytes and platelets are labeled. RBCs and platelets are removed with sedimentation and settling agents early in the labeling procedure.

Notes

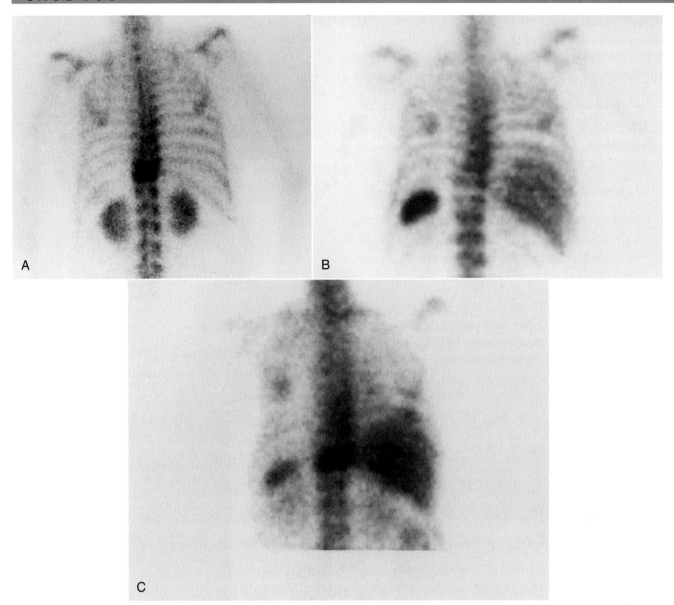

A 67-year-old patient has low-grade fever, back pain, and suspected osteomyelitis of the lumbar spine. A, ^{99m}Tc-MDP bone scan; B, ^{111}In-oxine leukocytes; C, ^{67}Ga citrate.

1. Describe the scintigraphic findings of these three studies.

2. Provide a differential diagnosis for the combined ^{111}In-leukocyte study and bone scan.

3. Interpret the three studies together.

4. Explain the discrepancy between the ^{111}In-leukocyte and ^{67}Ga studies.

Inflammatory Disease: Osteomyelitis of the Spine

1. Bone scan (A) shows increased uptake in the T11 vertebra. ^{111}In-oxine leukocyte study (B) shows decreased uptake in the same region. ^{67}Ga (C) shows increased uptake that matches the bone scan in relative intensity.

2. Osteomyelitis, fracture, infarction, metastasis, orthopedic hardware, surgical defect, information related to localized radiation therapy, myelofibrosis, Paget's disease.

3. Suggestive of osteomyelitis.

4. The ^{111}In-oxine leukocyte study has a false-negative rate as high as 40% in the spine. This was the reason that the ^{67}Ga study was obtained.

Reference

Palestro CJ, Kim CK, Swyer AJ, et al: Radionuclide diagnosis of vertebral osteomyelitis: indium-111-leukocyte and Tc-99m MDP scintigraphy, *J Nucl Med* 32:1861–1865, 1991.

Cross-Reference

Nuclear Medicine: THE REQUISITES, 3rd ed, pp 404–411.

Comment

Vertebral osteomyelitis usually occurs in adults and most commonly in the lumbar spine, followed by thoracic and cervical locations. *Staphylococcus aureus* is the most common causative organism. Predisposing conditions include urinary tract infection and instrumentation, intravenous drug abuse, cancer, and diabetes mellitus. Plain radiographs are not sensitive and may be nonspecific for the diagnosis in nonvirgin bone. Osteomyelitis originates as a septic embolus that lodges in an end arteriole of the vertebral body. The embolus propagates retrograde and circumferentially around the vertebral body, occluding other arteries and causing septic infarction and osteomyelitis.

Radiolabeled leukocyte studies have a high accuracy for diagnosis of osteomyelitis, except in the spine. The reason for decreased rather than increased uptake of leukocytes with vertebral osteomyelitis has not been well explained, but is a common finding (photopenia compared with adjacent vertebrae). The reason may be poor blood entry due to edema or infarction.

^{67}Ga citrate is sensitive for osteomyelitis but is not specific because uptake can be seen whenever bone remodeling occurs for any reason (e.g., previous trauma or infection, orthopedic hardware). The ^{67}Ga study result is interpreted as positive if the uptake is greater than the bone scan or in a different distribution. It would be interpreted as negative for osteomyelitis if ^{67}Ga uptake were less than bone. In this case, the ^{67}Ga uptake is approximately equal to bone, which is considered equivocal for osteomyelitis. However, in the presence of a normal x-ray and the strongly positive bone scan in the clinical setting of suspected osteomyelitis, this study would be considered highly suspicious.

Notes

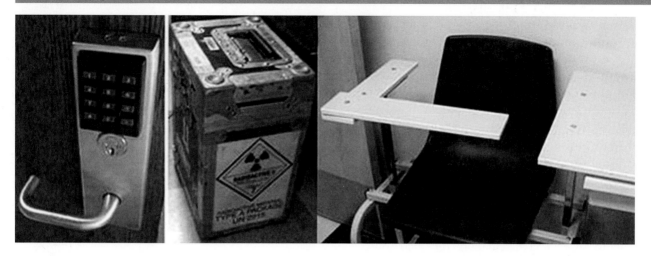

1. Which of the items shown should undergo routine tests versus random tests for radiation contamination?

2. What are the acceptable limits for dose rate at the surface the middle item (Yellow II)?

3. What are the three main forms of radionuclide radiation? Contamination?

4. What is generally considered an appropriate wipe test sample? How should wipe test samples be assayed?

Radiation Safety: Radiation Contamination—Wipe Test

1. The radiopharmaceutical carrier (*middle*) should be tested for contamination using a survey meter within 3 hours of its arrival in nuclear medicine during business hours. Neither the doorknob (*left*) nor desk (*right*) are areas that should be at high risk of contamination. They may undergo random testing for contamination.

2. At the surface, the package should measure no more than 200 mrem/hr (the same is true for a Yellow III package). A White I package should measure no more than 0.5 mrem/hour at the surface. If there is any reason to suspect contamination, the final source external container should undergo wipe testing.

3. Contamination is defined as dispersible radioactivity found in an undesirable location. It may be fixed, transferable (nonfixed), or airborne.

4. Wipe tests are performed to detect transferable contamination using a cotton swab, prep pad, filter paper, or other small tissue/paper. To be considered adequate, wipes should generally cover an area of approximately 100 cm^2 and be done in an S pattern.

References

Saha GP: *Physics and Radiobiology of Nuclear Medicine*, 3rd ed. New York: Springer-Verlag, 2006.

U.S. Nuclear Regulatory Commission: Regulatory Guide 10.8 and Title 10, *Code of Federal Regulations*.

Cross-Reference

Nuclear Medicine: THE REQUISITES, 3rd ed, pp 16–17.

Comment

Fixed contamination is that which cannot be easily removed from a surface by wiping, casual contact, or the like, and may only be released by disruption of the surface through grinding, use of volatile liquids, or the like. Fixed contamination may leach or weep from a surface over time and become airborne or transferable (e.g., contamination in the walls of containers used for radioactive transport or storage). Transferable contamination is that which may be easily spread by contact, wiping, washing, etc. (e.g., radioactivity found on the surface of a countertop caused by a spill). Airborne contamination is suspended in air (e.g., radioactive gas that escapes during performance of a pulmonary ventilation study).

Wipe tests are done as part of random contamination testing performed on a weekly basis in nuclear medicine departments. The person carrying out the wipe test should wear gloves to prevent hand contamination. Each wipe test sample should be numbered or labeled and put in an individual container or vial. Wipe test samples should be assayed using a G-M survey meter, liquid scintillation counter, etc., as appropriate. A dose calibrator is not sensitive enough to be used for wipe test assays.

The local radiation safety officer is an invaluable resource for information regarding appropriate protocols to minimize and monitor contamination and can provide additional documentation regarding current guidelines and requirements in your state and institution.

Notes

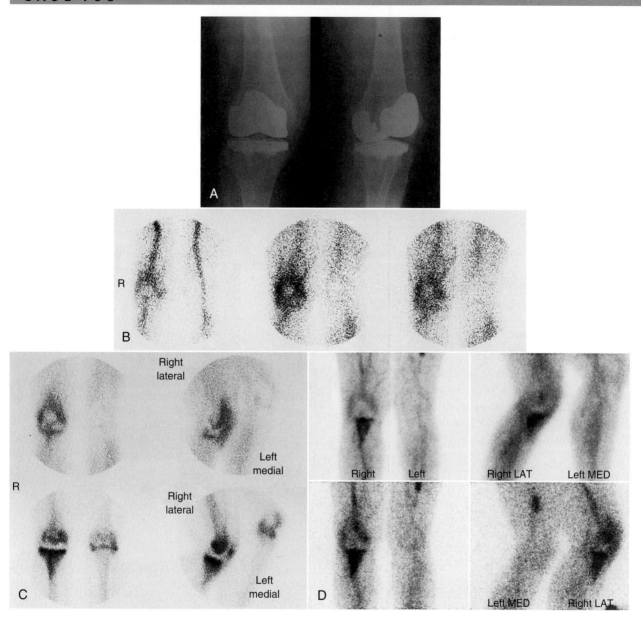

Rule out infected right knee prosthesis. A, Radiograph is shown.

1. Describe the three-phase bone scan findings. B, Blood flow; C, immediate blood pool (*top*), and delayed images (*bottom*).

2. Describe the ^{99m}Tc-HMPAO leukocyte study (D, *top*) and ^{99m}Tc-SC study (D, *bottom*).

3. What is the purpose of the ^{99m}Tc-SC study?

4. Interpret the study.

C A S E 1 6 8

Inflammatory Disease: Knee Arthroplasty— Rule Out Infection: Bone, Leukocyte, and Marrow Scans

1. Increased blood flow to the right knee (B), most prominently to the superior region of the prosthesis. Increased blood pool (C, top) in a similar pattern in the anterior view. The right lateral blood pool suggests a soft-tissue/joint distribution and no definite increase in the region of the proximal tibia. Delayed bone images (C) show increased uptake in the proximal tibia.

2. Increased uptake in the right proximal tibia on both studies.

3. Serves as a template for the patient's bone marrow distribution. Absence of infection would demonstrate similar uptake of radiolabeled leukocytes and ^{99m}Tc-SC. Infection would show increased uptake of radiolabeled leukocytes in a region of normal or reduced ^{99m}Tc-SC marrow uptake.

4. Suggestive of soft-tissue/joint infection. Negative for osteomyelitis. The increased flow/blood pool in the distal femur does not match the increased uptake in the proximal tibia. The marrow study is similar to the HMPAO study (i.e., increased proximal tibia uptake, probably due to surgery).

Reference
Love C, Marwin SE, Palestro CJ: Nuclear medicine and the infected joint replacement, *Semin Nucl Med* 39:66–78, 2009.

Cross-Reference
Nuclear Medicine: THE REQUISITES, 3rd ed, pp 411–412.

Comment
The role of ^{99m}Tc-MDP bone scanning in the diagnosis of total knee arthroplasty infection is limited because of persistent periprosthetic uptake of radiotracer for some time after prosthetic implantation. The intensity of uptake cannot be used to differentiate an infected from an uninfected prosthesis.

Radiolabeled leukocyte studies, whether ^{111}In-oxine or ^{99m}Tc-HMPAO, are sensitive for the diagnosis of infected prostheses. However, specificity is a problem because implantation of an orthopedic prosthesis produces alterations in the distribution of bone marrow. The distribution of radiolabeled leukocytes in a noninfected knee is similar to that seen with ^{99m}Tc-SC. Thus, regions of increased marrow may exist that could be interpreted as infection with a leukocyte-only study, but when interpreted alongside with a bone marrow study,

the pattern is that of altered distribution, not infection. Although marrow is often not present in the normal bones of the knee, one study of patients with knee prostheses found normal marrow in 50% of noninfected knees. When infection is severe, the marrow scan may show decreased uptake at the site of infection. The radiolabeled leukocyte study should be performed first. If no increased periprosthetic activity is visible, a marrow study is not needed. The combined leukocyte-marrow study has proved particularly valuable for hip prostheses.

Notes

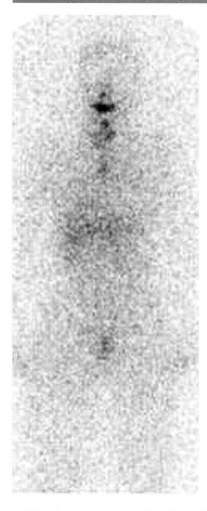

A 27-year-old woman is referred for radioiodine therapy for thyroid remnant ablation 4 weeks after thyroid-ectomy for papillary thyroid cancer using 100 mCi of ^{131}I. She lives at home with 2 children, ages 6 months and 3 years.

1. What safety practices should be implemented to minimize the dose of radiation to technologists and/or physicians administering therapy to this patient?

2. What additional considerations are necessary in handling the therapeutic dose of ^{131}I that would not be of concern for the diagnostic dose of ^{123}I?

3. Under what circumstances can the patient be released after outpatient treatment with ^{131}I?

4. Give standard precautions to minimize radiation exposure to the public from outpatients treated with ^{131}I.

C A S E   1 6 9

Radiation Safety: Radioiodine Therapy

1. Standard radiation safety practices are based on time, distance, and shielding. The dose should be transported in a closed container, gloves worn, and the ^{131}I kept in its container until ingestion.

2. Radioactive iodine ^{131}I is a mixed beta and gamma ray emitter, whereas ^{123}I emits only gamma rays. Lead shielding is used for ^{123}I. Plastic/Plexiglas (low Z material) is used for ^{131}I beta particles. Care should be taken to guard against possible volatility (including capsules if loaded with liquid ^{131}I).

3. Release eligibility based on administered activity, measured dose rate, or patient-specific dose calculations.

4. NRC regulations recommend precautions for patients receiving ^{131}I doses greater than 33 mCi: (a) maintain distance of 6 feet from others; (b) minimize contact with pregnant or nursing women and children; (c) use separate bath linens or dishes from others; (d) flush the toilet twice with the lid down after use; (e) wash hands with each use of the bathroom; (f) shower daily; (g) avoid trips that would require close contact with others; (h) use a separate bathroom.

References

Tuttle WK, Brown PH: Applying Nuclear Regulatory Commission guidelines to the release of patients treated with sodium iodine-131, *J Nucl Med Technol* 28:275–279, 2000.

U.S. Nuclear Regulatory Commission: *Regulatory Guide 8.39: Release of Patients Administered Radioactive Materials*, 1997.

Cross-Reference

Nuclear Medicine: THE REQUISITES, 3rd ed, p 101.

Comment

NRC guidelines for outpatient treatment of patients with ^{131}I-NaI are designed to minimize the radiation dose to the public. Patients may be released after being treated if (a) measured dose rate at 1 m is no more than 7 mrem/ hour or (b) administered ^{131}I activity is no more than 33 mCi or (c) maximum likely dose to an individual exposed to the patient is no more than 500 mrem in 1 year. Some patients must be treated as an inpatient (e.g., patient inability to be in isolation for the required time due to the presence of dependent children or others in the home), high likelihood of unavoidable or unacceptable radiation exposure to caregivers or members of the public (e.g., urinary incontinence), or inability to follow radiation safety practices. For inpatients, precautions must be exercised by nursing and health care personnel with patient contact, including (a) being aware of concurrent medical problems and plans for addressing these while hospitalized; (b) admitting patient to designated room/floor on which nurses and staff are trained in radiation precautions; (c) covering the room and bathroom floor with absorbent material for ease of clean up; (d) covering the toilet seat and sink handles with plastic; (e) requiring those entering the room to wear protective equipment (disposable gowns, gloves, shoe covers, masks); (f) limiting entrance into patient's room, no-visitor policy once the patient has been dosed; (g) designating a storage container for nondisposable/ reusable items whose level of radiation should be allowed to decay to background levels before further use or processing.

Notes

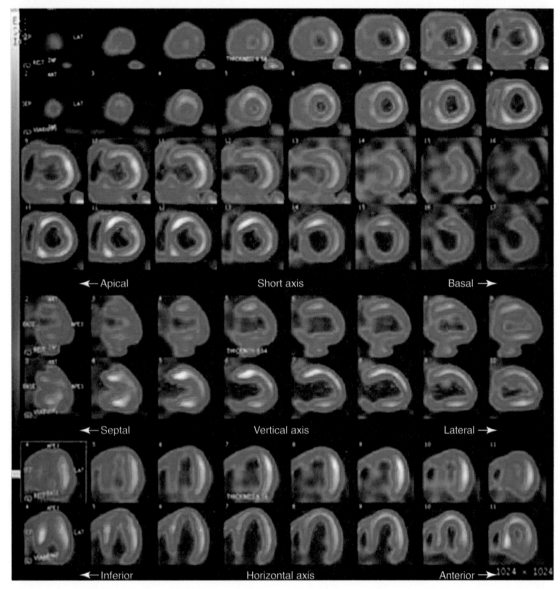

^{82}Rb-Cl

^{18}F-FDG

A 67-year-old man with CAD and an LVEF of 34% was referred to differentiate hibernating from scarred myocardium for possible revascularization. ^{82}Rb-Cl PET rest perfusion images (*top*) and ^{18}F-FDG-PET metabolism images (*bottom*).

1. What is hibernating myocardium and when should it be suspected?

2. What is the clinical significance of hibernating myocardium?

3. What is the physiologic explanation for performing combined resting perfusion and FDG metabolism imaging? What would hibernating images look like?

4. Is there evidence of hibernating myocardium? If so, where?

Cardiovascular System: FDG-PET—Hibernating Myocardium

1. Hibernating myocardium is a low myocardial blood flow state of chronic ischemia. It is suspected in CAD patients with poor ventricular function and a stress-rest myocardial perfusion study showing a fixed defect, caused by either myocardial infarction or hibernating myocardium.

2. Revascularization will improve ventricular function and long-term survival in patients with hibernating myocardium.

3. Under normal fasting conditions, the myocardium uses free fatty acids as its primary source of energy. However, in the setting of ischemia, glucose utilization increases. Thus, with chronic ischemia, there will be a mismatch between perfusion (reduced) and FDG metabolism (increased).

4. Yes. Hibernating myocardium is seen in the septum and anterior wall and to a lesser extent in the distal inferior wall. The perfusion defect in the inferior wall is mostly fixed—infarcted.

References

Bengel FM, Higuchi T, Javadi MS, Lautamäki R: Cardiac positron emission tomography, *J Am Coll Cardiol* 54:1-15, 2009.

Krombach GA, Niendorf T, Günther RW, Mahnken AH: Characterization of myocardial viability using MR and CT imaging, *Eur Radiol* 17:1433-1444, 2007.

Cross-Reference

Nuclear Medicine: THE REQUISITES, 3rd ed, pp 488-490.

Comment

Hibernating myocardium is the term used for chronic ischemia that manifests as ventricular contractile dysfunction. Under normal fasting conditions, the myocardium uses free fatty acids mobilized from adipose tissue as its main source of energy via mitochondrium-localized β-oxidation. Fatty acid use declines rapidly in the setting of ischemia, and myocardial metabolism becomes increasingly dependent on nonoxygen-requiring processes. In this setting, glycolysis is exploited for the supply of energy to chronically ischemic although viable (hibernating) myocardium. Imaging with FDG detects this increased use of glucose and is able to define myocardium that is viable even though there is resting hypoperfusion on perfusion imaging.

Multidetector CT and MRI are being used increasingly for assessment of myocardial viability, as manifested by delayed enhancement and hyperenhancement of nonviable regions after contrast injection. The mechanism is believed to be increased extracellular volume in damaged myocardium. MRI provides better spatial resolution than PET, but the prognostic implication of findings on MRI is not established. CT compares well with MRI in sensitivity for the detection of viable myocardium and affords the possibility of also obtaining angiographic images in the same imaging session. Given the emergence of hybrid PET/CT (and perhaps PET/MRI in the future), multimodality cardiovascular imaging will likely exploit the strengths of each study in an effort to best evaluate patients with ischemic cardiomyopathy.

Notes

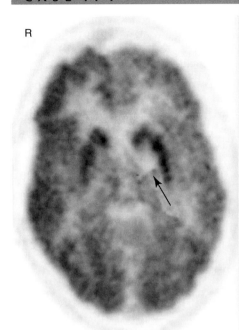
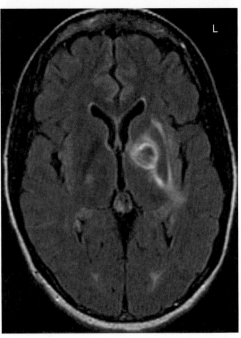

A 28-year-old patient has AIDS.

1. Describe the ^{18}F-FDG-PET and MRI findings.

2. What is the differential diagnosis based on MRI?

3. What is the diagnosis for this patient?

4. What other radiopharmaceutical can be used for this differentiation?

Inflammatory Disease: Brain FDG-PET—Malignancy versus Infection in an HIV Patient

1. A small rounded area of photopenia on FDG-PET (*arrow*) corresponds to a ring-enhancing lesion with surrounding edema in the region of the left basal ganglia on MRI.

2. Malignancy (e.g., lymphoma) versus infection (e.g., toxoplasmosis).

3. Negative for malignancy. Consistent with inflammatory/infectious etiology.

4. ^{201}Tl with SPECT.

References

Bakshi R, Ketonen L: Imaging of the central nervous system complications of HIV and AIDS related illnesses. In: *NeuroAids.* New York: Nova Science Hauppauge, 2006, pp 199–223.

Hoffman JM, Waskin HA, Schifter T, et al: FDG-PET in differentiating lymphoma from nonmalignant central nervous system lesions in patients with AIDS, *J Nucl Med* 34:567–575, 1993.

Kita T, Hayashi K, Yamamoto M, et al: Does supplementation of contrast MR imaging with thallium-201 brain SPECT improve differentiation between benign and malignant ring-like contrast-enhanced cerebral lesions? *Ann Nucl Med* 21:251–256, 2007.

Cross-Reference

Nuclear Medicine: THE REQUISITES, 3rd ed, p 432.

Comment

The diagnostic and therapeutic dilemma of an intracerebral mass in patients with HIV is challenging. Biopsy is diagnostic; however, surgeons are reluctant to operate on these patients. Conventional imaging with CT and MRI cannot distinguish between malignant and nonmalignant causes. Imaging with ^{18}F-FDG or ^{201}Tl-Cl can be a great help in the management of these patients. If the study suggests malignancy, biopsy is indicated. If the study is negative, therapy for infection is indicated, usually for toxoplasmosis.

There is a larger base of supportive literature on the use of ^{201}Tl; however, the reported accuracy of FDG-PET and ^{201}Tl seems to be similar, approximately 90%. The image resolution of PET is superior.

Central nervous system involvement is seen in as many as 90% of individuals with HIV. One potential sequela from central nervous system HIV infection is AIDS dementia complex, which is a progressive cognitive-motor disorder that can cause damage to neural tissues, particularly in the basal ganglia, a common location for central nervous system lesions in this patient population. Perfusion imaging with SPECT or metabolic imaging with FDG-PET is sensitive for AIDS dementia complex, which has a typical pattern of patchy, multifocal cortical and subcortical regions of hypoperfusion.

Notes

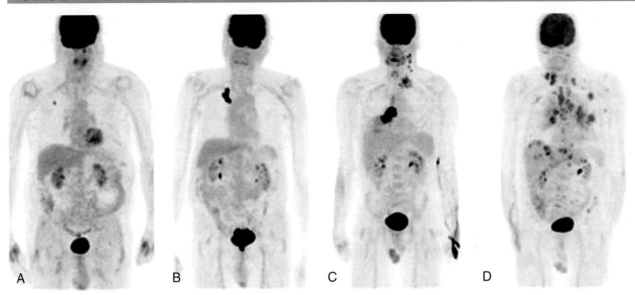

A, ^{18}F-FDG-PET MIP image from a patient presenting with a solitary pulmonary nodule (SPN). B to D, Three other patients with studies for staging of non-small cell lung cancer.

1. A, What are common causes of false-positive and false-negative findings on ^{18}F-FDG-PET for SPN?

2. B, Describe the pattern of uptake. What tumor characteristics would make this tumor unresectable?

3. Stage patients C and D and give an explanation.

4. What are common sites of metastasis from non-small cell lung cancer?

Oncology: FDG-PET—Lung Cancer

1. False positives: infection, inflammation, granulomatous disease; false negatives: small size (<1 cm), bronchoalveolar or carcinoid tumors, non-FDG-avid tumors (e.g., mucinous histology).

2. Single focus of intense FDG uptake in the patient's right upper lobe primary lung cancer without evidence of nodal disease or metastasis (N_0M_0). Unresectable if there is invasion into the mediastinum, heart, great vessels, esophagus, trachea, vertebral body, recurrent laryngeal nerve, or carina (T4 and therefore stage IIIB).

3. C: $T_2N_3M_1$ (stage IV): SPN larger than 3 cm but less than 7 cm (T2), ipsilateral mediastinal nodes (N2), contralateral supraclavicular and cervical node metastases (M1). D, $T_1N_3M_1$ disease (stage IV): primary tumor less than 3 cm (T1) contralateral mediastinal lymph node metastases (N3) diffuse metastases (liver, lungs, spine, nodes).

4. Adrenal glands, liver, contralateral lung, brain, and bone.

References

Behzadi A, Ung Y, Lowe V, Deschamps C: The role of positron emission tomography in the management of non-small cell lung cancer, *Can J Surg* 52:235–242, 2009.

Ung YC, Maziak DE, Vanderveen JA, et al: 18 FDG PET in the diagnosis and staging of lung cancer: a systematic review, *J Natl Cancer Inst* 99:1753–1767, 2007.

Cross-Reference

Nuclear Medicine: THE REQUISITES, 3rd ed, pp 314–323.

Comment

An SPN is defined as a single nonspiculated, rounded opacity 3 cm or smaller, in the absence of atelectasis or lymphadenopathy, surrounded by lung parenchyma. Clinical findings and standard radiography are indeterminate in 75%. Forty percent of SPNs prove to be malignant; adenocarcinoma is the most common histology. Infection and granulomas are the most common benign causes and are primarily due to tuberculous, fungal, nocardia, abscess, and parasitic infections. Although early reports found that SPNs with SUVs less than 2.5 (based on body weight) are benign, recent studies find that visual analysis performs as well as SUV and that the incidence of malignancy in lesions with low but detectable FDG uptake is significant (24%). Correlation of the PET findings with those of CT is important (e.g., is the lesion spiculated, growing?). Bronchoalveolar carcinoma has a 60% false-negative rate on FDG-PET.

Respiratory motion may lead to false-negative studies. Integrated PET/CT studies are obtained during "quiet" tidal breathing. Thus, lung lesions may move in and out of the plane of acquisition during respiration, especially if they are small (<8–10 mm) or located in the lower lobes and adjacent to the diaphragm. The presence of motion can blur uptake of small lesions, resulting in an underestimation of metabolic activity (i.e., partial volume effect). Respiratory gating of PET/CT may aid in more accurately accessing these lesions.

FDG-PET is more accurate than CT alone for the detection of nodal disease in patients with non-small cell lung cancer (sensitivity, 85% vs. 61%). FDG-PET can help to avoid unnecessary thoracotomy by identifying advanced disease not detected by other means in 20% of patients. FDG-PET can monitor and predict response to therapy.

Notes

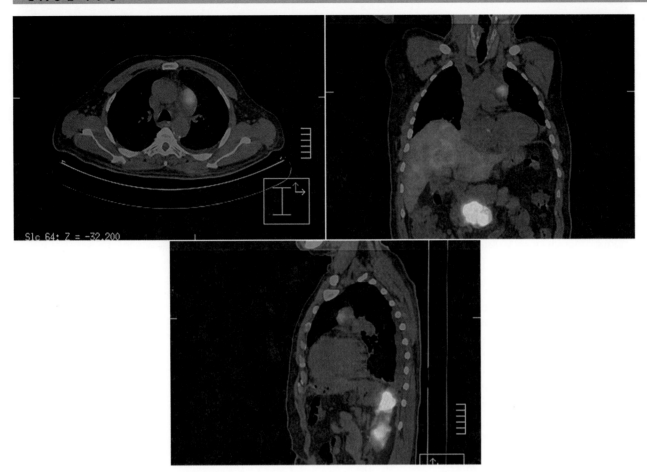

Slc 64: Z = -32.200

A 62-year-old patient had recent surgery diagnostic of a neuroendocrine tumor in the region of the pancreatic uncinate process. Selected SPECT/CT images are shown.

1. What is the likely radiopharmaceutical?

2. Describe the image findings.

3. What is your interpretation?

4. What other tumors would show uptake with this radiotracer?

Endocrine System: Pancreatic Neuroendocrine Tumor with Metastases— SPECT/CT

1. ^{111}In-pentetreotide (OctreoScan).

2. Improves specificity. Old fractures or surgery, degenerative changes, will not usually have increased flow.

3. In addition to the primary pancreatic tumor, there is evidence of probable retroperitoneal adenopathy seen on the sagittal view and metastasis to the prevascular lymph nodes seen on the coronal and transverse slices.

4. Carcinoid tumor, gastrinoma, glucagonoma, medullary thyroid carcinoma, insulinoma, vipoma, pituitary adenoma, pheochromocytoma, paraganglioma, pituitary adenoma.

References

Garin E, Le Jeune F, Devillers A, et al: Predictive value of ^{18}F-FDG PET and somatostatin receptor scintigraphy in patients with metastatic endocrine tumors, *J Nucl Med* 50:858–864, 2009.

Wong KK, Cahill JM, Frey KA, Avram AM: Incremental value of 111-In pentetreotide SPECT/CT fusion imaging of neuroendocrine tumors, *Acad Radiol* 17:291–297, 2010.

Cross-Reference

Nuclear Medicine: THE REQUISITES, 3rd ed, pp 279–283.

Comment

Neuroendocrine tumors arise from the upper airways, small intestine, and duodenopancreatic regions. They are often asymptomatic in early stages and discovered after metastatic spread. ^{111}In-pentetreotide has high sensitivity for detection of many of the neuroendocrine tumors that are well differentiated and larger than 1 cm. Sensitivity is 80% to 90% for most of the neuroendocrine tumors, except for insulinoma, and superior to that of other imaging modalities for identifying and staging these tumors. Numerous studies indicate that ^{111}In-pentetreotide changes management in 21% to 53% of patients. SPECT improves the sensitivity for detection due to improved contrast resolution. Specificity for neuroendocrine tumors is also high. The addition of CT to SPECT aids in anatomic localization. ^{111}In-pentetreotide sensitivity for detection is not as high in poorly differentiated tumors. PET/CT is preferable in poorly differentiated tumors. On the other hand, FDG-PET has low sensitivity for well-differentiated neuroendocrine tumors.

Notes

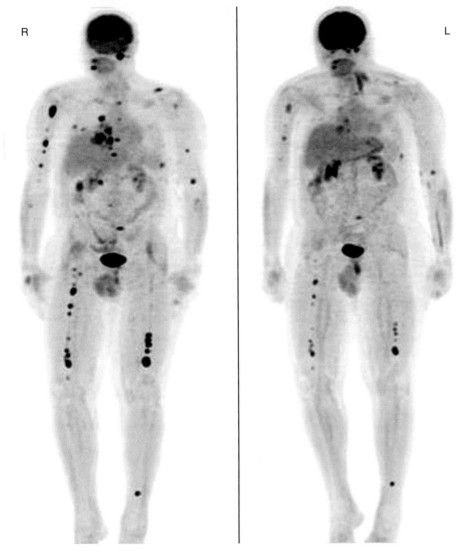

R

L

A 41-year-old man has multiple myeloma. ^{18}F-FDG-PET MIP images pre- and post-chemotherapy are shown.

1. Describe the change between the two FDG-PET studies and categorize the response as complete response, partial response, stable disease, or progressive disease.

2. What is the likely reason that the follow-up PET scan (image on right) was performed?

3. What is the usual time after chemotherapy to perform follow-up FDG-PET?

4. In the image on the right, what is the cause of uptake in the low left neck?

Oncology: FDG-PET—Multiple Myeloma

1. There is a reduction in the number, size, and intensity of the multiple FDG avid lesions. Partial response.

2. To determine whether the patient is responding to treatment and whether the same therapy should be continued or changed.

3. Three weeks after chemotherapy. Preliminary data suggest that imaging after two to three cycles may be adequate.

4. Physiologic uptake in neck muscles (e.g., scalene muscles).

References

Cheson BD: The International Harmonization Project for response criteria in lymphoma clinical trials, *Hematol Oncol Clin N Am* 21:841–854, 2007.

Young H, Baum R, Cremerius U, et al: Measurement of clinical and subclinical tumour response using F-18-fluorodeoxyglucose and PET: review and 1999 EORTC recommendations, *Eur J Cancer* 35:1773–1782, 1999.

Cross-Reference

Nuclear Medicine: THE REQUISITES, 3rd ed, pp 308–311.

Comment

Just as there are anatomic imaging criteria to evaluate response to therapy (e.g., the World Health Organization, Response Evaluation Criteria in Solid Tumors), criteria have also been established to evaluate metabolic FDG response to therapy. These criteria were outlined by the European Organization for Research and Treatment of Cancer in 1999, which incorporated SUVs: progressive disease—greater than 25% increase in SUV, visible increase in tumor size, or new lesions; stable disease—no visible increase in tumor size; partial response—less than 25% reduction in tumor size; complete response—resolution of abnormal FDG uptake.

There are currently no definitive guidelines as to when FDG-PET should be performed to determine response to therapy. However, general recommendations are at least 3 weeks after chemotherapy and 3 to 4 months after radiotherapy. Imaging should be delayed 4 to 6 weeks after surgery and for several days after a biopsy. This is because inflammatory uptake that can be seen as a result of the procedure may result in a false-positive interpretation. Performing the scan at a longer interval will presumably allow time for this inflammation to resolve. Studies now indicate that even after one cycle of chemotherapy, imaging can be performed to evaluate response to therapy and may aid in decisions regarding patient management. If a reasonable length of time has not elapsed, particularly after radiation therapy or surgery, a higher false-positive rate has been reported.

Notes

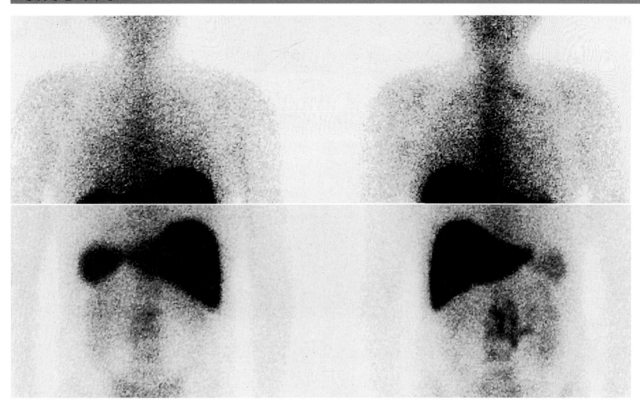

A 64-year-old man had prostatectomy for prostate cancer 3 years ago. The serum PSA is increasing. Bone scan and CT findings are negative. A ^{111}In-capromab pendetide (ProstaScint) scan is shown.

1. What is the mechanism of uptake?

2. Compare the sensitivity of CT and MRI with that of ^{111}In-capromab pendetide (ProstaScint) for detecting prostate cancer metastases after prostatectomy.

3. What are the abnormal imaging findings on this study? Give your interpretation.

4. How does the ^{111}In-capromab pendetide study affect the patient's therapy plan?

Oncology: ^{111}In-ProstaScint—Prostate Cancer

1. ^{111}In-labeled monoclonal antibody directed against the prostate-specific membrane antigen, a glycoprotein expressed by normal and cancerous prostate cells.

2. CT and MRI sensitivity ranges from 10% to 20%. Reported accuracy of ^{111}In-capromab pendetide (ProstaScint) is 70%.

3. Para-aortic upper abdominal uptake consistent with tumor adenopathy. Focal uptake in the left upper chest could be a metastasis; however, an inflammatory etiology is possible.

4. Recurrent tumor limited to the prostate bed or metastatic pelvic lymph nodes requires different radiation ports. Extrapelvic metastases require systemic therapy.

References

Blend MJ, Sodee DB: ProstaScint: an update. In: Freeman LM (ed): *Nuclear Medicine Annual 2001*. Philadelphia: Lippincott-Raven, 2001, pp 109–138.

Jana S, Blaufox MD: Nuclear medicine studies of the prostate, testes, and bladder, *Semin Nucl Med* 36:51–72, 2006.

Cross-Reference

Nuclear Medicine: THE REQUISITES, 3rd ed, pp 289–292.

Comment

Examination, histopathologic Gleason score, and serum PSA level are used to stage prostate cancer. After primary therapy for prostate cancer, the patient is monitored with the serum PSA level as a marker of tumor activity. Increasing PSA level suggests recurrence of tumor. Because bone metastases are common in metastatic prostate cancer, the ^{99m}Tc diphosphonate bone scan should be performed first. If the bone scan results are negative, CT or MRI may be performed; however, their sensitivity for the detection of recurrent prostate cancer is low because of small tumor size. ^{111}In-ProstaScint (capromab pendetide) is a monoclonal antibody directed against intact prostate cells. It is a murine immunoglobulin reactive with prostate-specific membrane antigen, a glycoprotein expressed by more than 95% of prostate cancers. Capromab pendetide (ProstaScint) is clinically indicated for the detection of soft-tissue metastases. Extrapelvic metastases in the abdomen sometimes can be diagnosed with planar imaging, as seen in this patient. However, SPECT is mandatory to detect prostate bed and pelvic tumor adenopathy. Capromab pendetide (ProstaScint) is less sensitive for bone metastases than the ^{99m}Tc diphosphonate bone scan. Capromab pendetide (ProstaScint) imaging has been interpreted in conjunction with ^{99m}Tc-RBC blood pool imaging to aid in anatomic localization. SPECT/CT or software fusion of CT/MRI with SPECT makes blood pool imaging unnecessary and is superior for anatomic localization.

Notes

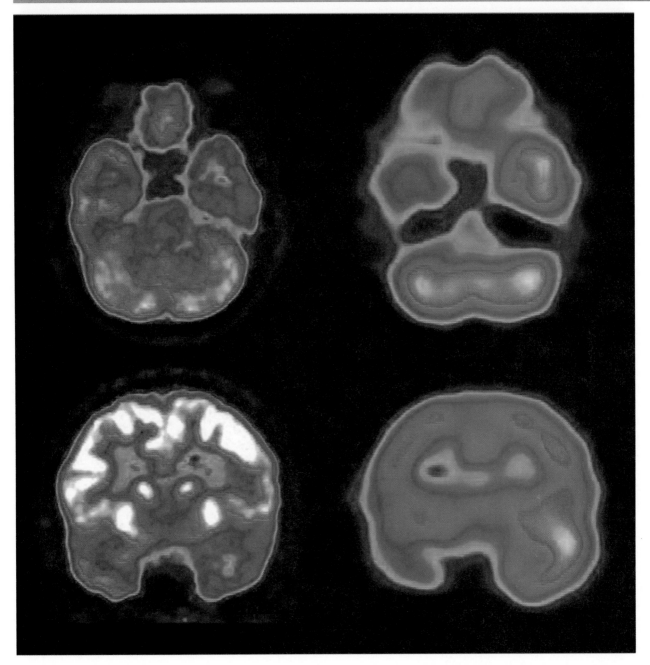

1. What radiopharmaceuticals are most frequently used for clinical PET (*left*) and SPECT (*right*) of the brain?

2. Describe the pattern of uptake on the PET images. What is the differential diagnosis?

3. Describe the pattern of uptake on the SPECT images. What is the differential diagnosis?

4. Describe a clinical setting in which both sets of images would have been obtained for the same patient.

Nervous System: FDG-PET—Seizure Localization

1. PET: ^{18}F-FDG. SPECT: ^{99m}Tc-HMPAO or Tc-99m-ECD.

2. PET: decreased uptake in the left temporal lobe. Atrophy, infarction, low-grade tumor, interictal seizure focus. Thus, the radionuclide studies must always be compared with anatomic imaging, MRI, or CT.

3. SPECT: increased uptake in the left temporal lobe. Herpes encephalitis, ictal seizure focus.

4. Combined interictal and ictal brain studies have a high accuracy for localization of a seizure focus. The typical mismatched pattern of uptake between FDG-PET interictal imaging (hypometabolism) and SPECT ictal imaging (hyperperfusion) is diagnostic for seizure focus localization in the left temporal lobe.

References

Goffin K, Dedeurwaerdere S, Van Laere K, Van Paesschen W: Neuronuclear assessment of patients with epilepsy, *Semin Nucl Med* 38:227–239, 2008.

Waxman AD, Herholz K, Lewis DH, et al: *Society of Nuclear Medicine Procedure Guideline for FDG PET Brain Imaging*. Reston, VA: Society of Nuclear Medicine, 2009.

Cross-Reference

Nuclear Medicine: THE REQUISITES, 3rd ed, pp 436–438.

Comment

Patients with complex partial seizures that are poorly controlled medically may benefit from surgical temporal lobectomy. Excision of the seizure focus, is usually related to mesial temporal sclerosis, eliminates the seizures or produces a marked improvement in pharmacologic control in 80% of patients. Although often the patient's seizure history, neurologic examination, electroencephalography, and MRI will be able to localize the seizure focus, at other times, its location remains uncertain. CT and MR have poor sensitivity for localizing a seizure focus. Electroencephalography is not always diagnostic, may show bilateral abnormalities, and requires confirmation. Depth electrodes can be placed surgically for localization; however, this is invasive and not without risk. If brain PET/SPECT imaging is concordant with clinical and electroencephalographic findings, surgery is performed at some centers without depth electrode placement.

Continuous video-electroencephalographic monitoring is recommended in anticipation of radiopharmaceutical injection for an ictal brain scan to ascertain that the patient is indeed having a seizure at the time of injection. The radiotracer should be injected as early as possible at the onset of seizure activity (within 2 minutes). Image quality is better with FDG-PET than the ^{99m}Tc radiopharmaceuticals. The short 2-hour half life of ^{18}F makes it logistically impossible to have the radiotracer on hand for injection during a seizure and would require patient imaging immediately thereafter. ^{99m}Tc-labeled brain radiotracers with a half-life of 6 hours fix irreversibly in the cerebral cortex, making them very useful for injection during an active seizure followed later by imaging, which may be delayed, if necessary. Interictal imaging is diagnostic for localization in approximately 70% of patients. Imaging after ictal injection is diagnostic in greater than 90%. The ictal study is considerably easier to interpret in conjunction with the interictal study than in isolation.

Notes

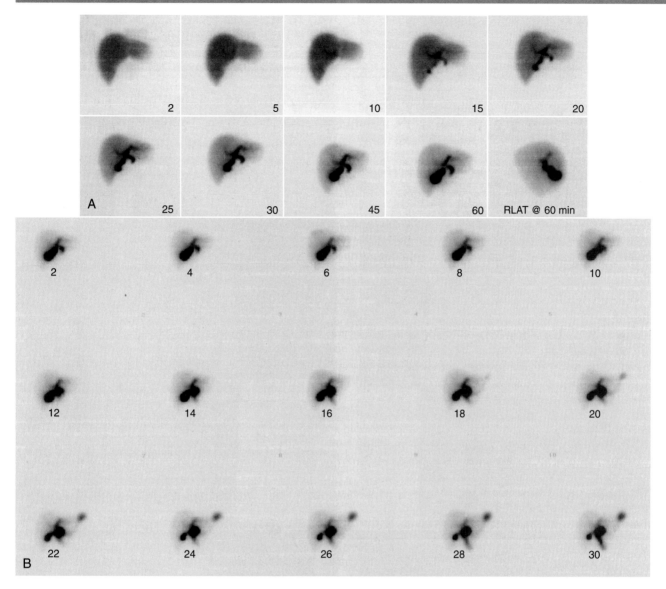

A, Initial routine cholescintigraphy for 60 minutes; B, 30-minute CCK-8 (sincalide) infusion.

An 8-year-old girl with acute abdominal pain. A, Initial routine cholescintigraphy for 60 minutes; B, 30-minute CCK-8 (sincalide) infusion. Ultrasonography showed a cystic mass in the region of the hepatic and common ducts.

1. Describe the cholescintigraphic findings.

2. What is the likely diagnosis?

3. What other clinical presentations are common in patients with this problem?

4. What is the anatomy and pathophysiology of this entity, and what is the appropriate therapy?

Hepatobiliary System: Choledochal Cyst

1. A, Good hepatic uptake and clearance into the gall-bladder, common hepatic, and common bile duct by 60 minutes. There is no biliary-to-bowel transit. B, With sincalide infusion, the gallbladder contracts; however, there is focal increasing accumulation of radiotracer just medial to the proximal portion of the common bile duct. The proximal common duct activity empties into the duodenum. Some enterogastric reflux is seen.

2. Choledochal cyst.

3. Cholangitis, sepsis, pancreatitis, or obstruction.

4. Congenital anomaly. Localized dilation of the biliary tract, either fusiform or diverticular outpouching. Surgery is the appropriate therapy.

References

Camponovo E, Buck JL, Drane WE: Scintigraphic features of choledochal cyst, *J Nucl Med* 30:622–628, 1989.

Kim OH, Chung HJ, Choi BG: Imaging of the choledochal cyst, *Radiographics* 15:69–87, 1995.

Cross-Reference

Nuclear Medicine: THE REQUISITES, 3rd ed, pp 180–183, 243.

Comment

A choledochal cyst is a congenital anomaly characterized by saccular dilation of the extrahepatic biliary tract. It is not a true cyst. The most common form is characterized by a fusiform dilation of the common bile duct. A second type is a diverticular outpouching of the common bile duct, and a third is a small saccular dilation of the distal common bile duct. Less common intrahepatic ductal dilation is referred to as Caroli's disease.

Recognition and appropriate early treatment of a choledochal cyst are critical because of the risk of severe cholangitis, obstruction, and adenocarcinoma (10% occurrence rate) if the cyst is left untreated. The diagnosis is made preoperatively in only 27% to 80% of patients in different published reports. A lower surgical morbidity is associated with a preoperative diagnosis. Ultrasonography is the best screening method for small children; CT has been advocated for older children and adults. Cholescintigraphy is used to noninvasively confirm the diagnosis (i.e., to ensure that the cystic structure connects with the biliary tract and sometimes to help identify the type). In this patient, imaging during sincalide infusion demonstrated filling of the choledochal cyst. Delayed images rather than sincalide would have shown the same thing, but probably would have taken longer. Definitive diagnosis is made by endoscopic retrograde cholangiopancreatography or intraoperative cholangiography.

Notes

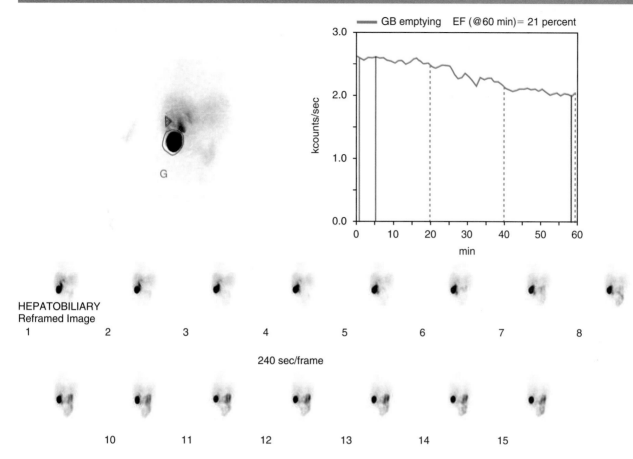

GB emptying   EF (@60 min) = 21 percent

kcounts/sec

min

HEPATOBILIARY
Reframed Image

1   2   3   4   5   6   7   8

240 sec/frame

10   11   12   13   14   15

This patient has a history of recurrent, biliary colic–like pain and repeated negative gastrointestinal workups that included ultrasonography. Sincalide (CCK-8) cholescintigraphy was ordered to confirm or exclude the diagnosis of chronic acalculous gallbladder disease. Images were acquired during sincalide infusion.

1. What is chronic acalculous gallbladder disease?

2. Why is sincalide cholescintigraphy required to make the diagnosis?

3. What is your diagnosis based on the images?

4. What is the accuracy of sincalide cholescintigraphy for chronic acalculous gallbladder disease?

Hepatobiliary System: Chronic Acalculous Gallbladder Disease

1. Chronic acalculous gallbladder disease is in most cases clinically and histopathologically identical to chronic calculous cholecystitis, except for the absence of gallstones.

2. Anatomic imaging diagnosis depends on gallstone visualization; however, there are no stones with this disease. Sincalide infusion evaluates gallbladder contraction. Diseased gallbladders do not contract.

3. Poor gallbladder contraction (normal, >35%). Consistent with chronic acalculous gallbladder disease.

4. A low gallbladder ejection fraction has a positive predictive value of more than 90% that cholecystectomy will cure the patient's symptoms and confirm the diagnosis histopathologically.

References

Yap L, Wycherley AG, Morphett AD, Toouli J: Acalculous biliary pain: cholecystectomy alleviates symptoms in patients with abnormal cholescintigraphy, *Gastroenterology* 101:786–793, 1991.

Ziessman HA: Functional hepatobiliary disease: chronic acalculous gallbladder and chronic acalculous biliary disease, *Semin Nucl Med* 36:119–132, 2006.

Cross-Reference

Nuclear Medicine: THE REQUISITES, 3rd ed, pp 175–176.

Comment

Symptoms of chronic cholecystitis overlap with other causes for abdominal pain. Ten percent of patients with chronic cholecystitis have an acalculous form. Diagnosis is difficult in this group of patients because anatomic imaging shows no stones or other abnormality. Other terms for chronic acalculous gallbladder disease include *chronic acalculous cholecystitis, gallbladder dyskinesia*, and *cystic duct syndrome*. All refer to patients with recurrent biliary colic–like pain, poor gallbladder contraction, and symptom resolution with cholecystectomy.

Sincalide cholescintigraphy should be performed in outpatients with recurrent symptoms suggestive of the disease who have been evaluated to exclude other diseases and had follow-up allowing time for other diseases to manifest. The test should not be performed in acutely ill patients and patients taking drugs that inhibit gallbladder contraction (e.g., progesterone, nifedipine, atropine, and morphine).

Proper methodology is critical. Sincalide infusions of 30 to 60 minutes are more reliable than short infusion of 3 to 15 minutes. Short infusions can result in poor contraction in one third of normal subjects, but show normal gallbladder contraction with a 30- to 60-minute infusion. As many as half of normal subjects receiving a 3-minute infusion have abdominal cramps and nausea caused by the rapid rate of infusion. With 30- to 60-minute infusions, no adverse symptoms occur. A 60-minute infusion of 0.02 µg/kg has the least variability and the best defined normal values and is now the recommended method of infusion (abnormal, <38%).

Notes

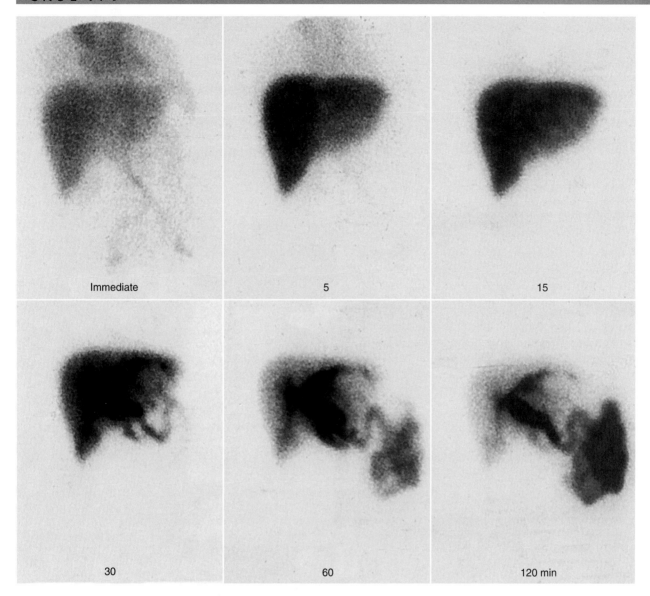

Immediate   5   15

30   60   120 min

A 46-year-old woman has recurrent upper abdominal pain since her cholecystectomy 15 months ago. Sequential images are shown over approximately 90 minutes.

1. Give the differential diagnosis for the postcholecystectomy syndrome.

2. Describe the cholescintigraphic findings.

3. Interpret the study.

4. What is the next diagnostic step?

Hepatobiliary System: Postcholecystectomy Syndrome—Biliary Stricture

1. Biliary causes include biliary duct stone, inflammatory stricture of the common duct, sphincter of Oddi dysfunction, inflamed cystic duct remnant.

2. Prompt hepatic uptake (blood pool clearance by 5 minutes), clearance into biliary ducts by 15 to 30 minutes, apparently dilated proximal hepatic and common ducts, some biliary-to-bowel clearance by 60 minutes, but retention of radiotracer in ducts. At 120 minutes, further small bowel clearance but prominent retention in common duct with apparent cutoff distally.

3. Retention of radiotracer in biliary ducts despite biliary-to-bowel clearance is suggestive of partial biliary obstruction.

4. Magnetic resonance cholangiopancreatography and, if necessary, endoscopic retrograde cholangiopancreatography to detect stones and stricture. If none, this suggests sphincter of Oddi dysfunction. The study patient had biliary stricture diagnosed by endoscopic retrograde cholangiopancreatography.

Reference

Ziessman HA: Functional hepatobiliary disease: chronic acalculous gallbladder and chronic acalculous biliary disease, *Semin Nucl Med* 36:119–132, 2006.

Cross-Reference

Nuclear Medicine: THE REQUISITES, 3rd ed, pp 182–187.

Comment

Recurrent abdominal pain symptoms occur in as many as 10% of patients after cholecystectomy (postcholecystectomy syndrome). The most common biliary cause is retained or recurrent stones and in some cases inflammatory fibrosis with stricture or sphincter of Oddi dysfunction. Cholescintigraphic findings are that of a partial biliary duct obstruction. Delayed biliary duct clearance is the dominant scintigraphic finding. Biliary-to-bowel transit may or may not be delayed. As many as 50% of patients with partial common duct obstruction have biliary-to-bowel transit by 60 minutes. In this case, nonclearance of the common hepatic and common bile duct at 2 hours is consistent with partial obstruction.

Cholescintigraphy is often used as a screening test. If results are positive, more invasive studies are indicated. Magnetic resonance cholangiopancreatography will detect ductal dilation but often cannot detect small stones. Stone and stricture must be excluded with endoscopic retrograde cholangiopancreatography. Sphincter of Oddi manometry demonstrating elevated pressure is more specific for making the diagnosis. However, manometry generally is not available and is technically demanding, and associated with a high rate of complications (e.g., pancreatitis). Cholescintigraphy can be used as a screening test to exclude the diagnosis of a biliary cause for the pain. Nonbiliary causes of pain would then be considered. A positive study requires further workup. The treatment for sphincter of Oddi dysfunction is sphincterotomy.

Notes

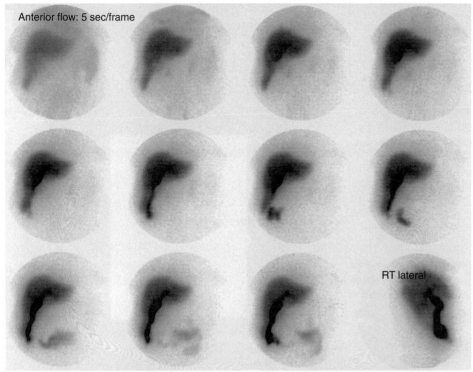

Anterior flow: 5 sec/frame

RT lateral

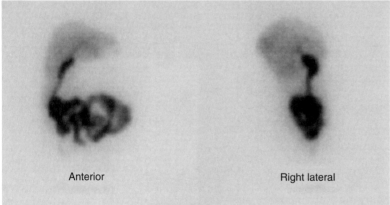

Anterior

Right lateral

A patient has a history of biliary-intestinal diversion of unknown type and now has abdominal pain.

1. Describe the scintigraphic findings.

2. What type of biliary diversion was most likely performed?

3. Are the study results normal or abnormal?

4. Could ultrasonography have provided the same information?

C A S E 1 8 0

Hepatobiliary System: Cholecystojejunostomy

1. Prompt hepatic uptake and rapid biliary-to-bowel clearance.

2. Cholecystoduodenostomy or cholecystojejunostomy.

3. Normal postoperative study results. Good biliary clearance into the intestinal tract.

4. Nondiagnostic examinations are frequent with sonography, occuring in 67% of patients, most often as a result of gas in the anastomotic bowel segment. Biliary dilation is often present without obstruction.

Reference

Ziessman HA, Zeman RK, Akin EA: Cholescintigraphy: correlation with other hepatobiliary imaging modalities. In: Sandler MP, Coleman RE, et al (eds): *Diagnostic Nuclear Medicine*, 4th ed. Baltimore: Lippincott Williams & Wilkins, 2002, pp 503–509.

Cross-Reference

Nuclear Medicine: THE REQUISITES, 3rd ed, pp 182–187.

Comment

Cholescintigraphy is useful for evaluating the postoperative biliary tract after creation of a biliary-enteric anastomosis. Evaluation of acute and early complications of surgery and long-term follow-up for biliary patency is possible. Knowledge of the postoperative anatomy of the patient is important when imaging the postoperative biliary tract. Biliary scintigraphy commonly is used to evaluate a choledochojejunostomy, which is a direct anastomosis of the extrahepatic portion of the common bile duct or the common hepatic duct to a Roux-en-Y of the jejunum. It is also used to evaluate intrahepatic cholangiojejunostomies. The latter is more complex, requiring direct anastomosis between small bowel and intrahepatic ducts that must be dissected out deep within the liver. Choledochoduodenostomy, cholecystoduodenostomy, and cholecystojejunostomy also can be studied. The latter two procedures frequently are used in benign disease states.

Many complications can occur postoperatively after creation of a biliary diversion. Biliary leakage is among the most common. Recurrent biliary obstruction is a major problem and is well suited for cholescintigraphic evaluation. Cholescintigraphy is the only noninvasive technique that can distinguish obstructed dilated ducts from those that are persistently dilated, but not obstructed.

Notes

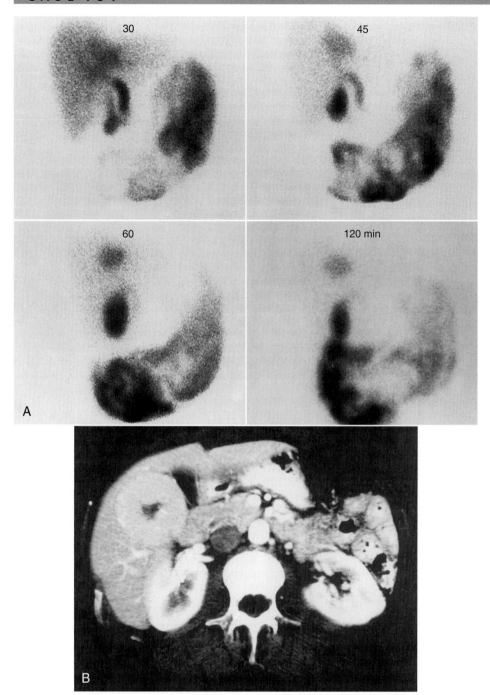

30

45

60

120 min

A

B

A 35-year-old woman has had intermittent acute abdominal pain. Cholescintigraphy (A) at 30 through 120 minutes. The CT scan (B) shows a large, circumscribed lesion at the juncture of the right and left liver lobes.

1. Describe the cholescintigraphic findings.

2. What is the differential diagnosis? What is the diagnosis in this case?

3. What is the appropriate therapy for each of these diagnoses?

4. What other radiopharmaceutical could confirm the diagnosis in this case?

Hepatobiliary System: Focal Nodular Hyperplasia (FNH)

1. Increased radiopharmaceutical uptake that corresponds to the CT lesion. The uptake is retained after liver washout.

2. Benign and malignant tumors (e.g., hepatic adenoma, hepatoma, FNH). FNH is the correct diagnosis in this case.

3. FNH usually requires no specific therapy. Hepatic adenoma requires discontinuation of oral contraceptives and surgical removal to prevent bleeding, and hepatoma requires resection.

4. ^{99m}Tc-SC.

Reference

Boulahdour H, Cherqui D, Charlotte F, et al: The hot spot hepatobiliary scan in focal nodular hyperplasia, *J Nucl Med* 34:2105–2110, 1993.

Cross-Reference

Nuclear Medicine: THE REQUISITES, 3rd ed, pp 187–190.

Comment

FNH and hepatic adenoma are benign liver tumors that occur as solid intrahepatic lesions in young and middle-aged women. The natural history of the two is quite different. Although hepatic adenomas may manifest as a mass, often the initial presentation is an abdominal crisis caused by intraperitoneal hemorrhage. Hepatic adenoma has a strong association with contraceptive use. Pathologically, adenomas consist of sheets of hepatocytes without structure, bile ducts, or Kupffer cells. FNH has only a weak association with contraceptive use, usually produces no symptoms, is discovered incidentally, and requires no specific therapy. This patient's pain was not related to the tumor and the finding was incidental. Pathologically, FNH tumors have a stellate fibrous core (see CT) and contain all three liver cell types.

On cholescintigraphy, FNH has a characteristic appearance: increased flow, normal or increased uptake, and delayed clearance compared with adjacent uninvolved liver, probably as a result of immature biliary canaliculi. In this case, a flow study was not obtained, but the findings are still rather specific. Hepatic adenomas, although made up exclusively of hepatocytes, have no uptake; the reason for this is uncertain. With hepatocellular carcinoma (hepatoma), images during the first hour demonstrate a cold defect; however, delayed imaging at 2 to 4 hours shows uptake within the tumor as the normal liver washes out. This pattern occurs because hepatocellular carcinoma cells are hypofunctional compared with normal liver, with delayed uptake and clearance. The low-level uptake within the hepatoma also is easier to visualize when the normal liver has washed out. Sensitivity for the detection of FNH with cholescintigraphy is greater than 90%. Although the diagnosis can often be made with anatomic imaging and ultimately biopsy, in uncertain cases, cholescintigraphy can be helpful.

Notes

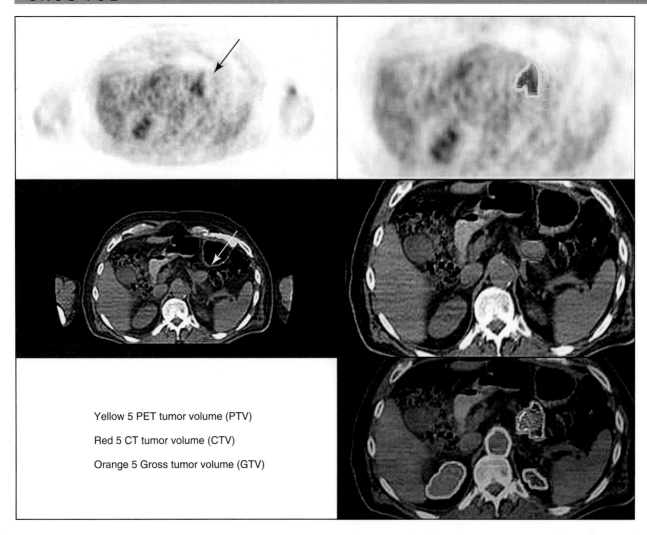

Yellow 5 PET tumor volume (PTV)

Red 5 CT tumor volume (CTV)

Orange 5 Gross tumor volume (GTV)

A 56-year-old man with recently diagnosed pancreatic cancer presents before radiation therapy.

1. What methods are currently used for calculation of tumor volume based on FDG-PET images?

2. Describe how the addition of PET data in the above patient altered the gross tumor volume.

3. What are benefits/limitations of using FDG-PET tumor volumes in radiotherapy treatment planning?

4. Other than ^{18}F-FDG, which other PET tracer(s) is(are) used in imaging tumors in the setting of radiotherapy?

Oncology: FDG-PET/CT—Radiation Therapy Planning

1. Threshold SUV centered on CT-delineated tumor site (e.g., all pixels with $SUV_{max} \geq 2.5$); isocontours to include pixels with a fixed percentage of the maximum pixel SUV (e.g., 40% of maximum pixel); pixels within a set standard deviation of maximum pixel SUV (e.g., standard deviation of 2.5); pixels with a fixed target: background ratio and subjective/visual "halo" evaluation. None of these methods is proven superior to the others.

2. Gross tumor volume was larger due to the addition of FDG-PET.

3. Benefits are decreased gross tumor volume by delineating uptake in normal structures; decreased interobserver variability in the definition of target treatment volumes; improved mapping of residual active tumor over the course of radiation therapy; increase in tumor volume to include metastasis/local spread not appreciated on anatomic imaging; identification of areas having the most metabolically active tumor for possible radiation therapy "boost." Limitations are interobserver and intermethod variability in tumor volume definition without standardization across imaging centers; variability in SUVs based on body weight in patients with significant changes in weight over the course of therapy. SUV based on lean body mass may prove superior.

4. ^{18}F-fluoride-misonidazole (^{18}F-FMISO), [64]Copper-diacetyl-bis(N4-methylthiosemicarbazone) (^{64}Cu-ATSM).

References

Nestle U, Weber W, Hentschel M, Grosu AL: Biological imaging in radiation therapy: role of positron emission tomography, *Phys Med Biol* 54:R1–R25, 2009.

van Baardwijk A, Baumert BG, Bosmans G, et al: The current status of FDG-PET in tumour volume definition in radiotherapy treatment planning, *Cancer Treat Rev* 32:245–260, 2006.

Cross-Reference
Nuclear Medicine: THE REQUISITES, 3rd ed, p 304.

Comment
FDG-PET as part of radiation therapy planning should be imaged on a flat bed similar to that used by radiation oncology for the radiation therapy treatment-planning CT. Mountable fiducial markers or patient braces/casts should be used to ensure that the patient and area-of-interest are positioned correctly during PET imaging to allow for rigid fusion of PET with the treatment-planning CT performed separately in the radiation oncology suite.

Tumor hypoxia is inversely correlated with prognosis. Radiation therapy is less effective in hypoxic tumors owing to the lack of available oxygen for radiation-produced lethal free radicals. ^{18}F-FMISO and ^{64}Cu-ATSM are tumor hypoxia imaging agents that can delineate hypoxic tumor burden and guide fractionated radiotherapy or radiation-sensitizing chemotherapy. Other molecular imaging agents in addition to hypoxic agents under investigation and of potential clinical use include tracers of protein synthesis such as [11]Carbon-methionine (^{11}C-MET). ^{11}C-MET shows promise in demarcating areas of residual active tumor after radiotherapy, and persistent uptake on ^{11}C-MET likely portends a worse prognosis and shorter survival.

Notes

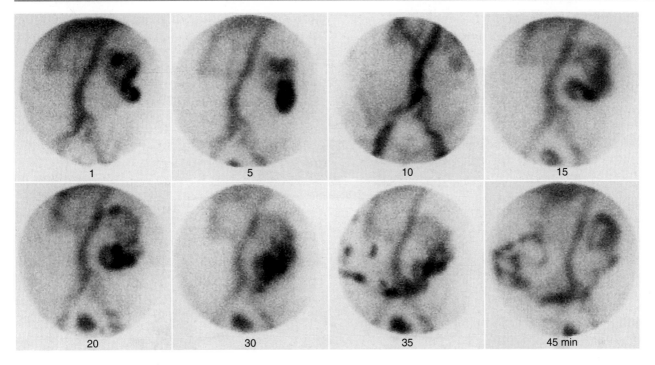

A 46-year-old man with recent onset of gastrointestinal bleeding.

1. What is the radiopharmaceutical? What is the preferred method for radiolabeling?

2. Describe the scintigraphic findings.

3. Provide a diagnosis.

4. List common causes for bleeding from this portion of the gastrointestinal tract.

Gastrointestinal System: ^{99m}Tc-Labeled RBCs—Small Intestine Bleeding

1. ^{99m}Tc-labeled RBCs. The in vitro method of labeling was used because of its high labeling efficiency (>97%).

2. Evidence of active bleeding, first seen at 5 minutes, starting in the left upper quadrant and moving in a serpiginous pattern across the mid- to lower abdomen to the right lower, then right mid-abdomen.

3. Bleeding originating from the proximal small bowel, probably the jejunum, in the left upper quadrant seen on the first image. There is retrograde reflux into the duodenum as well as antegrade flow, both seen on the second image.

4. Arteriovenous malformations and tumors.

References

Howarth DM: The role of nuclear medicine in the detection of acute gastrointestinal bleeding, *Semin Nucl Med* 38:133–146, 2006.

Mariani G, Pauwels EK, Al Sharif A, et al: Radionuclide evaluation of the lower gastrointestinal tract, *J Nucl Med* 49:776–787, 2008.

Cross-Reference

Nuclear Medicine: THE REQUISITES, 3rd ed, pp 364–374.

Comment

Major bleeding from the small intestine is uncommon and often difficult to localize because of the organ's length and circuitous overlapping path, its free intraperitoneal location, and the nature of the lesions that bleed in the small bowel. The most common etiology of small bowel bleeding is duodenal ulcer disease. Less common causes include arteriovenous malformation, tumors (e.g., leiomyosarcoma, leiomyoma, adenocarcinoma), Meckel's diverticulum, and Crohn's disease. In approximately 5% of patients with gastrointestinal bleeding, no cause for the bleeding is evident after an extensive evaluation. Almost 30% of these patients have lesions in the small bowel.

The pattern of movement of bleeding in this case is characteristic of the small bowel. It is important to distinguish this pattern from colonic bleeding. Frequent image acquisition until the site of origin is certain is mandatory. The most common error is premature study termination resulting in erroneous conclusions regarding a large versus small bowel origin. Although the images displayed in this case are at 5- to 10-minute intervals, the study was acquired on the computer at a framing rate of 1 minute per frame. Reviewing the cinematic display on the computer is helpful in confirming the site of the bleeding. The in vitro method of radiolabeling erythrocytes is optimal with labeling efficiency greater than 97%. The modified in vivo method, performed by drawing the patient's blood back into a syringe containing ^{99m}Tc-pertechnetate after intravenous injection of tin, is an alternative method with labeling efficiency of approximately 85% to 90%.

Notes

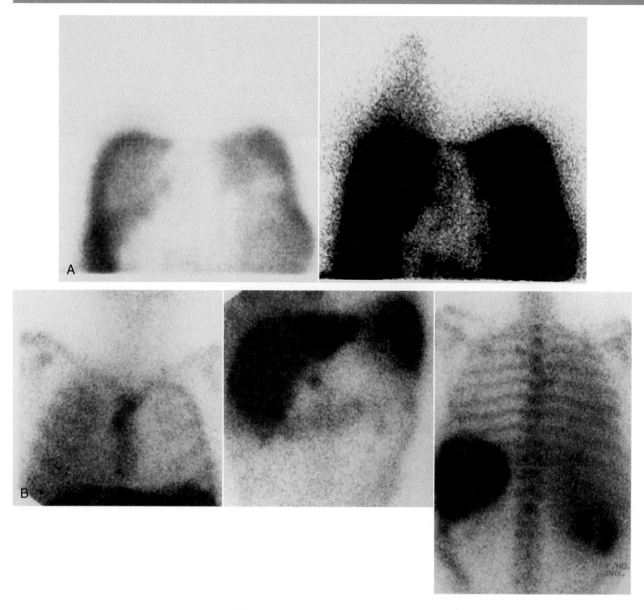

Patient A has cirrhosis and ascites with increasing shortness of breath and a right pleural effusion (immediate and 30 minutes). Patient B, with a peritoneovenous (Denver) shunt for intractable ascites, is experiencing increasing abdominal girth.

1. What clinical questions can scintigraphy address in these two patients?

2. Describe the procedure.

3. Which radiopharmaceuticals can be used? Which one was used in patient B?

4. Provide a conclusion for each study.

Gastrointestinal System: Peritoneal Scans and the Denver Shunt

1. A, Is there a connection between the pleural effusion and the ascites? B, Is the shunt patent?

2. Inject radiotracer into the peritoneum in an area where ascites is present. Ultrasound guidance is helpful. Immediate and delayed images are obtained to evaluate transit from the peritoneum to the pleural space, confirming transdiaphragmatic flow.

3. ^{99m}Tc-SC or ^{99m}Tc-MAA. The particles will stay below the diaphragm unless there is a connection. ^{99m}Tc-SC in patient B confirmed by liver, spleen, and marrow uptake.

4. A, Yes, there is a connection between the effusion and ascites. B, The shunt is patent.

References

Stewart CA, Sakimura IT: Evaluation of peritoneovenous shunt patency seen by intraperitoneal Tc-99m macro-aggregated albumin: clinical experience, *AJR Am J Roentgenol* 147:177–180, 1986.

Verreault J, Lepage S, Bisson G, et al: Ascites and right pleural effusion: demonstration of a peritoneo-pleural communication, *J Nucl Med* 27:1707–1709, 1986.

Comment

Pleural effusion in cirrhotic patients is not uncommon. When other causes have been excluded (e.g., cardiac, pulmonary, or pleural), the term *hepatic hydrothorax* is used for the transudative effusion. Transdiaphragmatic passage of fluid is the most important mechanism explaining a hepatic hydrothorax. Postmortem exams have shown that defects exist in the diaphragm at its tendinous portion of the diaphragm, probably tears resulting from stretching caused by abdominal distention from ascites.

LeVeen or Denver-type peritoneovenous shunts are used to decompress the peritoneal cavity in patients with significant ascites refractory to medical management. The shunt drains into a large vein in the neck or thorax. The caudal end is located within the peritoneal cavity and contains a one-way valve that opens when increasing ascites results in increased intraperitoneal pressure. Fibrinous deposits at the valve in the peritoneal space may cause shunt obstruction, manifesting as increasing ascites. Flow through the shunt requires sufficient pressure to open the valve; thus, the shunt is appropriate in patients who have limited ascites. A normally functioning shunt results in lung uptake within 10 minutes. ^{99m}Tc-MAA is advantageous in that the site of uptake (lungs) is removed from the site of injection (peritoneum), while ^{99m}Tc-SC demonstrates uptake (liver and spleen) near the site of injection.

^{99m}Tc-SC (0.1–1.0 μm) diffuses poorly through peritoneal surfaces; its appearance above the diaphragm confirms a pleural-peritoneal connection. ^{99m}Tc-MAA particles (10–90 μm) cannot be absorbed systemically because of their size. ^{99m}Tc-MAA is advantageous for peritoneal venous shunts because remote uptake in the lungs confirms venous access and patency.

Notes

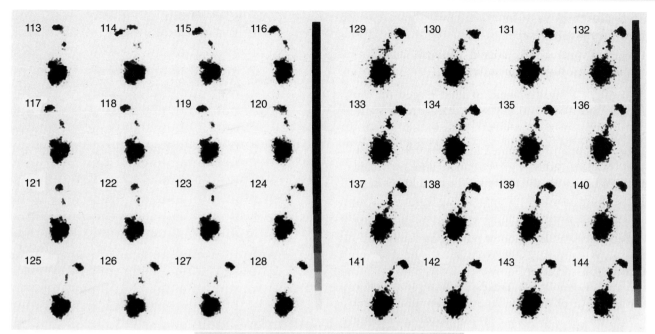

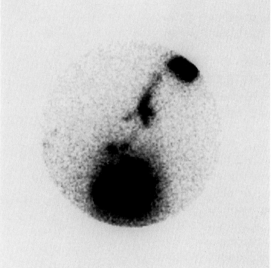

A 2-year-old child is referred for a salivagram (esophageal transit study) to diagnose suspected pulmonary aspiration. The result of a gastroesophageal reflux (milk) study was positive for reflux but negative for aspiration. Images are acquired in the anterior view.

1. What are the clinical symptoms of pulmonary aspiration in children?

2. What radiopharmaceutical is used for the salivagram, and what is the method of administration?

3. What are the scintigraphic findings in this case?

4. What is the advantage of the salivagram over the milk study?

Gastrointestinal System:
Pulmonary Aspiration

1. Recurrent pneumonia, cough, asthma, failure to thrive, apnea, sudden infant death.

2. ^{99m}Tc-SC in a small volume of fluid placed on the tongue and allowed to mix with oral secretions and swallowed.

3. Poor bolus progression noted in the dynamic esophageal swallow study with entrance into the main bronchi bilaterally and then into the right lower lobe.

4. The milk study is very sensitive for reflux; however, it is insensitive for aspiration. The salivagram is quite sensitive for the detection of pulmonary aspiration.

References

Bar-Sever Z, Connolly LP, Treves ST: The radionuclide salivagram in children with pulmonary disease and a high risk of aspiration, *Pediatr Radiol* 24(Suppl 1):S180–S183, 1995.

Heyman S, Respondek M: Detection of pulmonary aspiration in children by radionuclide "salivagram," *J Nucl Med* 30:667–679, 1989.

Cross-Reference

Nuclear Medicine: THE REQUISITES, 3rd ed, pp 354–356.

Comment

The aspiration of gastric contents can result in bronchospasm and severe bronchopneumonia that can be life-threatening. Aspiration often is seen in patients who have neurologic dysfunction or gastroesophageal reflux or after surgery to the upper airway or digestive tract.

Radionuclide milk studies are considerably more sensitive for diagnosing reflux than the barium swallow study. However, the sensitivity for diagnosis of aspiration is significantly lower, and the diagnosis is rarely made on the basis of a milk scan, even in patients with significant reflux. Many patients with aspiration have associated esophageal motor abnormalities and gastroesophageal reflux. The esophageal swallow portion of the salivagram study is acquired in a rapid dynamic mode (15- to 30-second frames) that allows visualization of esophageal swallowing physiology. To perform the test, 250 µCi ^{99m}Tc-SC in 10 mL of water is placed on the tongue or posterior pharynx. Once the transit study is completed, the remaining meal volume is fed and further imaging can be performed. Esophageal swallow studies also have been used to diagnose or follow the effectiveness of therapy in patients with achalasia, esophageal spasm, and scleroderma.

Notes

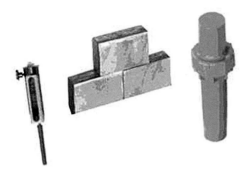

1. What common purpose do these objects provide? What are they called?

2. What factors determine how effective a shield is?

3. What are half-value layer (HVL) and tenth-value layer?

4. What is brehmsstrahlung radiation?

Radiation Safety: Shielding

1. Radiation shielding. Left to right: Lead-lined syringe holder with leaded glass for viewing, lead bricks, lead pigs to transport the radiotracer.

2. The effectiveness of a shield is determined by the density of the absorber medium, the thickness of the absorber, and the energy of the radiation source.

3. The HVL is the thickness of an absorber required to reduce the radiation source intensity by a factor of two. The tenth-value layer is the absorber thickness required to reduce radiation intensity by a factor of 10.

4. Brehmsstrahlung is German for "braking radiation" or "deceleration radiation." This is electromagnetic radiation produced by deceleration of a charged particle when deflected by another charged particle.

References

Cherry SR, Sorenson JA, Phelps ME: *Physics in Nuclear Medicine*, 3rd ed. Philadelphia: WB Saunders, 2003, pp 88-88, 431, 433, 435-436, 439-440.
Saha GB: *Physics and Radiobiology of Nuclear Medicine*, 2nd ed. New York: Springer, 2001, pp 54-63.

Cross-Reference

Nuclear Medicine: THE REQUISITES, 3rd ed, p 14.

Comment

Brehmsstrahlung is also sometimes termed *secondary radiation* since it is produced as a result of slowing the primary radiation such as beta particles. The loss of energy produces a spectrum of x-rays (approximately 40–100 keV) called brehmsstrahlung, most often of significance in heavy metals such as lead. Therefore, this form of radiation is best stored or shielded with low Z materials such as plastic and glass (low-density materials).

The HVL is smaller for high Z materials and larger for high-energy photons and is related to the linear attenuation coefficient (how well a particular absorber "absorbs" the radiation). Example for HVL: For a gamma-radiation source with an exposure rate of 100 mR/hour, the HVL of an absorber will reduce this exposure to 50 mR/hour. Example for tenth-value layer: When applied to positron emitters to shield against radiation from annihilation, the thickness should be 13.4 mm for the 511 keV photons.

The effectiveness of a shield is demonstrated by the following equation:

$$I = I_o\, e^{-\mu x}$$

I_o = number of photons per unit area or originating radiation intensity

I = radiation intensity after passing through absorber medium

μ = linear absorption coefficient

x = absorber thickness

Notes

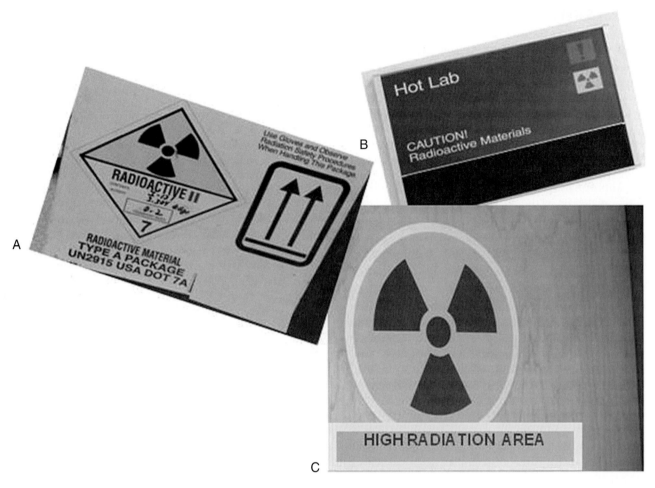

A

B

C

1. A, The package is specified as a type A. What does this mean? What federal agency governs the labeling of radioactive packages/materials for shipment?

2. B, "Hot Lab": This sign is mounted outside the Hot Lab in nuclear medicine departments. Which of the following would be an inappropriate function of the Hot Lab given the information on the sign? (a) Storage of food and drinks for use in the cardiac stress lab, (b) preparation and handling of patient doses before administration, (c) measurement of background radiation for comparison during routine contamination surveys.

3. C, What is a "high radiation area," as shown on this door?

4. In 2007, the International Atomic Energy Agency and the International Organization for Standardization developed a revised symbol intended as a supplement to the classic trefoil sign to increase awareness of potential radiation sources, designed to convey the warning "Danger—Keep away." What are the components of this symbol? Where is it intended to be used?

Radiation Safety: Signage

1. Type A packaging is used for most radiopharmaceuticals and is sufficient to prevent leakage during normal transport or minor accidents. Large amounts/activities require type B packaging, which is more accident resistant. The U.S. Department of Transportation governs the labeling and transport of radioactive materials.

2. (a) Inappropriate. Food and drink should not be kept where radioactive materials are being stored or used. (b) Appropriate. Sign denotes the presence of radioactive materials in the area. (c) Inappropriate. Background radiation measurements should be made in areas remote from radiation sources.

3. A high radiation area is a place where radiation levels could result in an individual receiving greater than 0.1 rem (1 mSv) in 1 hour at 30 cm from the radiation source or from any surface that the radiation penetrates.

4. The "Danger—Keep away" symbol consists of the classic trefoil from which rays emanate toward a skull and a person running away. This symbol is found on devices housing a radioactive source defined as dangerous by the International Organization for Standardization because of its potential to cause injury/death.

References

IAEA Safety Standards: Categorization of Radioactive Sources. Safety Guide No. RS-G-1.9. Nuclear Regulatory Commission. Title 10 Code of Federal Regulations 20.1003.

Saha GP: *Physics and Radiobiology of Nuclear Medicine*, 3rd ed. New York: Springer-Verlag, 2006.

Cross-Reference

Nuclear Medicine: THE REQUISITES, 3rd ed, p 14.

Comment

A *radiation area* is where radiation levels could result in an individual receiving a dose equivalent in excess of 0.005 rem (0.05 mSv) in 1 hour at 30 cm from the radiation source. *Very high radiation area* is where radiation levels could result in an individual receiving an absorbed dose in excess of 500 rad (5 Gy) in 1 hour at 1 m.

When public routes, including highways, waterways, and/or airways, are used to transport radioactive materials, the U.S. Department of Transportation rules and regulations apply. These rules are designed to protect members of the public who are not radiation workers from accidental exposure. Radioactive materials with specific activity less than or equal to 0.002 μCi/g are not governed by the Department of Transportation transport requirements, but are subject to NRC regulations for labeling and safety. A type A package is most often used in nuclear medicine. The type A package maximum depends on the specific isotope and its form (encapsulated vs. powder or liquid).

Notes

Ang: 0.00	Ang: 10.00	Ang: 20.00	Ang: 30.00	Ang: 40.00	Ang: 50.00	Ang: 60.00	Ang: 70.00

Ang: 80.00	Ang: 90.00	Ang: 100.00	Ang: 110.00	Ang: 120.00	Ang: 130.00	Ang: 140.00	Ang: 150.00

Ang: 160.00	Ang: 170.00	Ang: 180.00	Ang: 190.00	Ang: 200.00	Ang: 210.00	Ang: 220.00	Ang: 230.00

Ang: 240.00	Ang: 250.00	Ang: 260.00	Ang: 270.00	Ang: 280.00	Ang: 290.00	Ang: 300.00	Ang: 310.00

A 29-year-old man has a recent onset of fever and headache, but no previous medical problems.

1. Describe the ^{99m}Tc-HMPAO SPECT reconstructed volume display in this patient. Angle 0 is the anterior projection; angle 90, the left lateral view; and so forth.

2. What is the physiologic correlate of this scintigraphic pattern?

3. What is the differential diagnosis of this scintigraphic pattern in this patient?

4. What is the likely diagnosis considering the patient's history?

C A S E 1 8 8

Central Nervous System: ^{99m}Tc-HMPAO SPECT—Herpes Encephalitis

1. Increased uptake in the left temporal lobe.

2. Increased blood flow to the left temporal lobe.

3. Seizure focus (ictal injection), infection, tumor.

4. Herpes encephalitis.

References

Ackerman ES, Tumeh SS, Charon M, et al: Viral encephalitis: imaging with SPECT, *Clin Nucl Med* 13:640–643, 1988.

Meyer MA, Hubner KF, Raja S, et al: Sequential positron emission tomography evaluations of brain metabolism in acute herpes encephalitis, *Neuroimaging* 4:104–105, 1994.

Cross-Reference

Nuclear Medicine: THE REQUISITES, 3rd ed, pp 436–437.

Comment

Because of its poor prognosis and rapid progression, early diagnosis and treatment of herpes encephalitis is critical. The disease is life-threatening and may result in permanent memory and cognitive brain dysfunction for those who survive. The clinical diagnosis is based on nonspecific neurologic signs indicating temporal lobe dysfunction and focal electroencephalographic abnormalities. MRI is the initial diagnostic imaging method because of its high sensitivity and anatomic resolution of limbic structures. However, when inconclusive, brain perfusion SPECT or FDG-PET may be diagnostic. Increased tracer accumulation in the medial and lateral portions of the temporal lobe is characteristic of herpes encephalitis, although extratemporal sites sometimes may be seen.

Primary and secondary brain tumors generally have increased metabolism that can be seen on FDG-PET imaging. Although blood flow usually follows metabolism and is increased with most tumors, ^{99m}Tc-HMPAO SPECT cerebral perfusion studies rarely show increased uptake with tumors. The reason for this is uncertain; perhaps it is due to a lack of receptors. Seizure foci have increased uptake on FDG-PET and brain perfusion SPECT during the ictal phase but have decreased uptake during the interictal phase.

Notes

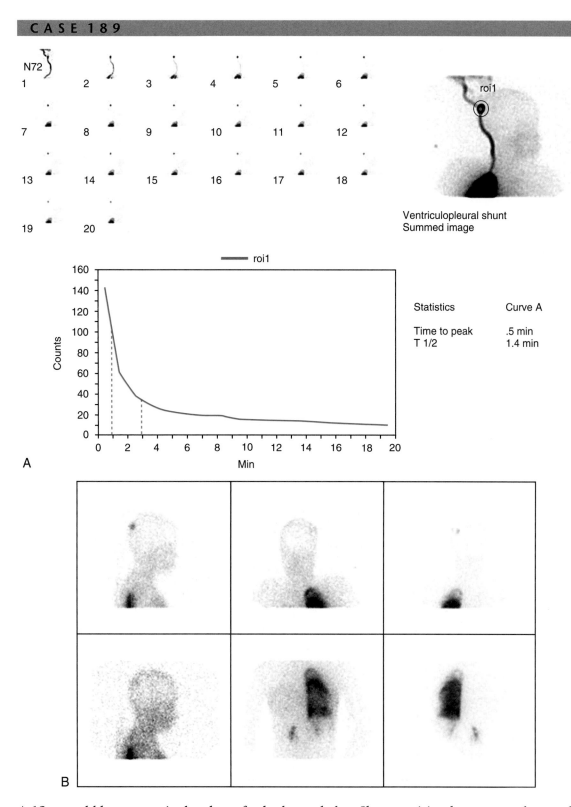

Ventriculopleural shunt
Summed image

— roi1

Statistics   Curve A

Time to peak   .5 min
T 1/2   1.4 min

A

B

A 12-year-old has a ventricular shunt for hydrocephalus. Shunt revision has occurred several times. A, Initial 20 minutes dynamic after injection of the radiopharmaceutical in the scalp shunt reservoir with images and time-activity curve. B, Static images after a dynamic study.

1. What is the likely radiopharmaceutical?

2. Describe the scintigraphic findings on images A (dynamic flow) and B (immediately post-flow).

3. What is your interpretation?

4. What other types of shunts are placed for this condition?

Central Nervous System: Ventriculopleural Shunt Study

1. The radiopharmaceutical could be either ^{99m}Tc-DTPA or ^{111}In-DTPA.

2. A, Rapid clearance of the shunt reservoir and tubing into the pleural cavity. B, Clearance of tubing and all radiotracer in the pleural space.

3. Patent ventriculopleural shunt.

4. Ventriculoperitoneal is the most common shunt used. Ventriculoatrial shunts and ventriculopleural shunts are sometimes placed after a ventriculoperitoneal shunt has become nonfunctional.

References

Uvebrant P, Sixt R, Bjure J, Roos A: Evaluation of cerebrospinal fluid shunt function in hydrocephalic children using 99mTc-DTPA, *Childs Nerv Syst* 8(2):76–80, 1992.

Vernet O, Farmer JP, Lambert R, Montes JL: Radionuclide shuntogram: adjunct to manage hydrocephalic patients, *J Nucl Med* 37(3):406–410, 1996.

Cross-Reference

Nuclear Medicine: THE REQUISITES, 3rd ed, pp 446–449.

Comment

Ventricular cerebrospinal fluid (CSF) shunts are surgically placed to treat symptoms associated with hydrocephalus or idiopathic intracranial hypertension. Approximately 98% of shunts inserted are ventriculoperitoneal because they have a low complication rate. Ventriculoatrial shunts account for less than 1% of CSF shunts, usually in patients who have had previous abdominal surgeries or peritoneal infection. Even less common are ventriculopleural shunts.

Shunt malfunction is suspected when a patient's symptoms recur or worsen after initial improvement after shunt placement. Malfunction may be due to obstruction of the proximal or distal catheter, infection, or mechanical failure.

The physician, nurse, or physician's assistant measures the intracerebral pressure, withdraws a small amount of CSF, and then injects the radiotracer within a small fluid volume into the shunt reservoir. Sometimes, attempts are made to reflux the tracer into the ventricles to evaluate proximal patency by temporarily occluding the distal catheter. The lack of reflux would suggest obstruction. Prompt clearance distally from the reservoir and tubing is consistent with a nonobstructed distal shunt. With a ventriculoperitoneal shunt, tracer can be seen to flow through the tubing and freely diffuse throughout the peritoneal cavity. With a ventriculoatrial shunt, activity normally clears from the tubing rapidly. Any holdup in the shunt suggests obstruction. Similarly with a ventriculopleural shunt, activity normally clears rapidly into the pleural cavity.

Notes

T
RESLCD

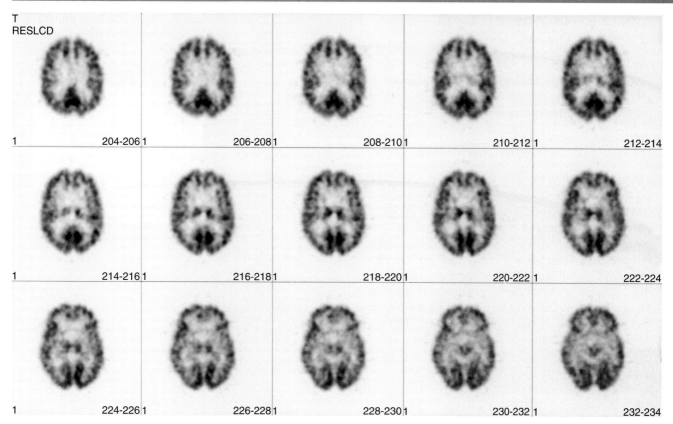

1	204-206	1	206-208	1	208-210	1	210-212	1	212-214
1	214-216	1	216-218	1	218-220	1	220-222	1	222-224
1	224-226	1	226-228	1	228-230	1	230-232	1	232-234

A 33-year-old man with a neurologic disorder was referred for this ^{18}F-FDG-PET scan.

1. What is the FDG-PET scan abnormality?

2. What symptoms are likely?

3. What is the pathologic condition?

4. What is the diagnosis?

Central Nervous System: FDG-PET—Huntington's Disease

1. Hypometabolism of the basal ganglion.

2. Progressive motor abnormalities of involuntary choreiform movements and akinetic rigidity with progressive cognitive deterioration.

3. Neuronal degeneration in the striatum, with the caudate more involved than the putamen.

4. Huntington's disease.

References

Boecker H, Kuwert T, Langen KJ, et al: SPECT with HMPAO compared to PET with FDG in Huntington's disease, *J Comput Assist Tomogr* 18:524-528, 1994.

Marshall VL, Reininger CB, Marquardt M, et al: Parkinson's disease is overdiagnosed clinically at baseline in diagnostically uncertain cases: a 3-year European multicenter study with repeat [123I]FP-CIT SPECT, *Mov Disord* 24:500-508, 2009.

Cross-Reference

Nuclear Medicine: THE REQUISITES, 3rd ed, pp 440-441.

Comment

Huntington's disease is an autosomal dominant disorder of unknown origin that manifests in middle age. It is a progressive disease with symptoms and signs of involuntary choreiform movements and akinetic rigidity, behavioral changes, and dementia. CT and MRI often show no changes early in the disease, although in later stages, atrophy of the head of the caudate and frontal cortex may be seen. FDG-PET studies show hypometabolism in the caudate and putamen nuclei, which, as gray matter, should have uptake similar to that of the cortex. These changes precede atrophy seen on CT. Hypometabolism in the caudate nucleus is seen in one third of patients genetically at risk of the disease.

Parkinson's disease is another movement disorder, one that is caused by loss of the pigmented neurons in the substantia nigra and is characterized by bradykinesia, tremor, and rigidity. Dementia occurs in later stages in 20% to 30% of patients. No consistent characteristic SPECT or PET imaging pattern has been reported. However, patients with severe Parkinson's dementia late in the disease course may have scintigraphic findings indistinguishable from those of late Alzheimer's disease (i.e., bilateral hypoperfusion and hypometabolism of the posterior parietotemporal and frontal regions).

DaTSCAN (ioflupane I-123 injection) is expected to be approved by the U.S. Food and Drug Administration (FDA) in the near future for the diagnosis of Parkinson's disease. Ioflupane has a high binding affinity for presynaptic dopamine transporters. Patients with the disease have very reduced uptake in the basal ganglion.

Notes

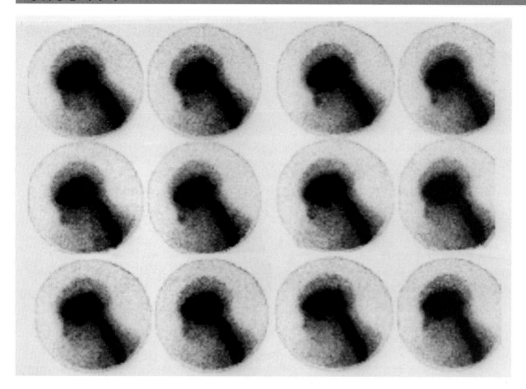

A 53-year-old woman has a history of head trauma and recent increasing headache and rhinorrhea. Left lateral views obtained over 1 hour are shown.

1. Name the appropriate radiopharmaceutical(s).

2. How is the radiopharmaceutical administered?

3. What is the imaging finding and interpretation?

4. How can the site of the abnormality be further defined?

Central Nervous System: CSF Leak

1. ^{111}In-DTPA.

2. Intrathecal injection.

3. Activity in the region of the nose, indicating CSF leak, probably at the cribriform plate.

4. Anterior views. With the use of nasal pledgets placed in the superior, middle, and inferior nasal turbinates.

References

Harbert JC: Radionuclide cisternography. In: Harbert JC, Eckelman WC, Neumann RD (eds): *Nuclear Medicine, Diagnosis and Therapy.* New York: Thieme, 1996, pp 396–398.

Lawrence SK, Sandler MP, Partain CL, et al: Cerebrospinal fluid imaging. In: Sandler MP, Coleman RE, Wackers FJTh (eds): *Diagnostic Nuclear Medicine*, 3rd ed. Baltimore: Williams & Wilkins, 1996, pp 1163–1176.

Cross-Reference

Nuclear Medicine: THE REQUISITES, 3rd ed, pp 446–449.

Comment

CSF rhinorrhea and otorrhea can be difficult diagnostic challenges. Most leaks produce a small volume of fluid and leak intermittently. Some patients have repeated bouts of meningitis, and patient recognition of fluid drainage may be minimal or absent. Often, imaging is required to confirm the CSF origin of rhinorrhea. Multiple modalities (e.g., CT with metrizamide and MRI) are also used for this purpose. The radionuclide method is an old, established technique and still useful in many cases.

Trauma and surgery are the most common causes of CSF rhinorrhea. Hydrocephalus and congenital defects are less common nontraumatic causes. CSF leak may occur at any site from the frontal sinuses to the temporal bone. The cribriform plate is the most susceptible to fracture. CSF otorrhea is a far less common result of CSF leak. Perforation of the dura with communication through the petrous bone is the usual cause of otorrhea, although diversion through the eustachian tube also has been observed.

The study is performed with pledgets of cotton placed in the superior, middle, and inferior nasal turbinates bilaterally. The purpose is to differentiate frontal, ethmoidal, and sphenoidal sinus leakage. The pledgets are counted in a well counter rather than imaged and thus are more sensitive than imaging for the detection of leakage. Although lateral and anterior imaging is done for rhinorrhea, posterior imaging is performed for otorrhea.

Notes

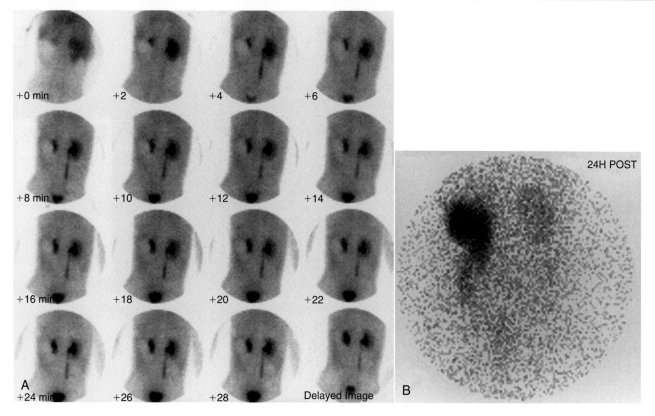

+0 min +2 +4 +6

+8 min +10 +12 +14

+16 min +18 +20 +22

A
+24 min +26 +28 Delayed Image

B 24H POST

A 55-year-old woman with a history of renal stones has a recent onset of flank pain. Renal scintigraphy with 30-minute dynamic renography (A) and 24-hour delayed image (B).

1. What are the scintigraphic findings?

2. Explain the changing imaging findings.

3. What is the diagnosis?

4. What is the likely cause?

Genitourinary System: Urinary Leak and Urinoma

1. A photopenic region, best seen on early images, involves most of the left renal fossa. Only the very upper pole is functioning. Urinary clearance into left renal pelvis is displaced medially by the photopenic defect. The right renal pelvis and upper two thirds of the ureter fill. There is poor clearance bilaterally. Delayed images show increased uptake in the region of the initial cold defect and inferior to it.

2. The cold defect is a urinoma with an attenuating mass effect. Over time, the radioactive urine enters this space and mixes with the nonradioactive urinoma. Activity in the region of the urinoma increases over time, whereas the kidney and background activity seen earlier have cleared.

3. Active urinary leak and urinoma.

4. Urinary tract obstruction.

Reference

Titton RL, Gervais DA, Hahn PF, et al: Urine leaks and urinomas: diagnosis and imaging-guided intervention, *Radiographics* 23:1133–1147, 2003.

Cross-Reference

Nuclear Medicine: THE REQUISITES, 3rd ed, pp 245, 253.

Comment

Rupture of the weakest portion of the collecting system, the calyceal fornix, occurs when renal pelvic pressure exceeds a critical level. Less commonly, the tear may affect the pelvis or ureter. Elevated pressure may occur during a bout of acute ureteral obstruction, retrograde pyelography, intravenous urography with abdominal compression, and massive VUR. Spontaneous extravasation (not caused by trauma, instrumentation, or surgery) is usually caused by a ureteral calculus and almost always is benign and self-limited. Continued leakage of urine in the presence of obstruction may lead to the formation of an encapsulated retroperitoneal urine collection, a urinoma. In adults, spontaneous urinomas are confined to the perinephric space.

Urinomas generally do not result from small perforations unless the leak is accompanied by obstruction distal to the exit point. Until they become very large, urinomas often are clinically silent. Eventually, a palpable tender mass may develop in conjunction with malaise, weight loss, nausea, and vague abdominal pain or back discomfort. The urinoma may worsen the obstruction because of its mass effect. Treatment consists of repair of the obstruction and excision and drainage of the urinoma.

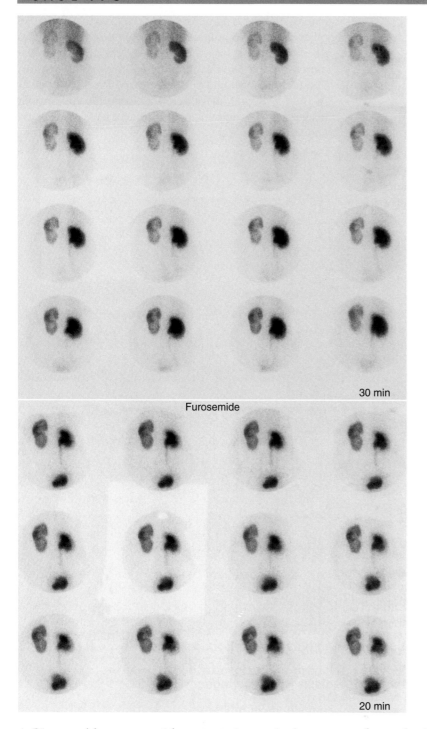

Furosemide

30 min

20 min

A 51-year-old woman with metastatic cervical cancer and new hydronephrosis noted on CT.

1. Describe the scintigraphic renal findings.

2. What imaging finding should you see before administering furosemide?

3. What is the diagnosis before and after the administration of diuretic (furosemide)?

4. How is differential renal function calculated?

Genitourinary System: Diuretic Renography—Bilateral Obstruction

1. Left kidney: delayed and decreased cortical uptake, no clearance into the calyces or pelvis. Right kidney: prompt uptake and clearance into the collecting system, faint persistent visualization of the right ureter, and poor response to furosemide.

2. Filling of the renal collecting system.

3. Before furosemide: high-grade obstruction on the left and hydronephrosis on the right, suspicious for obstruction. After furosemide: high-grade obstruction on the left and obstruction on the right.

4. Percentage of renal uptake by each kidney divided by total renal uptake between 1 and 3 minutes (cortical uptake before clearance into the calyces and pelvis).

References

Piepsz A, Ham HR: Pediatric applications of renal nuclear medicine, *Semin Nucl Med* 36:16–35, 2006.

Taylor AL: Radionuclide renography: a personal approach, *Semin Nucl Med* 29:102–127, 1999.

Cross-Reference

Nuclear Medicine: THE REQUISITES, 3rd ed, pp 234–244.

Comment

The administration of a diuretic is not indicated in high-grade obstruction because there is no collecting system radiotracer to challenge. Diuretic renography is useful in patients with lower grade obstructions (i.e., urinary excretion into the collecting system but retention in the renal pelvis). If the collecting system drains with diuretic, it is not obstructed (e.g., in patients with congenital hydronephrosis or hydronephrosis caused by ureteropelvic reflux). Other groups of patients in whom this technique is valuable are those who have had surgical correction of an obstruction but have persistent dilation and those with known partial obstruction (e.g., those with pelvic tumor compressing the ureters and new hydronephrosis noted on CT). The question is not whether an obstruction exists. Rather the question is whether urgent intervention is needed (e.g., stenting) to save the kidney and its renal function. Drainage after administration of a diuretic in these patients suggests that renal function will not deteriorate in the short term.

The rate of radiotracer washout may be quantified after furosemide. A common method is to calculate a half-time of emptying. As in all nuclear medicine, quantification must be interpreted in conjunction with image analysis. Normal values for the rate of emptying depend to some extent on the methodology used. In some clinics, diuretic is administered at the time that the radiopharmaceutical is administered and in others, as soon as the renal pelvis has filled. Still others administer the diuretic at the end of the initial 25- to 30-minute study. The technique should be standardized for the particular method. Postvoid images should be routine and upright images can be helpful in individual cases, particularly children.

Notes

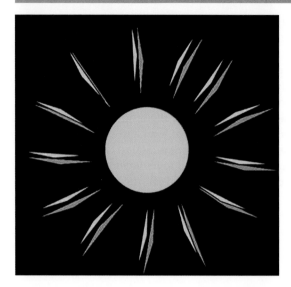

1. What are the main sources of radiation exposure?

2. What factors determine the extent of damage from radiation exposure?

3. Name some of the harmful effects of ionizing radiation overexposure.

4. What is the difference between a stochastic effect and a nonstochastic effect? Provide an example of each. Do these have thresholds?

Radiation Safety: Radiation Overexposure

1. Natural radiation (e.g., radon gas, cosmic rays, body [internal], external environment [rocks, soil, etc.]), and man-made (e.g., x-rays, gamma rays, consumer products).

2. Type of radiation delivered, amount and duration of radiation delivered, dose rate, exposed organs, and energy transfer to the exposed tissue.

3. *Somatic* effects include erythema, radiodermatitis, cataracts, and increased risk of cancer. *Teratogenic* effects occur in utero and are seen in the offspring of the individual who received the radiation (e.g., congenital malformations, mental retardation). *Genetic* effects occur before conception and in the offspring of the individual who received the radiation (e.g., asthma, diabetes mellitus, epilepsy, anemia).

4. *Stochastic* effect: there is no threshold, occurs randomly with the probability of experiencing an effect increasing with radiation dose. Usually occurs years after radiation exposure; the severity is independent of the dose given (e.g., cancer). *Nonstochastic* effect or deterministic effect: there is a threshold. The severity of an effect from radiation varies with the dose given (e.g., cataracts).

References

Graham DT, Cloke PJ: *Principles of Radiological Physics*, 4th ed. Philadelphia: Elsevier, 2003, p 343.

Stabin MG: *Radiation Protection and Dosimetry*. New York: Springer, 2007, p 92.

Wootton R: *Radiation Protection of Patients*. Cambridge, UK: Cambridge University Press, 1993, pp 24–25.

Cross-Reference

Nuclear Medicine: THE REQUISITES, 3rd ed, pp 15–18.

Comment

Acute radiation syndrome is an illness resulting from a radiation dose greater than 50 rad of penetrating radiation to the body in a short period of time. This most commonly affects the skin, central nervous system, hematopoietic tissues, and gastrointestinal tract. The first symptoms include nausea, vomiting, and diarrhea (prodromal phase) lasting from a few minutes up to several hours. The latent phase occurs after the prodromal phase, and the individual generally feels healthy over a period of a few hours to a few weeks. Next is the overt phase characterized by variable symptoms lasting from a few hours to several months. The final late stage is either recovery (several weeks to 2 years) or death.

The typical causes of death after radiation overexposure are hematopoietic failure, vascular injury, mucosal damage of the gastrointestinal tract, damage to the central nervous system, and infection. Central nervous system involvement is the most severe and can result in death within 3 days of radiation exposure.

Radiation doses greater than 600 to 800 cGy can cause permanent sterility in men and can affect women in the same manner at doses of 500 to 800 cGy. Manifestations of irradiation to the fetus include mental retardation or embryonic death and abortion.

Notes

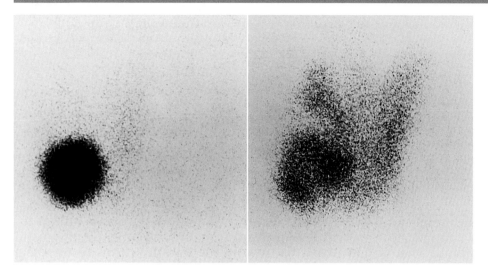

A 44-year-old woman had two ^{123}I thyroid scans performed 1 year apart. She is clinically thyrotoxic.

1. What is the likely diagnosis in the first scan (*left*)?

2. What has happened in the intervening time?

3. What is the patient's thyroid function and diagnosis at the time of the second scan (*right*)?

4. The patient has a low but not suppressed TSH level and normal thyroxine level. What is the diagnosis?

Endocrine System: Therapy of Toxic Thyroid Nodule

1. Toxic autonomous thyroid adenoma in the right lobe.

2. The patient has been treated with [131]I. The autonomous nodule is still hyperfunctional with cold areas, likely representing hemorrhage, necrosis, or both. It is no longer suppressing the remaining thyroid.

3. The patient is euthyroid.

4. Persistent functioning autonomous adenoma (nodule); incompletely treated.

References

Becker DV, Hurley JR: Radioiodine treatment of hyperthyroidism. In: Sandler MP (ed): *Diagnostic Nuclear Medicine*, 3rd ed. Baltimore: Williams & Wilkins, 1996, pp 943–958.

Sarkar SD: Benign thyroid disease: what is the role of nuclear medicine? *Semin Nucl Med* 36:185–193, 2006.

Cross-Reference

Nuclear Medicine: THE REQUISITES, 3rd ed, pp 88–94.

Comment

This patient became clinically euthyroid with ^{131}I therapy after the first scan. She returned for a repeat thyroid scan because of persistent right lower lobe thyroid nodule on examination and a suppressed serum TSH level. The second study shows that the palpable nodule is still hyperfunctioning compared with the rest of the thyroid but considerably less than before therapy. The effectiveness of radioactive iodine therapy for single autonomous nodules is high; however, occasionally a second treatment is needed. Effective therapy would have resulted in a totally cold (nonfunctioning) nodule.

Short- and long-term adverse effects of radioactive iodine are few. Radioactive iodine therapy has been given for hyperthyroidism for more than 50 years. It is safe and effective. The usual ^{131}I dose for autonomous nodule(s) is 20 to 30 mCi. This dose is typically greater than that given for patients with Graves' disease because thyroid nodules are more resistant to therapy. Many studies have sought to find adverse effects (e.g., second tumors, leukemia, infertility, abnormal offspring); however, no significant increase in these problems has been found in treated patients. Transient worsening of hyperthyroid symptoms and local pain may be noted in a minority of patients in the days after therapy. These are easily controlled with β-blocker and anti-inflammatory drugs. [131]I therapy is contraindicated if the patient is pregnant because iodine crosses the placenta. The fetal thyroid traps and organifies iodine after 10 weeks; therefore, congenital hypothyroidism will result if ^{131}I is administered to the mother.

Notes

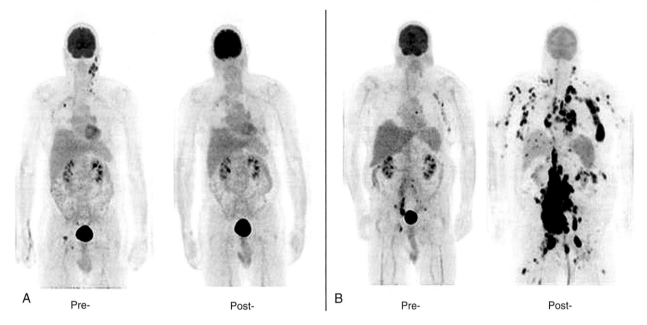

A Pre- Post- B Pre- Post-

Pre- and postradioimmunotherapy FDG-PET studies in two patients (A and B) with recurrent follicular lymphoma.

1. Which radiopharmaceuticals are available for radioimmunotherapy in non-Hodgkin's lymphoma? What is the antigen target?

2. Classify the therapy response in patient A versus patient B. What are reasons for the difference in response?

3. What is the dose-limiting organ/system for radioimmunotherapy? How should side effects be monitored?

4. Is radioimmunotherapy effective for patients in whom rituximab is ineffective? Explain.

Oncology: FDG-PET—Response to Radioimmunotherapy

1. ^{131}I-tositumomab (Bexxar) and yttrium-90 ibritumomab tiuxetan (Zevalin). Both target the CD20 antigen present on the cell surface of B lymphocytes.

2. Patient A had good partial response, with disease persisting only in a single right subpectoral lymph node. Patient B had disease progression.

3. Hematologic toxicity. Mild to moderate thrombocytopenia and neutropenia will develop in the majority of patients and must be monitored through count nadir, typically occurring at 4 to 7 weeks until recovery is confirmed, often 30 days.

4. Yes, patients in whom rituximab has not been effective can still receive anti-CD20 radioimmunotherapy, often with good outcomes. The therapeutic radionuclide produces a "cross-fire" effect in which cells at the center of the tumor not directly bound by antibody may be killed by the emitted beta particles.

References

Cheson BD, Leonard JP: Monoclonal antibody therapy for B-cell non-Hodgkin's lymphoma, *N Engl J Med* 359:613–626, 2008.

Jacene HA, Filice R, Kasecamp W, Wahl RL: ^{18}F-FDG PET/CT for monitoring the response of lymphoma to radioimmunotherapy, *J Nucl Med* 50:8–17, 2009.

Cross-Reference

Nuclear Medicine: THE REQUISITES, 3rd ed, pp 293–296.

Comment

Platelet counts less than 100,000 or bone marrow involvement of ≥25% precludes treatment with CD20-directed radioimmunotherapy. Pretherapy imaging is necessary. With ibritumomab tiuxetan (Zevalin), imaging is performed to detect altered biodistribution and is done with an ^{111}In conjugate of ibritumomab tiuxetan rather than [90]Y (a pure beta emitter). Once normal biodistribution is confirmed, the patient receives a weight-based dose of ^{90}Y-ibritumomab tiuxetan, also adjusted for mild thrombocytopenia. With ^{131}I-tositumomab (Bexxar), imaging is performed with low-dose ^{131}I-tositumomab to calculate a total-body residence time and, thereby, determine a therapeutic dose.

[90]Y-ibritumomab tiuxetan (Zevalin) and ^{131}I-tositumomab (Bexxar) are both murine IgG monoclonal antibodies. They both were initially approved by the FDA for use in patients with relapsed/refractory low-grade or follicular non-Hodgkin's lymphoma. Data suggest that anti-CD20 may be useful as a first-line single agent. ^{90}Y-ibritumomab tiuxetan has recently been approved by the FDA for first-line therapy of non-Hodgkin's lymphoma as part of a multiagent consolidation chemotherapy regimen.

Available evidence suggests that Bexxar and Zevalin may perform similarly. The efficacy of ^{131}I-tositumomab (Bexxar) and ^{90}Y-ibritumomab tiuxetan (Zevalin) in patients with high-grade lymphomas such as mantle cell lymphoma has been shown to be less effective than that seen in patients with low-grade lymphomas (31% overall response rate compared with 63–70%). FDG-PET has been shown to be an effective method for monitoring response to radioimmunotherapy. Patients having more than a 50% decrease in SUVs at 3 months tend to have a longer disease-free survival.

Notes

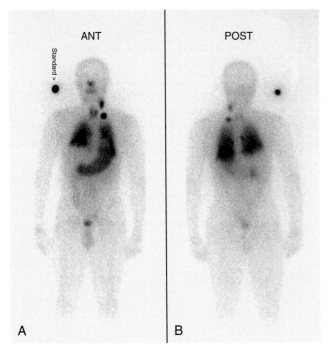

A 53-year-old woman with papillary, follicular varian, thyroid cancer after near-total thyroidectomy.

1. What is the study? What is the radiopharmaceutical?

2. Describe the pattern of uptake and give your interpretation.

3. What dose of ^{131}I is used for thyroid uptake for a scan in a patient with suspected substernal goiter (A) and for a thyroid cancer patient after thyroidectomy (B)?

4. Explain why ^{131}I therapy but not ^{123}I is effective for Graves' hyperthyroidism, toxic nodules, and thyroid cancer.

Endocrine System: Thyroid Cancer
Whole-Body Scan

1. ^{123}I whole-body thyroid cancer scan. ^{131}I is most commonly used, but the excellent image quality and similar biodistribution indicate that this is ^{123}I.

2. Abnormal diffuse uptake in the lungs, uptake in the midline neck, left supraclavicular, and lower cervical regions, all consistent with metastatic tumor.

3. Thyroid uptake, 10 µCi; thyroid scan, 50 µCi; thyroid cancer scan, 2 to 4 mCi. Be careful to distinguish between millicuries (mCi) and microcuries (µCi).

4. The beta particle emissions of ^{131}I are taken up by thyroid follicular cells and are responsible for its therapeutic effect.

References

Freitas JE: Therapy of differentiated thyroid cancer. In: Freeman LM (ed): *Nuclear Medicine Annual 1998*. Philadelphia: Lippincott–Raven, 1998.

Hurley JR, Becker DV: Treatment of thyroid cancer with radioiodine (131-I). In: Sandler MP, Coleman RE, Wackers FJTh, et al (eds): *Diagnostic Nuclear Medicine*, 3rd ed. Baltimore: Williams & Wilkins, 1996, pp 959–989.

Cross-Reference
Nuclear Medicine: THE REQUISITES, 3rd ed, pp 94–98.

Comment

^{131}I has been used for whole-body thyroid cancer scintigraphy for decades; however, there are a high total-body radiation dose (0.5 rad/mCi) and the potential for thyroid stunning (i.e., decreased uptake of the subsequent therapeutic dose). Thus, ^{123}I is now being used as an alternative to ^{131}I and provides similar diagnostic information. Disadvantages of ^{123}I are its short physical half-life (13 hours), which limits delayed imaging to 24 hours (^{131}I imaging is usually at 48 hours), and its greater expense. The administered dose for thyroid cancer scans is approximately 1.5 mCi, compared with 200 µCi for routine thyroid scans.

The only accepted clinical indication for a ^{131}I thyroid scan other than thyroid cancer is substernal goiter. The higher gamma energy photopeak (364 keV) allows better detectability compared with possible attenuation of ^{123}I (159 keV) by the sternum. The radiation dose to the normal thyroid from ^{131}I is high, 1 rad/µCi, resulting in approximately 50 rad from a typical thyroid scan dose. Most patients referred for this indication are elderly patients with goiter. Many clinics use ^{123}I first and reserve ^{131}I as a second-line evaluation for a substernal gland.

Notes

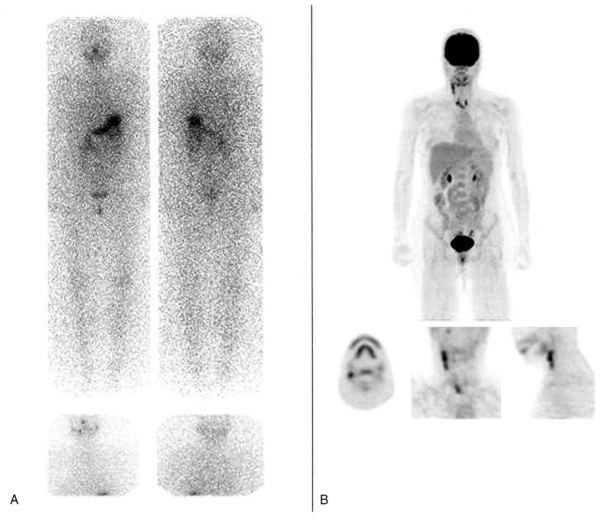

A   B

A 32-year-old woman with papillary thyroid carcinoma, thyroidectomy, and radioiodine remnant ablation 2 years ago. Now with an increasing serum thyroglobulin. A, Whole-body ^{123}I study; B, FDG-PET 2 weeks after image A was performed.

1. Describe the uptake/distribution pattern in study A. Is this normal or abnormal?

2. Describe the findings and interpret study B.

3. What are clinical indications for FDG-PET in patients with thyroid cancer?

4. What can you infer about the molecular properties of the patient's thyroid cancer given the findings in study B?

Oncology: FDG-PET—Thyroid Cancer

1. Normal whole-body radioiodine scan. Uptake and clearance in the oropharynx, salivary glands, stomach, bowel, bladder, and genital region.

2. FDG uptake in the thyroid bed. Evidence of metastases with focal uptake in the right cervical region suggests lymph node metastases.

3. Detection and localization of recurrent disease in serum thyroglobulin–positive/whole-body radioiodine scan–negative patients. FDG-PET is also useful for patients with poorly differentiated thyroid cancer and medullary thyroid cancer.

4. The lack of radioiodine uptake by the tumor with FDG uptake on PET suggests that the tumor has diminished ability to trap and organify iodine, consistent with dedifferentiation and transformation to a higher grade.

References

Finkelstein FE, Grigsby PW, Siegel BA, et al: Combined [^{18}F] fluorodeoxyglucose positron emission tomography and computed tomography (FDG-PET/CT) for detection of recurrent, ^{131}I-negative thyroid cancer, *Ann Surg Oncol* 15:286–292, 2008.

Lind P, Kohlfürst S: Respective roles of thyroglobulin, radioiodine imaging, and positron emission tomography in the assessment of thyroid cancer, *Semin Nucl Med* 34:194–205, 2006.

Cross-Reference

Nuclear Medicine: THE REQUISITES, 3rd ed, pp 95–97.

Comment

After ingestion, radioactive iodine is absorbed primarily in the small intestine, where it enters the bloodstream, is taken up by the follicular cells of the thyroid gland, and is ultimately concentrated. It is similarly taken up by well-differentiated thyroid cancer.

As many as 30% of differentiated thyroid cancers lose their ability to trap and organify iodine while retaining their ability to secrete thyroglobulin. Patients with elevated serum thyroglobulin and negative whole-body radioiodine scan results have a poorer overall survival than those with iodine-avid tumor and present a clinical challenge for therapy. In the past, these patients were often treated with high-dose radioiodine therapy and serum thyroglobulin was followed to determine response to therapy.

FDG-PET/CT is reported to be 93% accurate in the detection of the tumor in this subset of patients with negative iodine scan results. The FDG-PET findings result in management change in a significant number of patients compared with conventional imaging and lab values alone. Localization of the tumor allows for potential surgical resection and then radioiodine therapy. It also serves as a baseline study for follow-up evaluation.

Notes

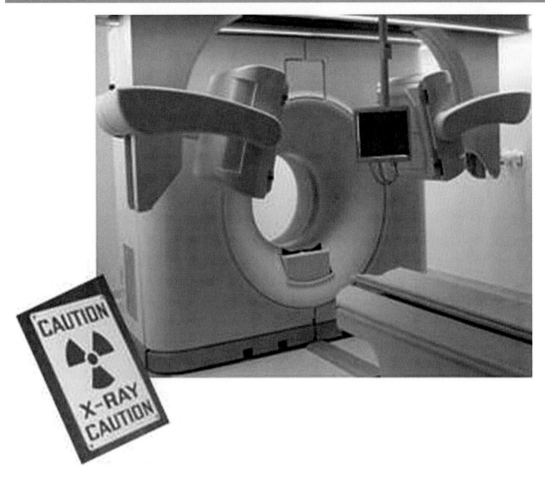

A 35-year-old woman with recurrent carcinoid syndrome referred for an ^{111}In-pentetreotide (OctreoScan) study. Whole-body planar scintigraphy revealed focal uptake in the chest. You request a chest SPECT-CT.

1. What are potential benefits and challenges of hybrid SPECT/CT imaging?

2. For a given set of CT parameters used during a SPECT/CT exam (e.g., 120 kVp, 400 mAs), would the effective dose (effective dose equivalent) to a child be higher or lower than that to an adult and why?

3. What are the strategies for reducing/limiting radiation dose from the CT portion of the SPECT/CT study?

4. What quality control issues must be addressed in SPECT/CT cameras compared with a gamma camera only?

Radiation Safety: Transmission CT

1. SPECT/CT imaging improves reader confidence and specificity over SPECT alone and postacquisition software SPECT and CT fusion. The fused image allows correlation of radiotracer uptake with its anatomic source and makes CT-based attenuation correction possible. Problems include physiologic motion (cardiac, respiratory, bowel peristalsis, filling of the bladder, movement of contrast), which may cause misregistration of the data sets.

2. Higher, due to their smaller size (mass) undergoing an exam using the same parameters.

3. Determine whether CT is a necessary portion of the study, reduce the x-ray beam energy (reduce kVp), decrease the photon fluence (flux), increase total beam width on multidetector CT, limit CT coverage to the field required to answer the clinical question, adjust settings based on body region (e.g., chest vs. pelvis), consider breast shielding, minimize use of multiple scans per examination (e.g., is CT necessary at both 4 and 24 hours?), use available technology that automatically reduces dose during scanning, adjust settings based on body weight, adjust table pitch while preserving image quality (pitch is inversely proportional to dose).

4. SPECT quality control. CT quality control: CT air/water calibrations in Hounsfield units, gantry alignment to determine offset to be incorporated into the fused image display to ensure image alignment.

References
Chowdhury FU, Scarsbrook AF: The role of hybrid SPECT-CT in oncology: current and emerging clinical applications, *Clin Radiol* 63:241–251, 2008.
McNitt-Gray MF: AAPM/RSNA Physics Tutorial for Residents: topics in CT. Radiation dose in CT, *Radiographics* 22:1541–1553, 2002.

Cross-Reference
Nuclear Medicine: THE REQUISITES, 3rd ed, pp 16–17.

Comment
In the performance of nuclear medicine and CT procedures in children, it is important to be aware that (1) pediatric tissues are more radiosensitive, (2) any given level of radiation results in a larger effective dose to pediatric patients, and (3) children have a longer period of time over which to develop cancers from radiation exposure. These issues may warrant discussion with the referring physician and the parents.

Radiation dose minimization should be used in all patients when possible, not only in female, reproductive-age, or pediatric patients. It is up to the physician to determine the point at which efforts to reduce radiation dose must be weighed against the acquisition of high-quality, interpretable images.

Notes

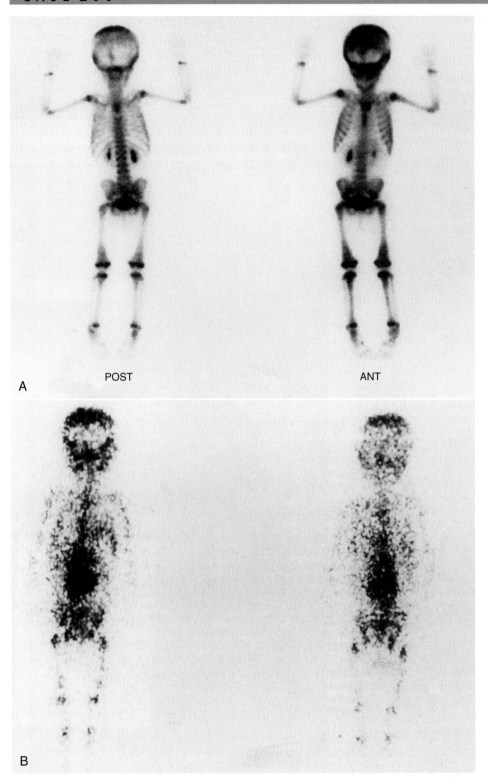

A

POST ANT

B

A 3-year-old boy with a retroperitoneal mass seen on CT.

1. Describe the imaging findings of the ^{99m}Tc-MDP bone scan (A) and the ^{131}I-MIBG study (B).

2. What is your interpretation of the two studies?

3. What are the most common tumor causes of extraosseous uptake of bone radiotracers in this age group?

4. What is the most sensitive imaging method for detection of bone metastases in this disease?

Oncology: Bone and MIBG Scans—Neuroblastoma

1. Bone scan shows symmetrical uptake in distal femurs and cranial and facial bones. MIBG shows a large midline area of abdominal uptake. Corresponding region on the bone scan shows a soft-tissue left peri-renal density, best seen in the anterior view. Diffuse MIBG marrow/bone uptake is seen.

2. The prominent midline uptake of MIBG is consistent with neuroblastoma. Subtle bone uptake is seen there. Symmetrical bone uptake in the distal femurs and cranial and facial bones is suggestive of tumor. The study confirms metastatic disease with extensive tumor in marrow/bone from skull to feet.

3. First, primary neuroblastoma. Osteosarcoma metastatic to the lung is another. Metastases of various tumors to the lung, colon, and breast is occasionally seen on bone scan.

4. Combination of ^{99m}Tc bone scan and ^{131}I-MIBG or ^{123}I MIBG.

References

Gelfand MJ: Metaiodobenzylguanidine in children, *Semin Nucl Med* 23:231–242, 1993.

Shulkin BL, Shapiro B: Current concepts on the diagnostic use of MIBG in children, *J Nucl Med* 39:667–688, 1998.

Cross-Reference

Nuclear Medicine: THE REQUISITES, 3rd ed, pp 109–112.

Comment

Neuroblastoma commonly manifests at an advanced stage, and bone scans are used routinely for the detection of metastatic lesions. Because the metastatic lesions of neuroblastoma originate in the bone marrow cavity, bone scans may underestimate the early stages of spread. The propensity of metastatic neuroblastoma to localize in metaphyseal regions adjacent to hot growth plates can also hinder early detection. The relatively subtle bone scan changes in this case contrast with the very abnormal MIBG study. The combination of both studies is required for the highest detection rate of metastases.

MIBG is taken up and localized in presynaptic adrenergic nerves, adrenal medulla, and neuroblastic tumors. On scintigraphy, normal MIBG uptake is seen in the liver, soft tissue, and blood pool but not in normal bones or bone marrow. Normal uptake also may be seen in organs with adrenergic intervention (e.g., heart, salivary glands, spleen). Normal bilateral adrenal uptake is seen in 10% of patients. MIBG commonly is ordered for staging and monitoring the effectiveness of therapy. Response to therapy is seen on the MIBG study before it is seen on the bone scan.

^{123}I-MIBG has been FDA approved and is now commercially available. It is the preferred agent because of its higher count rate and better image quality. ^{131}I-MIBG is under investigation as a therapeutic agent for neuroblastoma.

Notes

Note: Page numbers followed by f indicate figures and t indicate tables.